baby & child
healthcare

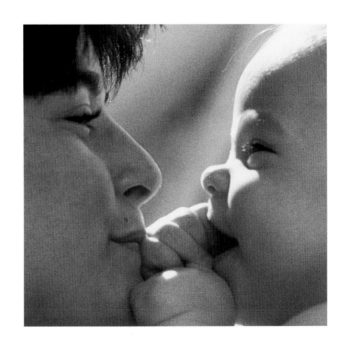

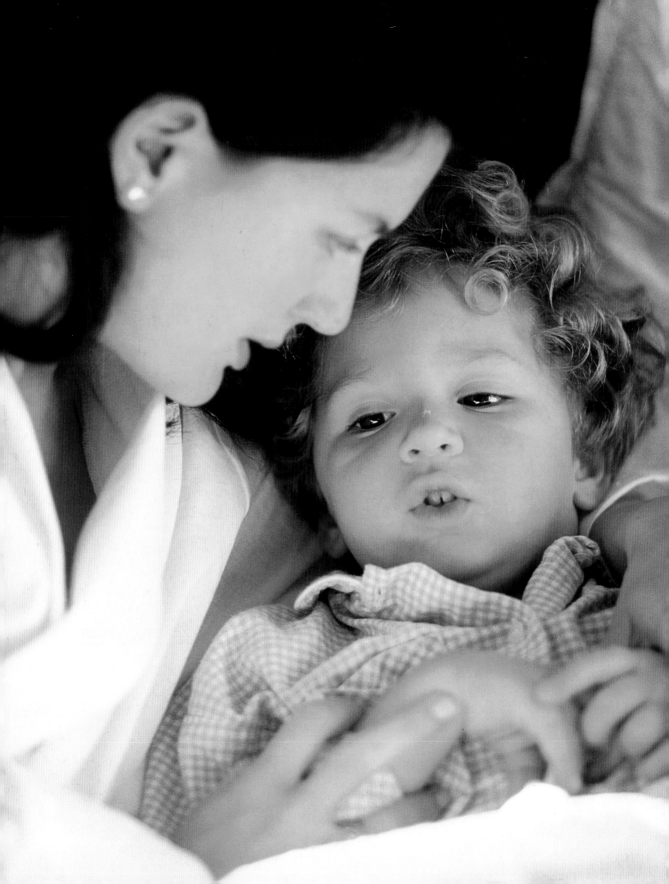

baby&child
healthcare

The essential A–Z home reference to children's
illnesses, symptoms and treatments

Dr. Miriam Stoppard

A Penguin Company

LONDON, NEW YORK, SYDNEY, DELHI, PARIS,
MUNICH and JOHANNESBURG

For Eden and Violet

This edition
Design and Editorial Edward Kinsey and Claire Cross
Senior Managing Art Editor Lynne Brown
Art Editor Glenda Fisher
DTP Karen Constanti
Production Louise Daly

Original edition
Senior Editor Fiona MacIntyre
Editors Charyn Jones, Jemima Dunne
Designers Mark Evans, Roger Priddy
Senior Art Editor Anne-Marie Bulat
Managing Editor Daphne Razazan

Originally published in Great Britain as
The Baby & Child Medical Handbook in 1986

First published as a Dorling Kindersley paperback in 1987

This edition first published in 2001
by Dorling Kindersley Limited
80 Strand, London WC2R 0RL

A CIP catalogue record for this book is available from the British Library.

ISBN-13: 978 0 7513 3348 0

Reproduced by Colourscan, Singapore
Printed and bound by Star Standard in Singapore

see our complete catalogue at
www.dk.com

Contents

Note: we use the masculine pronoun "he" when referring to the baby or child, unless the child shown in a photograph is female. This is for convenience and clarity and does not reflect a preference for either sex.

Preface

I WROTE THIS BOOK WHEN I WAS bringing up four little boys and quite often found myself tending to a sick child in the middle of the night. Those nightly vigils convinced me that an anxious parent, faced with a sick child, needs straight, uncomplicated information and advice, and so I arranged the book in a way that I would have found most helpful when I was in that position. I am delighted to update the book for today's parents.

The A–Z of childhood complaints is the mainstay of the book. All the information is given in simple terms that are easy to understand. Parents are directed to possible courses of action in a clear, logical way, and advice is given step by step. Emphasis on speed is always made when time is of the essence and a doctor should be contacted immediately or an ambulance sought.

It can be difficult to tell exactly what is wrong with a child from the various symptoms – fever, pain, redness, swelling, vomiting – and on most occasions a doctor is required to make an accurate diagnosis. However, to help the parent determine the most likely causes of the child's complaint, a section is devoted to the analysis of symptoms.

For some parents, having an ill child is not a transient event, but one that stretches into

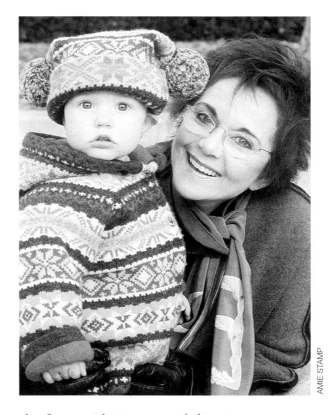

AMIE STAMP

the future. Their responsibility is to cope with a chronically ill child. I have tried to cover the main conditions, giving information on possible causes, the expected course of the disease, and how to make life easier for your child, yourself and the rest of your family. Long-term prognosing is always difficult, and sometimes dangerous, but I have attempted to indicate what the future might hold so that parents can accumulate practical experience and knowledge for the future. I apologize for those conditions that could not be included.

Baby and Child Healthcare is full of illustrations – both drawings and photographs; in some chapters, the text is in the form of annotation to the illustrations. This is because one of my main aims is to give information in a readily accessible form, almost at a glance. There is, of course, ample opportunity to use the book as a straightforward reference book so that you gain knowledge gradually.

I don't have any personal axes to grind, but the book is opinionated and I make no apologies for that. For instance, despite controversy in the U.K. about the possible association of the MMR vaccination and autism, I continue to advocate vaccination as there is no robust scientific evidence of a cause and effect relationship. Where such an opinion is given, it is based on controlled research studies, or the lack of them, not out of personal bias. Throughout the book I hope to give parents enough clear, up-to-the-minute information to learn to trust their own instincts and to know when to be their own family nurse or doctor and when it is essential to get medical help.

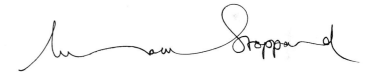

How to use this book

WHEN YOUR CHILD IS ILL, you need to know what to do – whether to call the doctor, or whether you can safely treat your child at home yourself. You may also be unsure of what is wrong with him and need help in determining what the matter is.

How your child's body works

An illustrated guide to the skeleton, muscles, organs and glands of your child's body is given on pages 12 to 22. This will help you to understand what the constituent parts of the body look like, where they are and how they function.

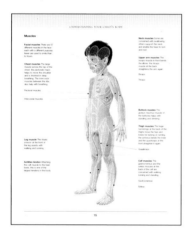

If your child is ill and you think you know what is wrong

Turn straight to the relevant article in the A–Z of Common complaints, pages 52 to 264. This is an alphabetical listing of the most common complaints affecting children – from bruises to bronchitis, stings to styes. There, you will find an explanation of the illness, with a list of the symptoms most likely to appear. The circumstances under which you should call the doctor are clearly defined, followed by the

probable treatment. There is advice, too, on what you yourself can do to help your child (both treatment and nursing tips). There are special charts to aid diagnosis for diarrhoea, fever and vomiting.

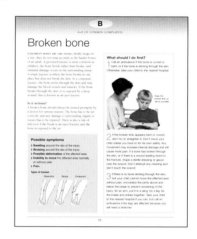

If you are not sure what is wrong

If your child has an obvious symptom, but you are not sure which A–Z entry to look up, turn to the Visual diagnosis guides, pages 43 to 48. Although it is hard to give a diagnosis from one or two symptoms, these guides should help to point you in the right direction.

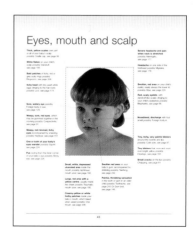

If you are looking after a sick child

The section on pages 24 to 40 gives tips on caring for a sick child, and shows, with step-by-step illustrations, how to take a temperature and give medicines. It also provides practical advice on how to reduce fevers and make your child comfortable, how and what to feed him, how to keep him amused and, should the need arise, how to prepare him for a stay in hospital.

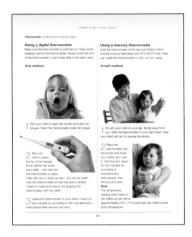

Complementary therapies

This section, on pages 316 to 318, outlines a safe approach to complementary medicine in children. There are guidelines on what to consider before embarking on a complementary therapy and where the possible pitfalls lie. Always consult your doctor for his advice before approaching a therapist.

Personal records

On pages 320 to 323 there are quick-reference charts for vaccinations – which ones your child needs and when; and infectious fevers – their symptoms, treatment and prevention. There is also a growth chart to give you reassurance that your child's growth is within normal limits.

How to prevent accidents
The most sensible precautions for safeguarding your child inside and outside—at home and at play—are shown on pages 266 to 282. Road and car safety are also dealt with.

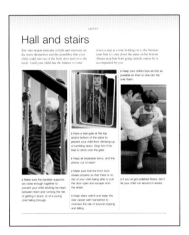

If your child has had an accident

If your child has an accident, you must be prepared to deal with it. Where possible, this preparation should involve going on a first-aid course, but you should frequently remind yourself of the basic, life-saving techniques by referring to the first-aid section on pages 284 to 314.

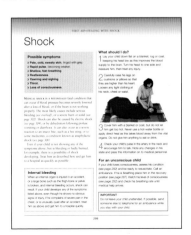

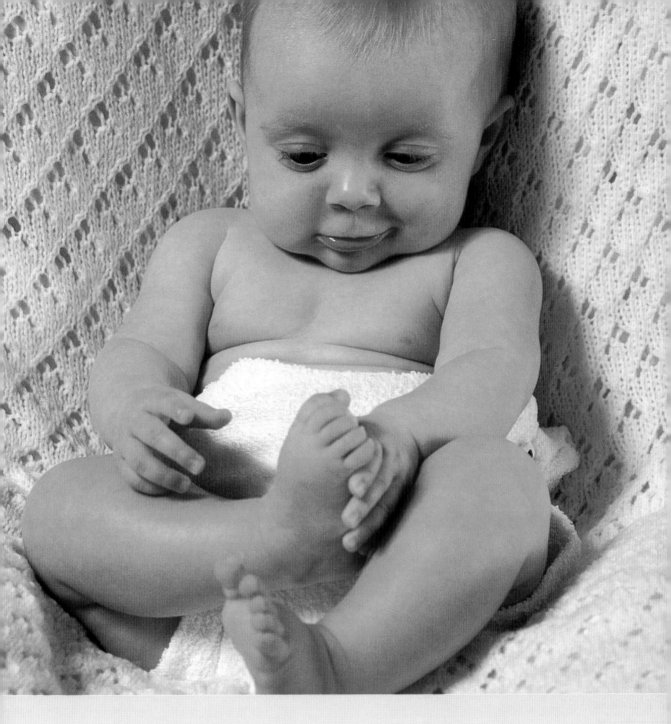

Understanding
your child's body

Bones

THE BODY IS BUILT on a framework of 206 bones called the skeleton. These bones act as levers for muscles to pull against, thus enabling movement, and they surround and protect the vital organs of the head, chest and abdomen.

How bones develop

Bones consist of a central shaft and two shaped ends. In a mature bone, the shaft and ends are hard structures, with a soft inner core of bone marrow (*see below*). In newborn babies, the bones are mostly made up of a soft, bendy material called cartilage, and, as your child develops, this cartilage is gradually converted to bone, a process known as *ossification*. In early childhood, the shaft is bone but the ends still consist largely of soft cartilage. By the time your child reaches adolescence, the bone formed in the ends joins the bone in the shaft and growth stops. Throughout childhood the bones are therefore fairly soft, which is why so-called "greenstick fractures", where the bone bends rather than breaks, can occur (*see page 70*).

What happens when your child grows

Your child grows in height as his bones lengthen. This growth does not take place over the whole length of a bone, but at each end. Growth occurs gradually throughout childhood. At puberty, however, both girls and boys put on a rapid growth spurt. With girls this normally begins when they are about 11 years old, and in boys about a year later. Girls stop growing when they are about 18; boys continue growing for one or two years longer, which accounts, at least in part, for the greater average height in boys.

Joints

The separate bones of the skeleton are connected by joints, and these joints are held together by strong bands of fibrous tissue called ligaments. There are several different types of joint – fixed, partly movable and freely movable. *Fixed joints* allow no movement; *partly movable joints* allow slight movement; *freely movable joints* allow movement in several directions, and there are several different types – hinge joints and ball-and-socket joints are two examples.

How bones are constructed

Each bone consists of a shaft and two ends. When fully developed, the shaft is largely made up of hard (or compact) bone with a soft central core of bone marrow. Most of the blood cells are made in the bone marrow – particularly in the large bones such as the thigh bone. The ends are made up of spongy bone and capped with cartilage to cushion them against the next bone.

Cross-section of mature bone

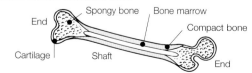

End · Cartilage · Shaft · Spongy bone · Bone marrow · Compact bone · End

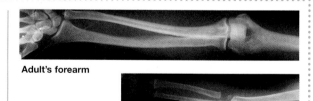

Adult's forearm

Child's forearm

Bone development
The x-rays above show what happens to bones as they develop. The shape of each bone is present at birth. The bones in each child's arm are made of areas of cartilage (not visible on the x-ray) and bone (visible as solid white areas). As a child develops the cartilage is converted to bone. By adolescence, this conversion is complete and the bones are solid.

Bones

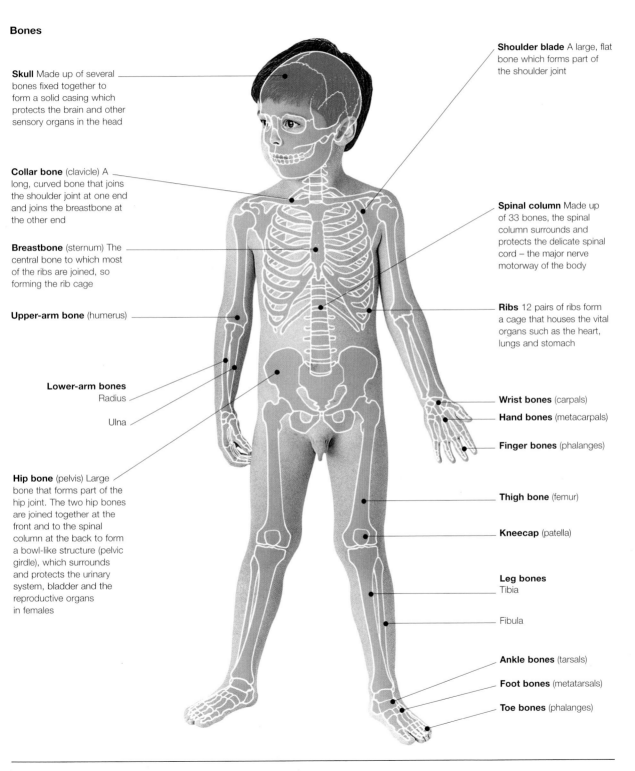

Skull Made up of several bones fixed together to form a solid casing which protects the brain and other sensory organs in the head

Collar bone (clavicle) A long, curved bone that joins the shoulder joint at one end and joins the breastbone at the other end

Breastbone (sternum) The central bone to which most of the ribs are joined, so forming the rib cage

Upper-arm bone (humerus)

Lower-arm bones
Radius

Ulna

Hip bone (pelvis) Large bone that forms part of the hip joint. The two hip bones are joined together at the front and to the spinal column at the back to form a bowl-like structure (pelvic girdle), which surrounds and protects the urinary system, bladder and the reproductive organs in females

Shoulder blade A large, flat bone which forms part of the shoulder joint

Spinal column Made up of 33 bones, the spinal column surrounds and protects the delicate spinal cord – the major nerve motorway of the body

Ribs 12 pairs of ribs form a cage that houses the vital organs such as the heart, lungs and stomach

Wrist bones (carpals)

Hand bones (metacarpals)

Finger bones (phalanges)

Thigh bone (femur)

Kneecap (patella)

Leg bones
Tibia

Fibula

Ankle bones (tarsals)

Foot bones (metatarsals)

Toe bones (phalanges)

Muscles

MUSCLES ARE MADE UP of long bands of closely interlocking fibres that cause movement by contracting and relaxing. There are two main types of muscle in the body – involuntary and voluntary. *Involuntary muscles* operate all the time without conscious control and include the muscles of the heart and the digestive system. *Voluntary muscles*, also known as skeletal muscles, can be consciously controlled and it is these muscles that cause the visible movement of the limbs.

Some muscles are designed to relax and contract quickly to make specific movements, for example, lifting an arm or kicking a ball, while others, such as the spinal muscles, are designed to remain in contraction for long periods of time. There are well over 600 named muscles in the body; illustrated opposite are some of the larger or most obvious ones.

How muscles grow

Although your baby can move quite vigorously at birth and all the muscles are present, they are not fully developed and will grow in length, breadth and thickness as your baby develops. The three most important factors affecting their development are the hormones present in the body, physical activity and diet. Before adolescence there is very little difference in the bulk and strength of boys' and girls' muscles. What difference there is is largely due to the tendency in boys to spend more time than girls on activities that require physical strength. After adolescence, however, the male hormones are important in the development of a boy's greater bulk and strength.

To develop properly, muscles must be used; if they are not used, they will actually decrease in size. A child who is encouraged to be active, and pursue physical activities requiring increasing stamina, will have larger, stronger and better-co-ordinated muscles than a child who is lethargic and takes little exercise or one who is discouraged from doing so by overprotective parents. Some children, however, have muscles that show great endurance while others seem to tire more easily, so try to let your child set his own limits. Don't expect your child to continue to the point of exhaustion; on the other hand, if he is full of energy, don't try to stop him continuing after other children have given up. Let him be the judge of his own limitations.

How muscles work

Muscles consist of a large central part known as the belly, which tapers at each end. The ends are attached to a bone, either directly, or by means of a narrow band of fibre called a tendon.

Most of the skeletal muscles work in pairs so that as one contracts, the other relaxes. To bend the elbow, the biceps muscle contracts and the triceps muscle relaxes; to straighten it, the triceps contracts and the biceps relaxes.

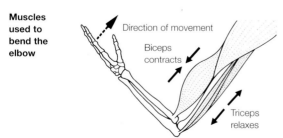

Muscles used to bend the elbow

Direction of movement

Biceps contracts

Triceps relaxes

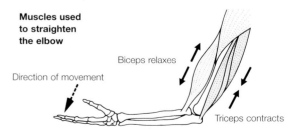

Muscles used to straighten the elbow

Biceps relaxes

Direction of movement

Triceps contracts

Muscles

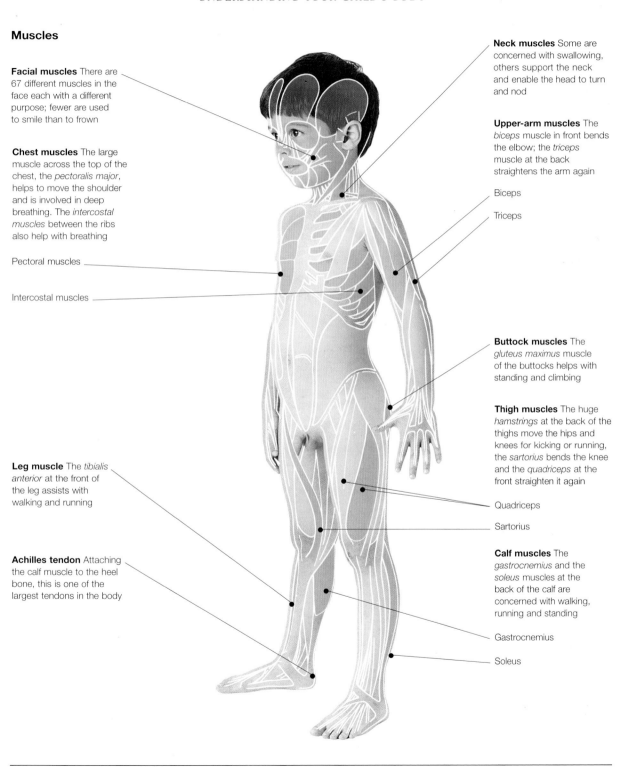

Facial muscles There are 67 different muscles in the face each with a different purpose; fewer are used to smile than to frown

Chest muscles The large muscle across the top of the chest, the *pectoralis major*, helps to move the shoulder and is involved in deep breathing. The *intercostal muscles* between the ribs also help with breathing

Pectoral muscles

Intercostal muscles

Leg muscle The *tibialis anterior* at the front of the leg assists with walking and running

Achilles tendon Attaching the calf muscle to the heel bone, this is one of the largest tendons in the body

Neck muscles Some are concerned with swallowing, others support the neck and enable the head to turn and nod

Upper-arm muscles The *biceps* muscle in front bends the elbow; the *triceps* muscle at the back straightens the arm again

Biceps

Triceps

Buttock muscles The *gluteus maximus* muscle of the buttocks helps with standing and climbing

Thigh muscles The huge *hamstrings* at the back of the thighs move the hips and knees for kicking or running, the *sartorius* bends the knee and the *quadriceps* at the front straighten it again

Quadriceps

Sartorius

Calf muscles The *gastrocnemius* and the *soleus* muscles at the back of the calf are concerned with walking, running and standing

Gastrocnemius

Soleus

The head

THE BRAIN AND THE MOST IMPORTANT sensory organs of the body (the eyes, ears, nose and mouth) are situated in the head. They are surrounded and protected by the skull. The skull is made up of several bones which, in older children and adults, are fused together.

The brain

The brain is a very important and complex structure. It is the main control centre of the nervous system – the system comprising the brain, spinal cord and the nerves – which controls all bodily functions. The brain receives information from the outside world through the various sensory organs, including the skin, and acts on this information by sending out instructions to the different parts of the body. Some parts of the body receive their instructions from nerves directly connected to the brain; others, such as the arms and legs, receive their messages via nerves branching off the spinal cord.

The brain is divided into three main parts – the cerebral hemispheres, the cerebellum and the brain stem. Each part controls a different body function. The brain is protected by three membranes called the meninges, and it is cushioned by fluid called cerebro-spinal fluid. This fluid, which is produced in the centre of the brain, flows between the two innermost membranes, and also surrounds the spinal cord.

Teeth

Your child's first teeth, known as milk teeth, will probably begin to come through when he is about six or seven months old. The full set of 20 teeth should have come through by the time he is about three years old. The permanent adult teeth will begin to appear when your child is about six, but the full set of 32 teeth will not be complete until he is about 17. The first permanent teeth to come through are the first molars. The milk teeth become loose and fall out one at a time and are normally replaced immediately by the permanent teeth. Sometimes, however, a permanent tooth begins to come through before the milk tooth has fallen out. This can cause pain and the dentist may have to extract the milk tooth.

Milk teeth

Age of appearance

2–3 years
12 months
18 months
7 months
6 months

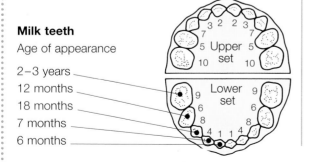

Permanent teeth

Age of appearance

17+ years
11–13 years
6–7 years
10–12 years
9–12 years
7–9 years
6–8 years

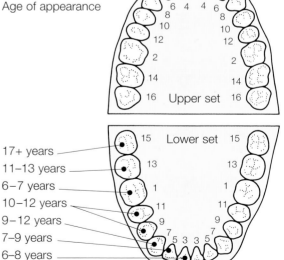

Areas of control

Certain areas of the brain are responsible for controlling specific bodily functions: for example, the occipital lobe for vision and motor cortex for voluntary movement. Memory cannot be localized in the same way but is thought to involve many different parts of the brain.

The brain

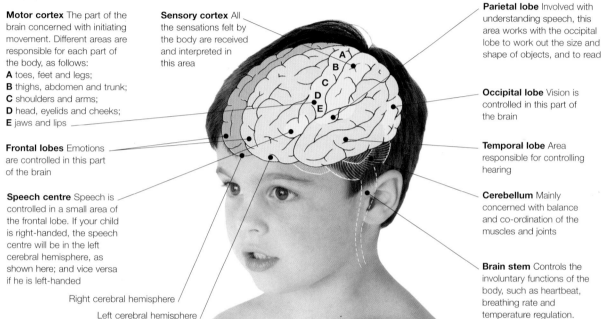

Motor cortex The part of the brain concerned with initiating movement. Different areas are responsible for each part of the body, as follows:
A toes, feet and legs;
B thighs, abdomen and trunk;
C shoulders and arms;
D head, eyelids and cheeks;
E jaws and lips

Sensory cortex All the sensations felt by the body are received and interpreted in this area

Frontal lobes Emotions are controlled in this part of the brain

Speech centre Speech is controlled in a small area of the frontal lobe. If your child is right-handed, the speech centre will be in the left cerebral hemisphere, as shown here; and vice versa if he is left-handed

Right cerebral hemisphere
Left cerebral hemisphere

Parietal lobe Involved with understanding speech, this area works with the occipital lobe to work out the size and shape of objects, and to read

Occipital lobe Vision is controlled in this part of the brain

Temporal lobe Area responsible for controlling hearing

Cerebellum Mainly concerned with balance and co-ordination of the muscles and joints

Brain stem Controls the involuntary functions of the body, such as heartbeat, breathing rate and temperature regulation.

Inside the brain

This cross-section of the brain shows the right cerebral hemisphere. It is joined to the left by a band of tissue called the corpus callosum. Each cerebral hemisphere is made up of two types of tissue: grey matter and white matter. Grey matter consists of the nerve cells, white matter consists of the nerve fibres. The hypothalamus is situated at the base of the brain and controls sleep and appetite. Under the central part of the brain is the pituitary gland, the gland that controls growth and development and ensures that all the glands in the endocrine system, the hormone-producing glands (*see page 21*), are functioning properly.

Cross-section of the brain

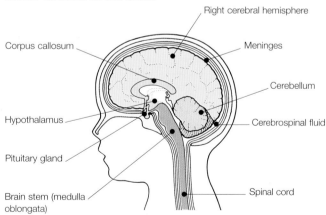

Corpus callosum

Hypothalamus

Pituitary gland

Brain stem (medulla oblongata)

Right cerebral hemisphere

Meninges

Cerebellum

Cerebrospinal fluid

Spinal cord

Continued on next page

The Head *continued from previous page*

The sense organs

The most important sense organs of the body (the nose, mouth, eyes and ears) are all situated in the head. Between them, they give us a great deal of information about the outside world.

The nose and mouth

The nose is the organ of smell and also forms the main entrance to the respiratory system. Air is breathed in through the nose and passes down into the lungs via the windpipe (trachea). The nose is lined with a hair-covered membrane that filters, moistens and warms air as it is taken into the body. The nose is also linked to the sinuses, which is why nasal infections can pass into the sinuses.

The mouth forms the entrance to the digestive system (*see page 21*); it is also involved (with the tongue, lips and larynx) in speech. The tongue is the organ of taste – different areas of the tongue distinguish the main types of flavour: salty, sweet, bitter and sour.

Cross-section of the nose and mouth

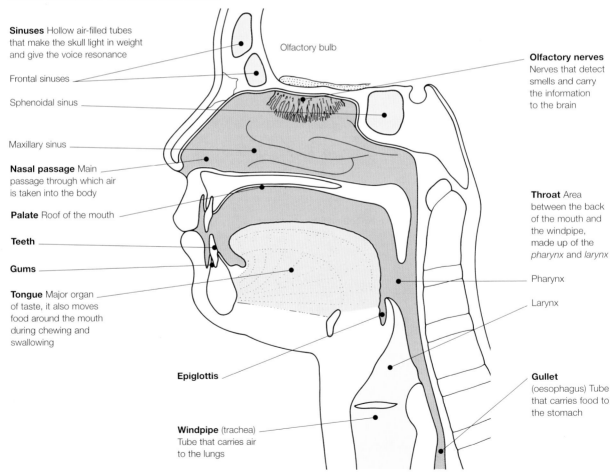

Sinuses Hollow air-filled tubes that make the skull light in weight and give the voice resonance

Frontal sinuses

Sphenoidal sinus

Maxillary sinus

Nasal passage Main passage through which air is taken into the body

Palate Roof of the mouth

Teeth

Gums

Tongue Major organ of taste, it also moves food around the mouth during chewing and swallowing

Epiglottis

Windpipe (trachea) Tube that carries air to the lungs

Olfactory bulb

Olfactory nerves Nerves that detect smells and carry the information to the brain

Throat Area between the back of the mouth and the windpipe, made up of the *pharynx* and *larynx*

Pharynx

Larynx

Gullet (oesophagus) Tube that carries food to the stomach

The eye

The eye works by focusing rays of light through a lens on to a sensitive layer in the back of the eye called the retina. The information is then sent to the brain via the optic nerve to be interpreted. Each eye sees an object from a different angle. The brain co-ordinates the image picked up by each eye so that a solid, three-dimensional object is seen. The eye is held in place by six muscles, which allow it to swivel and see in many directions.

Cross-section of the eye

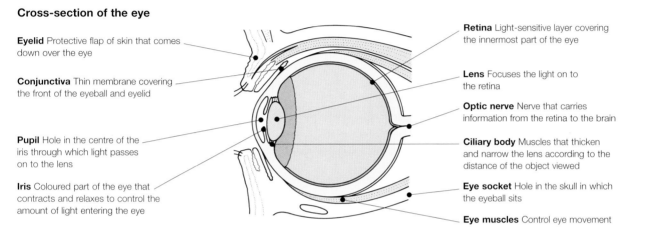

Eyelid Protective flap of skin that comes down over the eye

Conjunctiva Thin membrane covering the front of the eyeball and eyelid

Pupil Hole in the centre of the iris through which light passes on to the lens

Iris Coloured part of the eye that contracts and relaxes to control the amount of light entering the eye

Retina Light-sensitive layer covering the innermost part of the eye

Lens Focuses the light on to the retina

Optic nerve Nerve that carries information from the retina to the brain

Ciliary body Muscles that thicken and narrow the lens according to the distance of the object viewed

Eye socket Hole in the skull in which the eyeball sits

Eye muscles Control eye movement

The ear

The ear is an important organ, not only for hearing, but also for balance. The ear consists of three parts: the outer, middle and inner ear. The part of the ear that you see is the outer ear. All three sections of the ear are involved with hearing; balance is controlled in the inner ear alone.

Cross-section of the ear

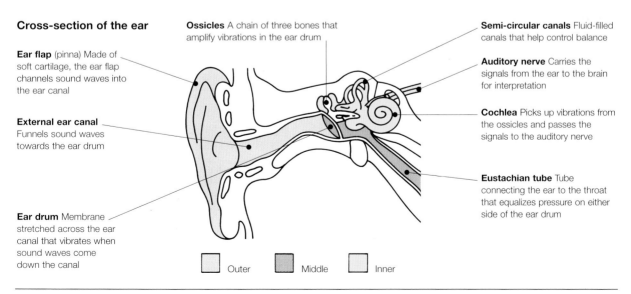

Ossicles A chain of three bones that amplify vibrations in the ear drum

Ear flap (pinna) Made of soft cartilage, the ear flap channels sound waves into the ear canal

External ear canal Funnels sound waves towards the ear drum

Ear drum Membrane stretched across the ear canal that vibrates when sound waves come down the canal

Semi-circular canals Fluid-filled canals that help control balance

Auditory nerve Carries the signals from the ear to the brain for interpretation

Cochlea Picks up vibrations from the ossicles and passes the signals to the auditory nerve

Eustachian tube Tube connecting the ear to the throat that equalizes pressure on either side of the ear drum

Outer   Middle   Inner

Organs and glands

HOUSED IN THE CENTRE of the body cavity are the organs that deal with digestion, breathing and blood circulation. The glands produce hormones, which control the functioning of the organs and growth and development.

Glands that swell

The glands that swell during an illness are not glands in the true sense because they do not secrete hormones. They are lymph nodes, part of the lymphatic system, which is responsible for helping the body to fight infection. When infection occurs, more white cells are produced all over the body and sent to the lymph nodes nearest the area of infection so that the germs can be destroyed. This causes the lymph nodes to swell and they may be slightly tender. Lymph nodes are sited all over the body; those in the neck are the most commonly activated by infection, but the other main sites are the armpit and groin.

Glands below the ear These glands swell if your child has an ear infection

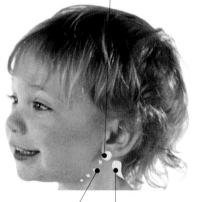

Glands below the ear and the jaw These are the glands most commonly affected by tonsillitis, for example

Glands in the back of the neck These swell if, for example, your child has German measles

Circulatory system

The blood, which consists of red and white blood cells suspended in a fluid called plasma, is the body's main transport system. It carries oxygen from the lungs and nourishment from digested food around the body, and carries waste matter, such as carbon dioxide (a by-product of breathing) away from the body cells.

There are two parts to the circulatory system: the *systematic circulation*, which carries blood to the tissues, and the *pulmonary circulation*, which carries blood from the heart to the lungs and back to the heart for oxygenation. Very simply, the circulatory system works as follows. Blood, bright red because it is loaded with oxygen, comes from the lungs into the left side of the heart. The heart pumps this blood out into the main artery, the aorta. This branches to carry blood to the head, neck and arms and to carry it to the abdomen and legs. These branches then subdivide into smaller and smaller arteries, ending in thin-walled capillaries in the body cells. It is in the capillaries that the nourishment and oxygen carried by the blood are passed into the cells, and waste matter, such as carbon dioxide, is picked up. The capillaries then join up to form veins, which carry the blood, now darker red because it contains less oxygen, back to the heart. The veins join up to form larger and larger veins and finally form two large veins, the superior vena cava from the head, neck and arms, and the inferior vena cava from the abdomen and legs. These both carry blood into the right side of the heart. From here, the blood is pumped to the lungs, where the carbon dioxide is given up to be breathed out of the lungs and a fresh supply of oxygen is collected.

Organs and glands

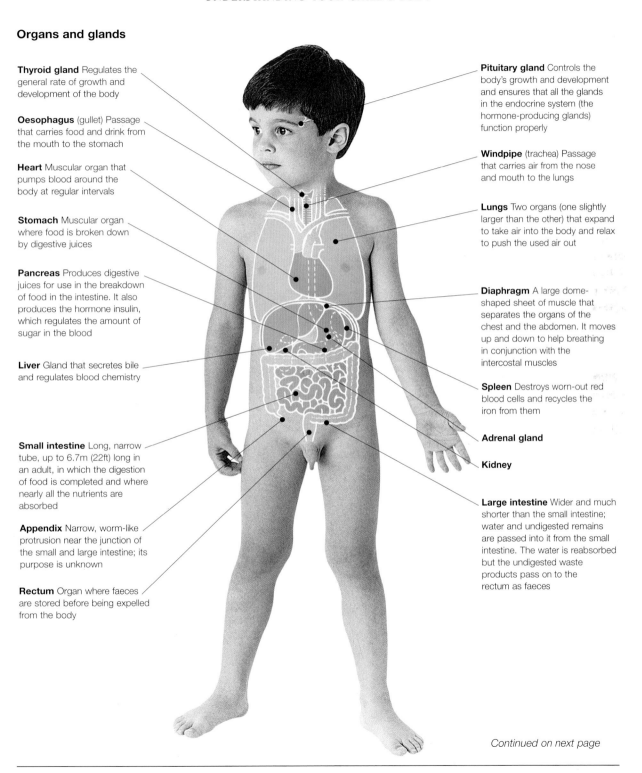

Thyroid gland Regulates the general rate of growth and development of the body

Oesophagus (gullet) Passage that carries food and drink from the mouth to the stomach

Heart Muscular organ that pumps blood around the body at regular intervals

Stomach Muscular organ where food is broken down by digestive juices

Pancreas Produces digestive juices for use in the breakdown of food in the intestine. It also produces the hormone insulin, which regulates the amount of sugar in the blood

Liver Gland that secretes bile and regulates blood chemistry

Small intestine Long, narrow tube, up to 6.7m (22ft) long in an adult, in which the digestion of food is completed and where nearly all the nutrients are absorbed

Appendix Narrow, worm-like protrusion near the junction of the small and large intestine; its purpose is unknown

Rectum Organ where faeces are stored before being expelled from the body

Pituitary gland Controls the body's growth and development and ensures that all the glands in the endocrine system (the hormone-producing glands) function properly

Windpipe (trachea) Passage that carries air from the nose and mouth to the lungs

Lungs Two organs (one slightly larger than the other) that expand to take air into the body and relax to push the used air out

Diaphragm A large dome-shaped sheet of muscle that separates the organs of the chest and the abdomen. It moves up and down to help breathing in conjunction with the intercostal muscles

Spleen Destroys worn-out red blood cells and recycles the iron from them

Adrenal gland

Kidney

Large intestine Wider and much shorter than the small intestine; water and undigested remains are passed into it from the small intestine. The water is reabsorbed but the undigested waste products pass on to the rectum as faeces

Continued on next page

Organs and Glands *Continued from previous page*

Organs of the lower abdomen

These include the two kidneys and the bladder (which, with the ureters and urethra, make up the urinary system), and the reproductive organs.

Male reproductive system

The male sex glands, the testes (testicles), are situated on the outside of the body in the scrotal sac.

They produce sperm and testosterone, the hormone that controls the development of the sex organs and the secondary sexual characteristics such as broad shoulders and well-muscled arms and legs.

From puberty onwards, all the organs of the reproductive system enlarge. The testes then begin to manufacture sperm, first in small quantities, then in increasingly larger amounts.

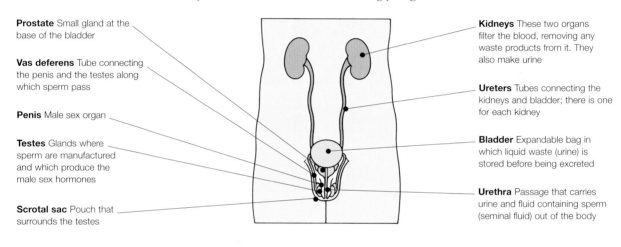

Prostate Small gland at the base of the bladder

Vas deferens Tube connecting the penis and the testes along which sperm pass

Penis Male sex organ

Testes Glands where sperm are manufactured and which produce the male sex hormones

Scrotal sac Pouch that surrounds the testes

Kidneys These two organs filter the blood, removing any waste products from it. They also make urine

Ureters Tubes connecting the kidneys and bladder; there is one for each kidney

Bladder Expandable bag in which liquid waste (urine) is stored before being excreted

Urethra Passage that carries urine and fluid containing sperm (seminal fluid) out of the body

Female reproductive system

At birth, the uterus is extremely small and it does not begin to grow until puberty. However, the ovaries already contain all the eggs that will ever be produced and released during a girl's fertile life.

Female sex hormones, oestrogen and progesterone, are manufactured by the ovaries. At puberty, their production begins to follow a monthly pattern, which stimulates the beginning of the menstrual cycle.

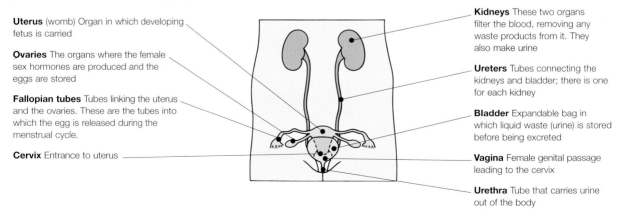

Uterus (womb) Organ in which developing fetus is carried

Ovaries The organs where the female sex hormones are produced and the eggs are stored

Fallopian tubes Tubes linking the uterus and the ovaries. These are the tubes into which the egg is released during the menstrual cycle.

Cervix Entrance to uterus

Kidneys These two organs filter the blood, removing any waste products from it. They also make urine

Ureters Tubes connecting the kidneys and bladder; there is one for each kidney

Bladder Expandable bag in which liquid waste (urine) is stored before being excreted

Vagina Female genital passage leading to the cervix

Urethra Tube that carries urine out of the body

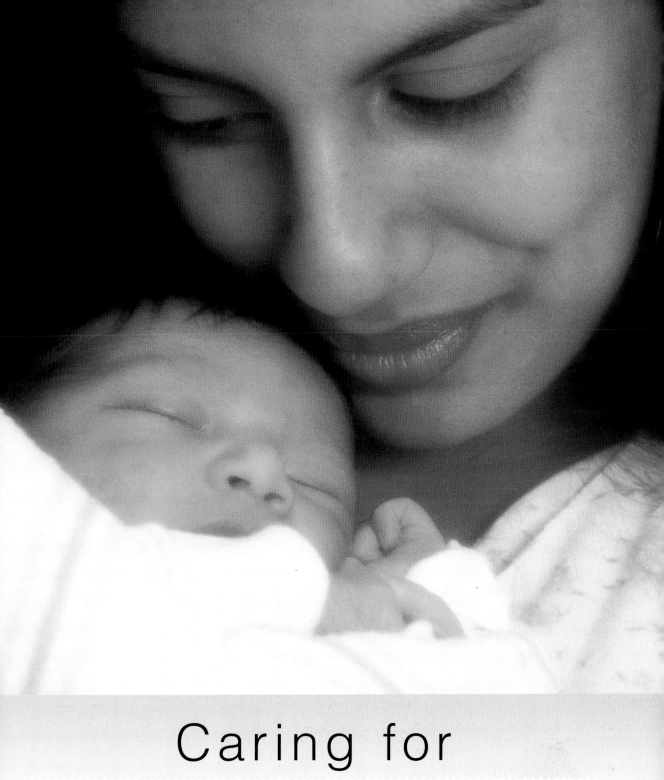

Caring for
a sick child

Calling the doctor

MOST PARENTS KNOW INSTINCTIVELY when their child is sickening for something: the child may not be as lively as usual; he may refuse his food; he may become clingy. However, the parent is not always able to diagnose exactly what is wrong, nor is he or she necessarily able to tell whether the child's symptoms are serious, or even potentially serious. An ill child is always distressing and the situation can be made even more tense if you cannot decide whether or not to call out the doctor.

There are some circumstances, after a serious injury, for example, when medical help must be sought immediately. For most parents, these situations are quite obvious. There are, however, many more situations where the seriousness isn't as clear-cut. This is where the worry comes in: "Are my child's symptoms quite normal or are they potentially serious?" What you must remember is that most doctors will not mind if you seek their advice. Always follow your instincts and, if you are ever in doubt, contact your doctor.

If your child is already undergoing treatment from your doctor and you are worried about his progress, call your doctor again. Don't take your child to a casualty department because the doctor in the casualty department will not be able to change your child's treatment without consulting your own doctor first.

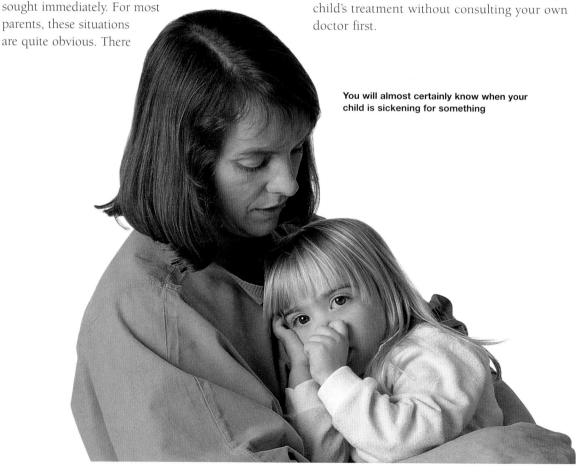

You will almost certainly know when your child is sickening for something

When to call your doctor

Listed below are the circumstances under which you should always call your doctor. The following are all important signs so never ignore them.

Temperature

◗ A raised temperature of over 39°C (102.2°F).
◗ A raised temperature accompanied by drowsiness and a purplish rash on the body, plus any other obvious signs of illness.
◗ A raised temperature accompanied by a convulsion, or a raised temperature if your child has had convulsions in the past.
◗ A raised temperature accompanied by a stiff neck and headache.
◗ A temperature below 35°C (95°F) accompanied by a cold skin surface, drowsiness, quietness and listlessness.
◗ A temperature which has dropped and then rises again suddenly.
◗ A temperature of more than 38°C (100.4°F) for more than three days.

Diarrhoea

◗ If your baby has diarrhoea for more than six hours.
◗ If diarrhoea is accompanied by pain in the abdomen, a temperature or any other obvious signs of illness.

Vomiting

◗ If your baby has been vomiting for a period of more than six hours.
◗ Prolonged, violent vomiting.
◗ Dizzy spells plus nausea and headaches.
◗ Nausea and vomiting accompanied by right-sided pain in the abdomen.

Loss of appetite

◗ If your baby goes off his food suddenly, or is less than six months old and doesn't seem to be thriving.
◗ If your child usually has a hearty appetite, but refuses all food for a day and seems listless.

Pain and discomfort

◗ If your child complains of headaches and feels sick and dizzy.
◗ If your child complains of blurred vision, especially if he's recently had a bang on the head.
◗ If your child has severe griping pains, which occur at regular intervals.
◗ If your child has a pain in the right side of his abdomen and feels sick.

Breathing

◗ If your child's breathing is laboured and his ribs are being sharply drawn in with each breath.

Emergencies

Always get your child to the nearest hospital by ambulance or car if you notice any of the following (see also pages 284–311):

◗ Your child has stopped breathing (see page 286).
◗ Your child is breathing with difficulty and his lips are going blue (see page 294).
◗ Your child is unconscious (see page 292).
◗ Your child has a deep wound that is bleeding badly (see page 300).
◗ Your child has a serious burn (see page 302).
◗ Your child has a suspected broken bone (see page 70).
◗ Your child has a chemical in his eyes (see page 130).
◗ Your child's ear or eye has been damaged (see pages 121 and 132).
◗ Your child has been bitten by an animal or a snake (see pages 65 and 221).
◗ Your child has eaten a poisonous substance (see page 305).

Continued from previous page

What to tell your doctor

Your doctor will need to know the answers to specific questions, both to help him make a diagnosis and to gauge the severity of the illness or injury. The doctor needs as much information as possible. If necessary, write down everything that you think might be helpful on a piece of paper and have it with you when you are speaking to the doctor so that you do not forget. He will probably need to know the following:

) Your child's age.

) Whether your child has a temperature. If so, what is it; did it come on quickly; how long has he had it; have there been any fluctuations and, if so, what were they?

) Are your child's neck glands swollen?

) Has your child vomited?

) Has your child had diarrhoea?

) Has your child complained of any kind of pain and, if so, where is the pain?

) Has your child suffered from dizziness or blurred vision (particularly if he's recently had a knock on the head)?

) Has your child had a convulsion? If so, how long did it last?

) Has your child lost consciousness?

) Did your child eat the last meal offered and has he eaten within the past three hours?

What to expect from your doctor

Whether you take your child to the doctor's surgery or arrange for a home visit, there are certain things you should expect your doctor to do. Make sure he gives you an honest opinion of what he thinks is wrong with your child and that he answers all your questions fully.

Taking your child's pulse

The pulse is the wave of pressure that passes along each artery every time the heart beats. You can feel the pulse wherever an artery lies close to the skin. The most common site for taking the pulse is at the wrist (radial pulse); it can also be taken on the inside of the upper arm (brachial pulse) or in the neck (carotid pulse), although this is normally only done if you suspect that the heart has stopped beating altogether (*see page 290*).

The pulse rate will vary with age. It is normally faster after exercise and slower after resting. A young baby's heart will beat about 160 times a minute; by the time he is one year old it will beat about 100–120 times per minute and by the time he is about seven or eight years old it will have slowed down to the adult rate of 80–90 beats per minute. A normal pulse is regular and strong; any abnormality, such as a fast, weak pulse or a slow pulse, may indicate that your child is ill.

If your child is under one, it is generally easier to take his pulse at the brachial artery, located on the inside of the upper arm.

Taking the radial pulse

1 Support your child's wrist with your thumb and place two fingers in the hollow below the palm of his hand on the thumb side, just below the wrist creases.

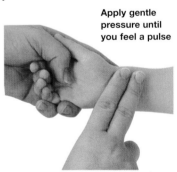

Apply gentle pressure until you feel a pulse

2 Count the number of beats you can feel in 15 seconds and multiply this figure by four to get the number of beats in a minute.

Your doctor should give your child a thorough examination. If, for example, your child has an earache, the doctor should examine his ears. If he has abdominal pain then your doctor should examine his abdomen without his clothes on. If he has got a sore throat and a cough, your doctor should listen to his chest as well as examining the throat and feeling his neck glands. You should not accept a prescription for your child without an examination first.

Here is a list of things you should expect your doctor to do or tell you, or that you should remember to ask him.

Expect your doctor to:

❱ Examine your child thoroughly.

❱ Give you an honest opinion of what is wrong. If your doctor does not know what is wrong, you should expect him to tell you that further investigations are necessary in order to obtain a clear diagnosis.

❱ Tell you the implications of the illness or condition. If, for example, your child has an acute attack of sinusitis or a middle-ear infection, your doctor should tell you that your child may need several courses of antibiotics to eradicate it completely.

❱ Not give you medicine if he is sure that there is nothing wrong. He would be wrong to give you something simply because you have gone into the surgery expecting to be treated. Respect him for not being pressurized into giving you a prescription.

❱ Answer all your questions – be persistent until you are completely satisfied.

❱ Give you as much information as possible about the medicines prescribed for your child – whether to give them before or after a meal, whether there are any side effects and whether there are any special precautions that you ought to take.

❱ Warn you of any possible complications and tell you what danger signs to look out for.

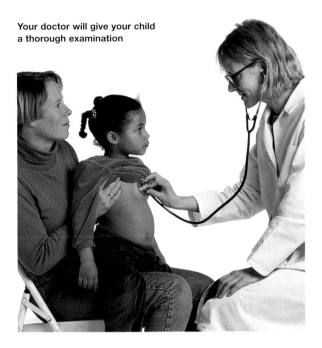

Your doctor will give your child a thorough examination

Things to ask your doctor

❱ If your child has a recurrent condition such as cold sores or boils, ask your doctor what you can do if you notice the symptoms recurring.

❱ Ask your doctor for home-nursing tips.

❱ If your child has a chronic condition, ask your doctor if there is anything that you can do yourself at home to help the condition. For example, if your child has infantile eczema, there's quite a lot you can do in terms of adding emollients to the bath water, using special soap, gently rubbing in moisturizing ointments and creams, even when the skin is clear. Avoiding synthetic clothes and bedding and using a non-biological laundry detergent may also help.

❱ If your child has an infectious disease, ask your doctor about the incubation period (for the benefit of your friends whose children have come into contact with your child), the length of time your child will be infectious and how long he will have to stay off school.

Temperature

IN CHILDREN, NORMAL BODY TEMPERATURE ranges from 36°C (96.8°F) to 37°C (98.6°F). Any temperature over 37.7°C (100°F) is classed as a fever. Hypothermia develops if the temperature falls below 35°C (95°F). Body temperature will vary according to how active your child has been and the time of day: it is lowest in the morning because there is little muscle activity during sleep, and highest in the late afternoon after a day's activity. It will also be high after your child has been running around.

An abnormally hot forehead may be the first indication that your child has a temperature. To be accurate, however, you must take your child's temperature with a thermometer (*see opposite and page 30*). Because the temperature-control centre in the brain is primitive in young children, the temperature can shoot up more rapidly than in adults. When a fever is present, you should take your child's temperature again after 20 minutes, just in case it was only a transitory leap. Never regard a high temperature as an accurate reflection of your child's health; it is only one sign of illness. A child can be very ill without a temperature or quite healthy with one.

Thermometers

The most accurate way to take your child's temperature is with a digital thermometer. Mercury thermometers are less likely to be accurate because children often will not keep them in place long enough. Digital thermometers can measure low as well as high temperatures, which is useful because babies and young children lose heat quickly and this can be dangerous (*see page 307*). Digital ear thermometers, which you insert very briefly into your child's ear, are probably the easiest type to use.

Digital thermometers are harder to break than mercury thermometers and are easy to use with children of all ages. They are, however, more expensive than other thermometers and require batteries to work. If you use a digital thermometer be sure to keep spare batteries on hand.

If you need to take your child's temperature using a mercury thermometer, place it under his armpit for three minutes (the result using this method will be 0.6°C, or 1°F, below body temperature). Once your child is about six or seven you can probably take his temperature orally using a mercury thermometer, as long as you can trust him not to bite the thermometer.

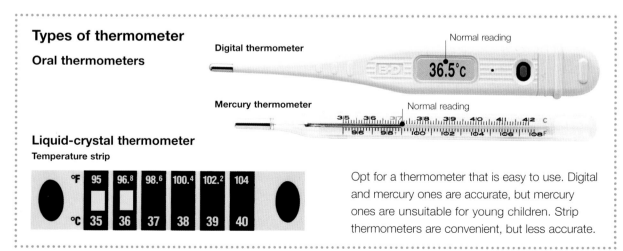

Types of thermometer

Oral thermometers

Digital thermometer

Normal reading

36.5°c

Mercury thermometer

Normal reading

Liquid-crystal thermometer
Temperature strip

| °F | 95 | 96.8 | 98.6 | 100.4 | 102.2 | 104 |
| °C | 35 | 36 | 37 | 38 | 39 | 40 |

Opt for a thermometer that is easy to use. Digital and mercury ones are accurate, but mercury ones are unsuitable for young children. Strip thermometers are convenient, but less accurate.

Liquid-crystal thermometers have a heat-sensitive panel on one side and panels with numbers on the other side. When the sensitive side is placed on the forehead, the numbers light up. Liquid-crystal thermometers are not as accurate as mercury or digital thermometers but they are safe and easy to use.

Reading thermometers

The temperature registered on a liquid-crystal thermometer is the number or panel that remains lit up. Mercury thermometers are more difficult to read. Hold the thermometer between your finger and thumb and turn it until you can see the point on the scale reached by the mercury. On a digital thermometer the number in the window is your child's temperature.

Using a forehead thermometer

Always read the manufacturer's instructions carefully.

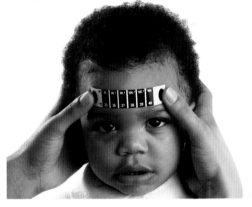

1 Hold the strip against your child's forehead with both hands, keeping your fingers clear of the numbered panels. Make sure the strip is flat against your child's forehead.

2 Leave it for about 15 seconds. Numbers and coloured panels will light up in sequence, as above, before coming to rest at the reading for your child's temperature.

Tips for taking your child's temperature

- Never take your child's temperature if he has just stopped running about.
- Never leave your child alone with a thermometer in his mouth.
- If there is an accident and a mercury thermometer breaks in your child's mouth, remove the pieces of glass quickly and carefully. The mercury is unlikely to spill from its tube but, if it does, tell your child to spit out as much as he can and mop up the rest with a dry tissue. If your child swallows any mercury, call your doctor.
- Make sure there is no break in the mercury inside the thermometer – it will affect the reading.
- If your thermometer is cracked, throw it away immediately.
- Wash the thermometer after use with soap and cold water.
- Always store the thermometer in its own case.

Continued on next page

Temperature *continued from previous page*

Using a digital thermometer

Make sure the thermometer is switched on. Keep spare batteries next to the thermometer. Always wash the end of the thermometer in cold water after it has been used.

Oral method

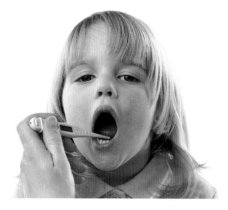

1 Ask your child to open her mouth and raise her tongue. Place the thermometer under her tongue.

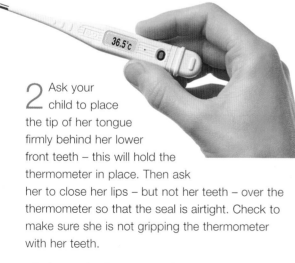

2 Ask your child to place the tip of her tongue firmly behind her lower front teeth – this will hold the thermometer in place. Then ask her to close her lips – but not her teeth – over the thermometer so that the seal is airtight. Check to make sure she is not gripping the thermometer with her teeth.

3 Leave the thermometer in your child's mouth for two minutes (or according to the manufacturer's instructions) then remove and read.

Using a mercury thermometer

Hold the thermometer at the top and shake it down until the mercury falls below the 35°C (95°F) mark. After use, wash the thermometer in cold, *not* hot, water.

Armpit method

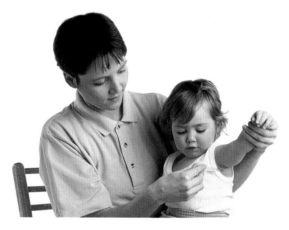

1 Sit with your child on your lap, facing away from you. With the thermometer in your right hand, raise your child's left arm to expose the armpit.

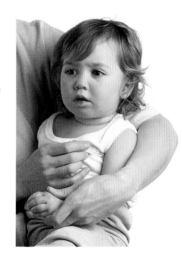

2 Place the thermometer into the armpit and lower your child's arm over it. Hold the arm down for two minutes (or according to manufacturer's instructions), then remove and read.

Note

The temperature reading when taken in the child's armpit will be approximately 0.6°C (1°F) lower than the child's actual body temperature.

Treating a raised temperature

The raised temperature that accompanies an illness is the body's way of responding to infection, and is a sign that the body is marshalling its defences (*see page 134*). While this is a good sign it is also important not to let your child's temperature get too high. If he has a high temperature, he will be very uncomfortable and irritable; moreover, high temperature, particularly in young children, can lead to convulsions (*see page 94*). So it is important that you lower his temperature.

Removing bedclothes

Remove your child's clothes and any blankets so that his body cools down by radiation, then leave him covered by only a cotton sheet. If his temperature rises over 39°C (102.2°F), he may be more comfortable left uncovered but wearing a short-sleeved cotton T-shirt and underpants or a vest and nappy.

Medicines

The most efficient way of reducing your child's fever is to give him medicine. Paracetamol is probably the best choice with children, as it has few side effects. It also has the advantage that it is available in syrup, or elixir, form so is much easier to give to young children. Paracetamol elixir can be bought at most chemists without a prescription and, as a child can develop a high temperature very quickly, it is a good idea to have a bottle in the medicine cabinet.

Whether you use junior paracetamol tablets or elixir, it is very important not to give your child more than the recommended dose – but don't give him less either – and do not give them to your child for longer than two days without consulting your doctor. To make it more palatable to a child, paracetamol elixir is usually sweetened so, if at all possible, make sure your child brushes his teeth after taking it.

Tepid sponging

If your child's temperature is over 40°C (104°F) for longer than half an hour, and removing her bedclothes hasn't helped, try tepid sponging. Always use tepid water, never cold. Tepid water causes the blood vessels in the skin to dilate, therefore aiding heat loss; cold water causes the blood vessels to contract and retain heat.

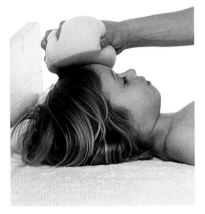

1 Half fill a bucket with water that is comfortable to your elbow or the inside of your wrist and put several clean flannels or sponges in it. Place dry towels around your child so that the bed does not get wet.

2 Wring one of the flannels or sponges out slightly so that it is still dripping. Starting from the head, and using brisk but gentle strokes, sponge the whole of your child's body. Change the sponge when it feels warm.

3 Take your child's temperature after five or 10 minutes. If it has dropped to 38°C (100.4°F), stop sponging. If her temperature has not dropped, continue with the sponging and take her temperature every five minutes. Stop when it has dropped.

4 Cover her with a cotton sheet, and watch her carefully. Be careful not to let her get too cold. Repeat tepid sponging if her temperature rises again. If her temperature does not drop, consult your doctor immediately.

Medicines

WHEN YOU TAKE YOUR CHILD to the doctor he may prescribe some form of medicine for your child. Ask your doctor to give you as much information as possible about the medicines: ask if there are likely to be any side effects, or whether there are foods that should be avoided, or special precautions that should be taken while your child is taking the medication (*see page 27*).

Most medicines for young children are made up in a sweetened syrup to make them more palatable, and can be given with a spoon, tube or dropper. Droppers, tubes and syringes are often more suitable for babies who haven't learned to swallow from a spoon. Some medicines for older children are supplied as tablets or capsules.

On most occasions your child will be co-operative but nearly everyone has been faced with the situation of trying to give medicine to a child who refuses to take it. It is very important that your child takes any medicine prescribed when he is ill. In fact, I think that this is one occasion when blackmail is justified. Be firm but never harsh, cruel or threatening and never punish your child for being difficult about taking the medicines. Very occasionally a child will resist physically. In this case there really is no alternative but for you to be forceful.

Giving medicines to a baby or young child

It can be more difficult to administer medicines to babies because they wriggle. You will need the help of another adult or older brother or sister. Position your baby so that he is slightly raised. Never lay him down flat while giving him medicine because he may inhale the medicine into his lungs.

Using a spoon

1 If the baby is very young, sterilize the spoon by boiling it or placing it in a sterilizing solution. Hold your baby in the crook of your arm. If he won't open his mouth, open it by gently pulling down his chin; if necessary get someone to do this.

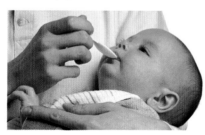

2 Place the spoon on his lower lip, raise the angle of the spoon and let the medicine run into his mouth.

Using a dropper

1 Hold your baby as described left and take up the specified amount of medicine into the glass tube.

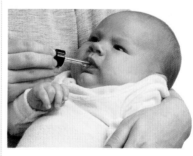

2 Place the dropper in the corner of your baby's mouth and release the medicine gently.

Using a medicine tube

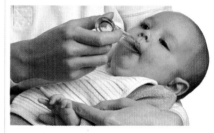

Pour the required dose into the tube. Hold your baby as described left. Place the mouthpiece on his lower lip and let the medicine run gently into his mouth.

Other methods

Measure the required dose into a container, dip your little finger in, then let your baby suck it off your finger. A plastic syringe can also be helpful. Ask your doctor to recommend one.

Giving medicines and tablets to older children

On the whole, children do not generally mind medicine too much and often want to pour medicine out for themselves rather than let you give it to them. I have listed a few tips below that may help if your child is difficult. For example, tablets can be crushed and mixed with jam, and medicines can sometimes be mixed with a favourite drink. Capsules, however, should not be broken.

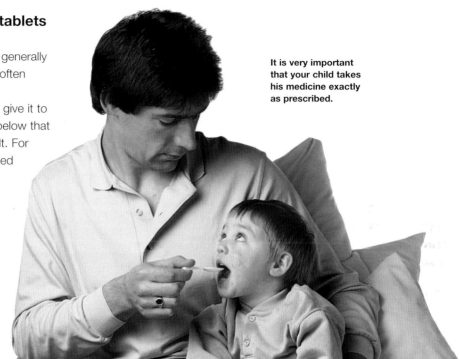

It is very important that your child takes his medicine exactly as prescribed.

Tips on giving medicines
Giving medicines to babies

◗ Get the help of another adult or older child.
◗ If you are on your own, wrap a blanket around your baby's arms so that you can stop him struggling and hold him steady.
◗ Only put a little of the medicine in his mouth at a time.
◗ If your baby spits the medicine out, get the other person to hold his mouth open while you pour the medicine into the back of his mouth and then, gently but firmly, close his mouth.

Giving medicines to older children

◗ Suggest that your child holds his nose while taking the medicine, thereby lessening the effect of the taste.

◗ Don't forcibly hold your child's nose as he may inhale some of the medicine.
◗ Mix liquid medicine with another syrup such as honey to dilute the taste.
◗ Don't add liquid medicine to a drink as it will just sink to the bottom of the glass or stick to the sides and you won't be sure that your child has had the whole dose.
◗ Show your child that you have his favourite drink ready to wash the taste of the medicine away, even if you would not normally allow your child to have it very often.
◗ Help your child to clean his teeth thoroughly after taking any liquid medicine to prevent syrup sticking to his teeth.
◗ Crush tablets between two spoons and mix the powder with honey, jam or ice cream.

Medicines *continued from previous page*

Giving drops

Ear, nose or eye infections may be treated with external drops. It is always easier to administer drops to a baby or young child if you lay him on a flat surface before you begin and enlist the help of another adult or an older child to keep him still and hold his head steady. An older child will probably be more co-operative and you will only need to ask him to tilt his head back or to the side while you put the drops in.

Ear drops

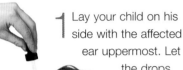
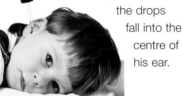

1 Lay your child on his side with the affected ear uppermost. Let the drops fall into the centre of his ear.

2 Hold your child steady until the drops have run into the canal.

Nose drops

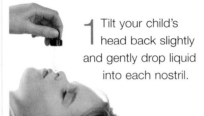

1 Tilt your child's head back slightly and gently drop liquid into each nostril.

2 Count the number of drops as you put them in. Two or three drops at a time are normally sufficient; any more will run down his throat and cause him to cough and splutter.

Eye drops

1 Tilt your child's head slightly so that his affected eye is lowermost. This way, no drops can run from the affected eye to the other. If this is difficult, get someone to hold him.

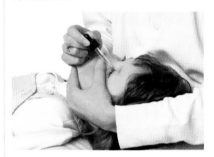

2 Very gently pull his lower eyelid down and let the drops fall between his eye and his lower lid.

Tips for giving drops

- Warm nose drops and ear drops by standing the container in warm, *not hot*, water for a few minutes, so that your child doesn't get a shock when they drop into his nose or ear.
- Do not let the dropper touch your child's nose, ear or eye, or you will transfer the

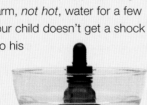

germs back to the bottle. If the dropper does touch your child, wash it thoroughly before putting it back in the bottle.
- Proprietary drops should not be used for longer than three days without consulting a doctor – they can actually cause worse irritation and inflammation than the condition you were treating in the first place.

Medicine chest

You should always keep some medicines in the house in case of an emergency in the middle of the night when you may not be able to get to a chemist easily. Keep them somewhere obvious so that you can find them quickly when you need them. Never mix pills up in the same container and never keep unused prescription medicines. Keep all medicines out of reach of children, in a locked cupboard, if necessary.

You should also have a first-aid kit (*see page 314*). Keep all the equipment in a clean, dry, airtight box and put it somewhere it can be found in an emergency.

Medicines to avoid

The following items, commonly given as useful, should be avoided:
▶ Any proprietary product containing a local anaesthetic, such as amethocaine or lignocaine, because they can cause allergies. They are generally found in creams for mouth ulcers or insect stings.
▶ Any skin creams containing antihistamines – unless prescribed by your doctor – they can cause skin allergies.
▶ Any proprietary product containing aspirin.
▶ Mouth washes, gargles, eye drops, nose drops and ear drops, unless recommended by your doctor.

Essential items

Medicine chest
▶ Digital thermometer – keep two in case one breaks.
▶ Forehead thermometer.
▶ Junior paracetamol tablets.
▶ Paracetamol elixir.
▶ Calamine lotion for soothing skin irritations, sunburn and stings.

First-aid kit
▶ Box of adhesive dressings.
▶ Wound dressings – cotton wool and gauze pad already attached to a bandage.
▶ Packet of skin closures.
▶ Cotton wool.
▶ Mild antiseptic cream.
▶ Gauze dressings – keep dry and paraffin-coated ones.
▶ Surgical tape.
▶ Crepe bandages for supporting sprains and strains.
▶ Open-weave bandages.
▶ Triangular bandage.
▶ Blunt-edged tweezers, safety pins and scissors.

Useful household items
▶ Packet of frozen peas, or ice cubes in plastic bags for cold compresses.
▶ Newspaper, folded to make a splint.
▶ Elastic belt to support a strain/sprain.
▶ Rehydration fluid to replace fluid lost after vomiting or diarrhoea.
▶ Bicarbonate of soda added to the bath water to relieve itching.
▶ Salt added to a bath to clean wounds.
▶ Vinegar mixed with water to soothe jellyfish stings.

Nursing a sick child

VERY FEW PARENTS ESCAPE being called upon to look after a sick child – all children fall ill at some time. Babies often become very clingy when they are ill and may cry more than normal because they do not understand what is happening to them. If a baby is being breastfed he will probably want to be fed more often, as much for the comfort of being near you as anything else. Bottlefed babies will also want to be cuddled and will want smaller feeds more often. If your baby has recently given up his bottle, you may find that he wants it back again.

Older children also become rather insecure when they are ill and want to be with one of their parents all the time. Nursing a child does not require any special skills, just love. Few things can go wrong and, if a child's condition takes a turn for the worse, most parents will spot it immediately. Simply use your common sense. If you are worried, take your child to your doctor or ask for a home visit (*see pages 24–7*). If any medicines are prescribed, make sure you give them exactly as directed (*see pages 32–4*), and follow any nursing tips your doctor gives you. Try to be cheerful and optimistic because children are often frightened by being ill and will be quick to sense your concern.

Should my child stay in bed?

Take your lead from your child. There's no need to keep a child with a fever in bed, although he should stay in a draught-free room where the temperature is constant. The room does not have to be particularly hot – if it is comfortable for you, it should be warm enough for your child. If your child is really ill, he will probably want to stay still and will sleep a lot but when he is awake he will want to be with you – make up a bed for him in the room where you are working so that he can see and hear you. This will also be easier for you as you won't have to keep running backwards and forwards to his room. If your child wants to be out of bed and playing, let him do so in the corner of the room where you are working. Leave his bed straightened so that he can go there if he wants to. If he is very tired, it is better to put him to bed, but remember to go and visit him regularly so that he does not feel neglected.

Should I isolate my child?

Evidence suggests that, in cases of infectious diseases, the degree of severity of the disease increases if there has been sustained close contact. Therefore it is advisable to keep other children away from the infected child as much as possible. Obviously, if your child has a more serious infection that does need isolation, such as hepatitis (*see page 160*) or meningitis (*see page 178*), your doctor will arrange for your child to be admitted to hospital or advise you on the necessary precautions. Also, if your child

Tips for nursing your child

- Use cotton sheets – they are more comfortable for a child with a temperature.
- Change his sheets regularly, particularly if he has a fever – clean sheets feel better.
- Put a jumper and socks or slippers on over his pyjamas if he does not want to stay in bed all the time.
- Leave a box of tissues on his bedside table.
- Leave a bowl or bucket beside your child's bed if he is feeling sick so that he doesn't have to run to the toilet.
- If your child vomits, hold his head and comfort him while he is being sick and give him a mint or strongly flavoured sweet, or help him clean his teeth, to take away the after-taste.

has German measles (*see page 142*), you should warn any women you think may be pregnant – or who may come in contact with someone who is pregnant.

Feeding a sick child

Most children with a fever don't want to eat, so while you should offer food, you should never force your child to eat. As long as he is getting plenty of liquid, your child can survive perfectly well for two or three days on very little to eat. When the illness is over, your child's appetite will return. As soon as it does, take advantage of it and let your child eat as heartily as he wants to. If he does want to eat, there is no particular food that is especially necessary when your child is ill, so forget the rules and spoil him a little by giving him his favourite foods until he is well again. I've always felt that there is no danger of a child slipping into bad habits as a result of special treatment while he is ill if he knows that the usual rules will be reinstituted as soon as he is well again.

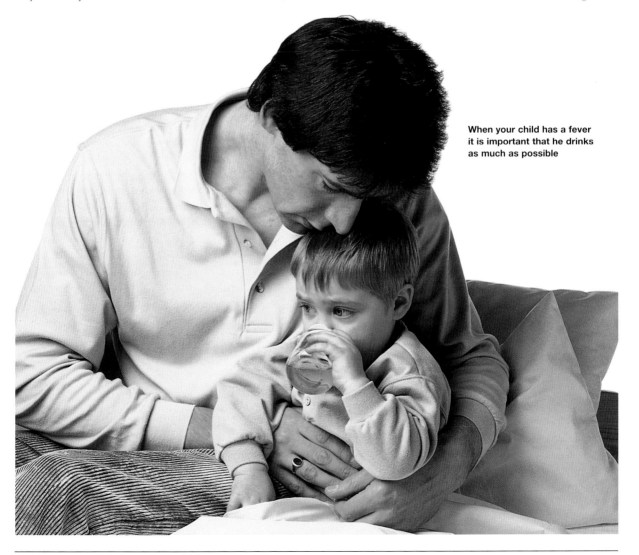

When your child has a fever it is important that he drinks as much as possible

Nursing a sick child *continued from previous page*

Getting a sick child to drink

While your child can survive without much food when he is ill, it is very important that he drinks as much as possible to replace any fluid lost in sweating and vomiting or diarrhoea. A child with a fever needs to drink at least 100–150ml (3–5fl oz) liquid per kilo (2.2lb) of body weight per day. This should be increased to 200ml (7fl oz) per kilo (2.2lb) if he is vomiting or has diarrhoea (*see page 109*). Get your child to drink as often as you can, even a little every half an hour while he's awake. Help an older child by leaving his favourite drink by the bed, and then remind him every so often to take a sip. Fizzy glucose drinks are not nutritious, nor are they necessary; I do not recommend them.

Occupying a sick child

When your child is ill you can legitimately spoil him. Let him play with games that previously have never been allowed in bed. Even messy activities like painting will not cause too much mess if you put a large sheet of polythene over the bed.

Be easy on yourself as well and relax all the rules on tidiness – you can always clear up later. Whatever you do, don't make a fuss and don't nag your child to be tidy. Sit down and spend time with him, read him stories, play games or sing him songs, and help him with his colouring, painting or building.

Let your child watch television or listen to the radio while he is ill – have the television in his room or in the room where you are both sitting. Buy him some new toys and give them to him one at a time. If he isn't feeling too ill, try wrapping them up and play a game with the parcel; ask him to guess what's in the packages and let him tear off the wrapping. Ask his friends to come and see him and let them play for a short time.

If your child is not in bed all the time, there's absolutely no reason to keep him indoors on a warm day, even if he has a mild fever, but don't let him

Tips on feeding and drinking

Feeding your child

- Give your child small meals more often than you would normally.
- Don't scold your child for not eating – he will eat again as soon as he gets better.
- Give your child his favourite foods.
- If your child has a sore throat, give ice cream or an ice lolly made with fruit juice or yogurt to soothe his throat.
- If your child is feeling slightly sick give him mashed potato.
- As soon as your child's appetite returns, take full advantage of it and let him eat as much as he can.

Making drinks more interesting

- Give your child a glass to drink out of which is normally reserved for adults.
- A sure ploy is to offer drinks in a tiny glass or egg cup. It is more fun and makes the quantities look smaller.
- Give your child fresh fruit juices such as pear, apple, orange or water melon. Dilute these drinks with fizzy mineral water to make them more interesting.
- Use an interesting straw such as a curly or bendy one.
- If your child does not like milk, make it more attractive by adding milkshake mixes or some ice cream.
- Vary the drinks as much as possible.
- With a young child or baby, get him to sip drinks from a teaspoon. Make it seem like a game by using a long-handled spoon.

**If your child is well enough, give
him toys to play with in bed**

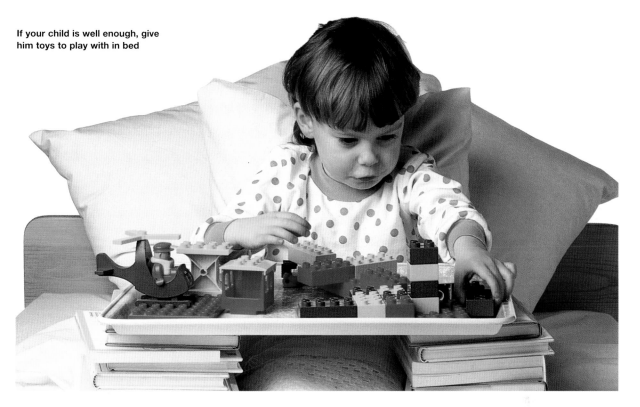

exercise too strenuously. If he wants to stay outside
for longer than a few minutes, he is probably getting
better anyway.

Getting better

As your child gets better his appetite will start to
come back and he will probably be more active.
As soon as his temperature is back to normal in the
morning and evening, he is probably ready to go
back to school, although, if he has been suffering
from an infectious illness, it may be wise to check
with your doctor first.

A young child may have regressed slightly while
he was ill. For example, if he was just out of nappies
you may have to start potty training again. Try not
to worry about this too much.

Your child in hospital

YOU WILL BE DOING YOUR CHILD a great favour if you always encourage him to think about hospitals as friendly places. Try to take him with you if you are visiting a family friend or relative – provided the person does not mind and that the visiting regulations allow it.

Preparing your child for hospital

If your child has to go into hospital, for an operation, for example, and you are given several weeks, or days, warning, prepare him by discussing as many aspects of his stay as possible. Talk about it with the whole family and get him generally used to the idea.

Answer all his questions honestly. Don't make promises that you can't keep and don't tell lies. If he is having an operation he will probably ask you if there will be any pain or discomfort after the operation. If you say that nothing is going to hurt and it does, he will simply get a shock and will not trust you again in the future. Explain that there will be some discomfort but that it won't last long.

Another good way to prepare him for a hospital stay is to read him a book about someone who goes into hospital. You could also buy him a toy stethoscope and play doctors and nurses with him. Encourage him to be the doctor or nurse and suggest that he makes up a hospital bed for his favourite teddy bear or toy.

When your child is in hospital

Few children's wards are frightening. However, it has been found that it is important for parents to be with their children as much as possible while they are in hospital. Because of this, almost all hospitals allow parents to stay in hospital with their child, particularly if he is very young. Many hospitals have sleeping facilities for parents with children up to the age of six.

When you are there, ask the ward sister and nurses how you can help with the daily routine. You will probably be encouraged to bath and change your child

What to take into hospital

If you can, you and your child should pack his case together a few days before he has to go in.

- Three pairs of pyjamas.
- Dressing gown and slippers.
- Three pairs of ankle socks.
- Hair brush and comb.
- Sponge bag with soap, flannel, toothbrush, toothpaste.
- Bedside clock.
- Portable radio or cassette player with headphones.
- Favourite books and portable games.
- Favourite picture or photograph.

and help with his feeding. You can read books and play games with him. If the ward has a ward teacher, ask if you can help with your child's schoolwork. If your child is well enough and will be in hospital for a while, ask his own schoolteacher to give you the work he would normally be doing at school.

If you cannot be with your child all day, try to arrange a rota so that someone he knows well is with him all the time.

Back home from hospital

It's quite normal for a child to behave a little oddly when he comes out of hospital. Firstly, your child's sleeping and eating patterns may have changed. Hospital meals, and certainly bedtimes, tend to be earlier than you'd have them at home. Secondly, because your child has been away from his domestic discipline, you may find that he will make a fuss about small points like brushing his teeth. Don't be too hard on him at first, give him time to readjust to being at home.

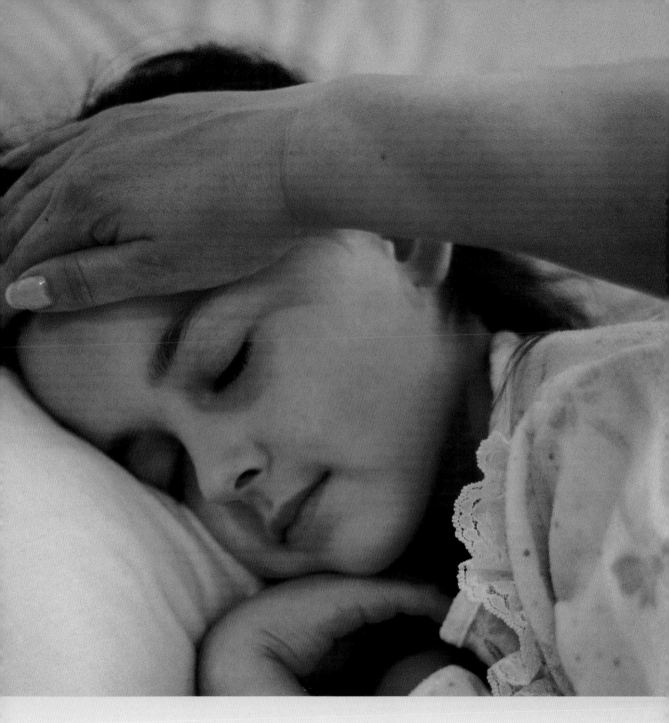

Visual
diagnosis guides

How to use this section

THIS SECTION IS DESIGNED to help if you don't know what has caused your child's symptoms, and are therefore unsure which A–Z entry to look up. Because it is impossible to give a definitive medical diagnosis from only one or two symptoms, this section instead helps you to make an educated guess as to the possible cause. For ease of reference, the body is illustrated in six sections (*see below*), and the symptoms relating to those parts are dealt with accordingly. To use the guide, turn to the page dealing with the affected part of the body and look for the symptom most similar to the one your child is suffering from (if your child

has more than one symptom, look up the major one first). Then turn to the A–Z entry suggested as a possible cause for more detailed information. If you cannot find the symptom that you are looking for, turn to the major index on page 331 and either look up the symptom itself (for example, headache) or the part of the body affected (head).

Listed below are the parts of the body that may be affected, and the page on which you will find them. Problems affecting the skin in general, such as rashes, are also listed.

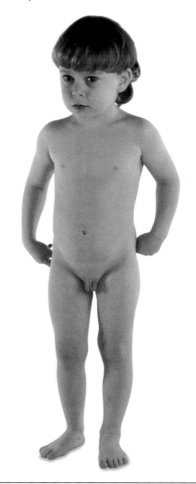

Eyes, mouth and scalp *page 43*
Eyes
Hair
Head
Scalp
Lips
Mouth
Teeth
Gums
Cheeks

Ears, nose and throat *page 44*
Ears
Nose
Throat
Neck
Cheeks

Abdomen, chest and back *page 45*
Chest
Lungs
Stomach
Groin
Abdomen
Shoulders
Back
Umbilicus (navel)

Genitals and bowels *page 46*
Penis
Vagina
Bowels

Arms, hands, legs and feet *page 47*
Arms
Hands
Fingers
Fingernails
Legs
Knees
Feet
Toes
Toenails

The skin *page 48*
Rashes
Lumps
Swellings
Paleness
Coldness
Itchiness
Dryness

Eyes, mouth and scalp

Thick, yellow scales over part or all of your baby's scalp *possibly* Cradle cap, see page 100.

White flakes on your child's scalp *possibly* Dandruff, see page 107.

Bald patches of itchy, red or grey scaly rings *possibly* Ringworm, see page 210.

Itchy head with tiny pearl-white eggs clinging to the hair roots *possibly* Lice, see page 175.

Sore, watery eye *possibly* Foreign body in eye, see page 131.

Weepy, sore, red eyes which may be gummed together in the morning *possibly* Conjunctivitis, see page 91.

Weepy, red-rimmed, itchy eyes accompanied by sneezing *possibly* Hayfever, see page 152.

One or both of your baby's eyes wander *possibly* Squint, see page 226.

Pus oozing from the inner corner of your baby's eye *possibly* Sticky eye, see page 228.

Severe headache and pain when neck is stretched *possibly* Meningitis, see page 178.

Headache on one side of the forehead *possibly* Migraine, see page 180.

Swollen, red area on your child's eyelid, nearly always the lower lid *possibly* Stye, see page 231.

Red, scaly eyelids, with dandruff-like scales clinging to your child's eyelashes *possibly* Blepharitis, see page 66.

Nosebleed, discharge with foul smell *possibly* Foreign body in nose, see page 191.

Tiny, itchy, very painful blisters around the nostrils and lips *possibly* Cold sore, see page 87.

Tiny blisters that ooze and crust over bright yellow *possibly* Impetigo, see page 166.

Small cracks on the lips *possibly* Chapping, see page 81.

Small, white, depressed ulcerated area inside the mouth *possibly* Aphthous mouth ulcer, see page 182.

Large, red area with a yellow centre, usually inside the cheek *possibly* Traumatic mouth ulcer, see page 182.

Creamy-yellow or white frothy patches inside your baby's mouth, which bleed when wiped *possibly* Oral thrush, see page 240.

Swollen red area on your baby's gum, accompanied by dribbling *possibly* Teething, see page 234.

Painful, throbbing sensation in the tooth or gum in an older child *possibly* Toothache, see page 245
Or Gum boil, see page 149.

Ears, nose and throat

Blotchy red rash that starts behind the ears and then spreads to the rest of the body, accompanied by swollen neck glands *possibly* German measles, see page 142.

Brownish-red rash of small spots that starts behind the ears then spreads to the rest of the body, usually preceded by a runny nose and red, sore eyes *possibly* Measles, see page 177.

Tiny white or yellow spots on and around a newborn baby's nose *possibly* Milia, see page 181.

Nasal speech and mouth breathing *possibly* Adenoids, see page 243.

Pain underneath the eyes *possibly* Sinusitis, see page 217.

Sneezing, with a runny nose and itchy eyes *possibly* Hayfever, see page 152.

A runny nose, often with a sore throat and fever *possibly* a Common cold, see page 90 *Or* Influenza, see page 167.

Bleeding nose *possibly* Nosebleed, see page 192 *Or* Foreign body in the nose, see page 191.

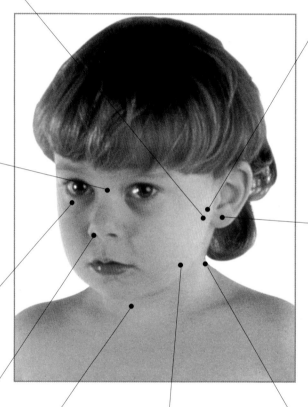

Pain in and around the ear *possibly* Otitis media, see page 198 *Or* Toothache see page 245 *see also* Earache, page 122.

Pussy discharge from the ear *possibly* Otitis media, see page 198.

Pain inside the ear canal, made worse when the earlobe is pulled *possibly* Otitis externa, see page 196.

Impaired hearing, accompanied by a sensation of fullness in the ear *possibly* Wax in the ears, see page 260 *Or* Glue ear, see page 145 *Or* Foreign body in the ear, see page 121.

Hoarse cough or loss of voice *possibly* Croup, see page 100 *Or* Laryngitis, see page 172.

Swelling on either or both sides of the face *possibly* Mumps, see page 182.

Swollen neck glands with a sore throat which may be accompanied by a fever *possibly* Tonsillitis, see page 243 *Or* Glandular fever, see page 143 *Or* Scarlet fever, see page 213.

Abdomen, chest and back

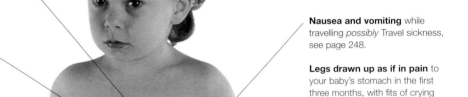

Intensely itchy, small blisters that appear in clusters on the trunk then spread to the rest of the body *possibly* Chickenpox, see page 82.

Flat, red or pink rash starting on the trunk and spreading to the neck and limbs, usually after a high fever *possibly* Roseola infantum, see page 211.

Rapid, difficult breathing in a baby under one year old, following a common cold *possibly* Bronchiolitis, see page 72.

Whooping sound during a coughing fit as air is breathed in *possibly* Whooping cough, see page 261.

Dry cough with a fever and rapid, laboured breathing, over the age of one *possibly* Bronchitis, see page 73.

Pain starting around the navel then moving to the lower right area of the groin in an older child *possibly* Appendicitis, see page 54.

Painless bulge in the groin that increases in size when your child coughs or strains *possibly* Inguinal hernia, see page 162.

Nausea and vomiting while travelling *possibly* Travel sickness, see page 248.

Legs drawn up as if in pain to your baby's stomach in the first three months, with fits of crying *possibly* Colic, see page 88.

Projectile vomiting in a newborn baby where milk shoots out forcefully from the mouth after a feed *possibly* Pyloric stenosis, see page 205.

Severe spasmodic cramps in a baby under 12 months with vomiting and red, jelly-like stools containing blood and mucus *possibly* Intussusception, see page 169.

Umbilical gramuloma (fleshy growth on umbilical stump) *possibly* due to infection, see page 251.

Nausea and vomiting and/or diarrhoea *possibly* Gastroenteritis, see page 140.

Painless bulge near the navel that increases in size when your child strains or coughs *possibly* Umbilical hernia, see page 162.

Weeping, umbilical cord stump in a newborn baby, which then crusts over *possibly* Umbilical cord infection, see page 251.

Genitals and bowels

Pimply red rash on area normally covered by your baby's nappy *possibly* Nappy rash, see page 187 *Or* Thrush, see page 240.

Persistent, involuntary soiling of the pants with loose bowel motions, in a child who has no other symptoms of illness and was previously toilet-trained *possibly* Encopresis, see page 127.

Small, thread-like worms around the anus, with intense itchiness *possibly* Worms, see page 263.

Hard, pebble-like stools and pain in the lower abdomen *possibly* Constipation, see page 92.

Red, swollen tip of penis *possibly* Balanitis, see page 62.

Loose, frequent bowel motions *possibly* Diarrhoea, see page 112.

Tight foreskin in a child over five years old *possibly* Phimosis, see page 201.

Red, jelly-like bowel motions containing blood and mucus, in a baby under one year, accompanied by severe abdominal pain *possibly* Intussusception, see page 169.

Smoky, dark-coloured or reddish-brown urine *possibly* Hepatitis, see page 160 *Or* Nephritis, see page 189.

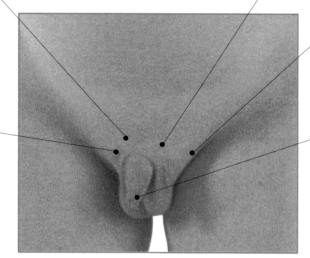

Loose, frequent bowel motions accompanied by vomiting, shortly after eating *possibly* Food poisoning, see page 137 *Or* gastroenteritis, see page 140.

Irritation of the vulva *possibly* Foreign body in the vagina, see page 253 *Or* Worms, see page 263.

Foul-smelling, pale stools *possibly* Coeliac disease, see page 85.

Frequent, painful passing of urine accompanied by fever *possibly* Urinary tract infection, see page 252.

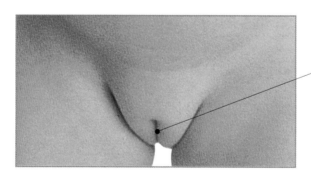

Arms, hands, legs and feet

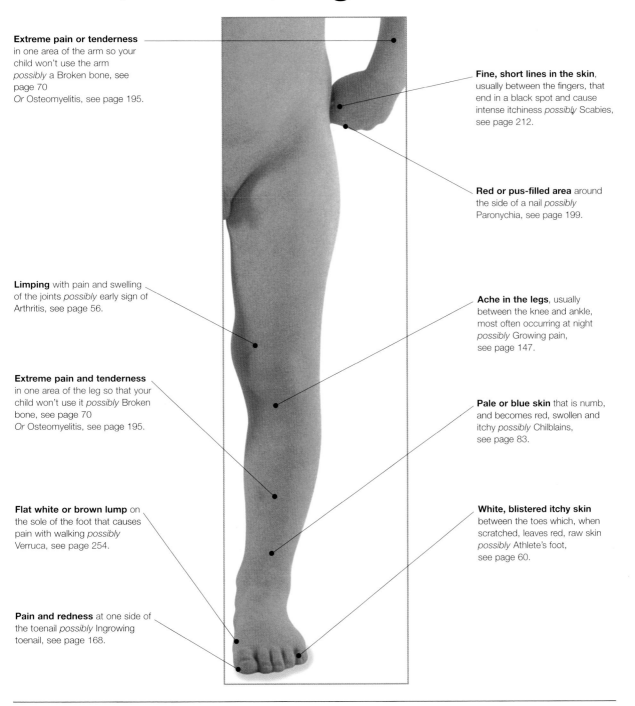

Extreme pain or tenderness in one area of the arm so your child won't use the arm *possibly* a Broken bone, see page 70 *Or* Osteomyelitis, see page 195.

Fine, short lines in the skin, usually between the fingers, that end in a black spot and cause intense itchiness *possibly* Scabies, see page 212.

Red or pus-filled area around the side of a nail *possibly* Paronychia, see page 199.

Limping with pain and swelling of the joints *possibly* early sign of Arthritis, see page 56.

Ache in the legs, usually between the knee and ankle, most often occurring at night *possibly* Growing pain, see page 147.

Extreme pain and tenderness in one area of the leg so that your child won't use it *possibly* Broken bone, see page 70 *Or* Osteomyelitis, see page 195.

Pale or blue skin that is numb, and becomes red, swollen and itchy *possibly* Chilblains, see page 83.

Flat white or brown lump on the sole of the foot that causes pain with walking *possibly* Verruca, see page 254.

White, blistered itchy skin between the toes which, when scratched, leaves red, raw skin *possibly* Athlete's foot, see page 60.

Pain and redness at one side of the toenail *possibly* Ingrowing toenail, see page 168.

The skin

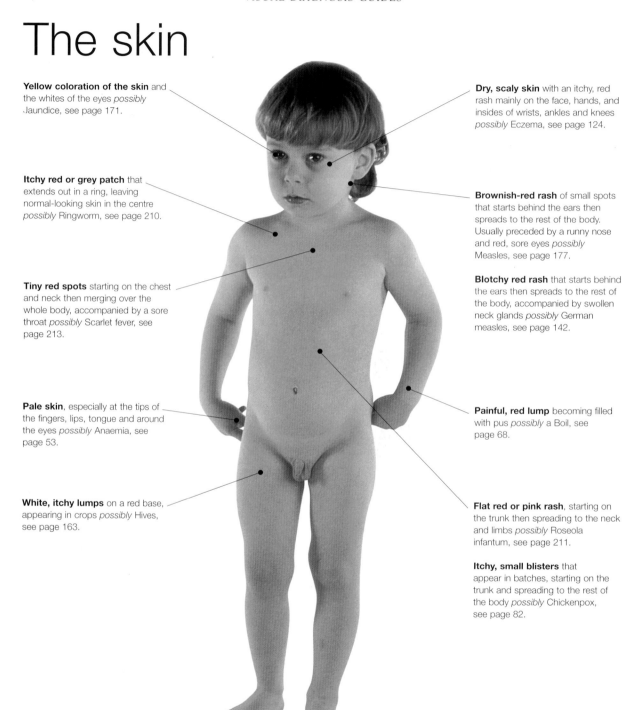

Yellow coloration of the skin and the whites of the eyes *possibly* Jaundice, see page 171.

Itchy red or grey patch that extends out in a ring, leaving normal-looking skin in the centre *possibly* Ringworm, see page 210.

Tiny red spots starting on the chest and neck then merging over the whole body, accompanied by a sore throat *possibly* Scarlet fever, see page 213.

Pale skin, especially at the tips of the fingers, lips, tongue and around the eyes *possibly* Anaemia, see page 53.

White, itchy lumps on a red base, appearing in crops *possibly* Hives, see page 163.

Dry, scaly skin with an itchy, red rash mainly on the face, hands, and insides of wrists, ankles and knees *possibly* Eczema, see page 124.

Brownish-red rash of small spots that starts behind the ears then spreads to the rest of the body. Usually preceded by a runny nose and red, sore eyes *possibly* Measles, see page 177.

Blotchy red rash that starts behind the ears then spreads to the rest of the body, accompanied by swollen neck glands *possibly* German measles, see page 142.

Painful, red lump becoming filled with pus *possibly* a Boil, see page 68.

Flat red or pink rash, starting on the trunk then spreading to the neck and limbs *possibly* Roseola infantum, see page 211.

Itchy, small blisters that appear in batches, starting on the trunk and spreading to the rest of the body *possibly* Chickenpox, see page 82.

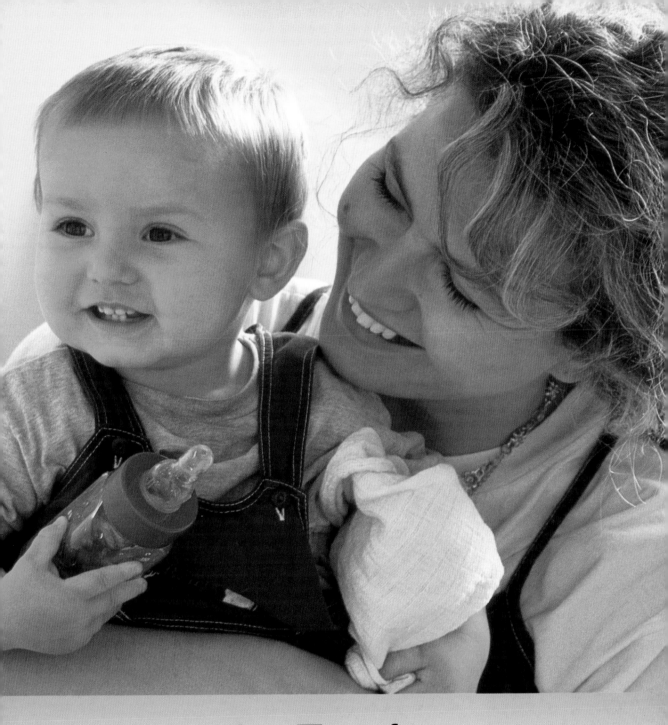

A–Z of
common complaints

How to use this section

THE A–Z OF COMMON COMPLAINTS is the core of the book, covering all of the most common childhood complaints. The entries take two basic forms. In the majority, a detailed description of the illness is given, with a possible symptoms box for easy reference, a list of what to check for first, and treatments that might be given. In some cases, such as bedwetting, no symptoms box is given because the symptom is the complaint's name.

Long-term complaints, such as cerebral palsy and spina bifida, are dealt with discursively. There is no check-list for What should I do first? nor do the headings Is it serious? or Should I call the doctor? appear. Instead, the treatments and procedures following diagnosis of a long-term ailment are given under the heading What can be done? An address to contact for help and advice is also given. Throughout the entries, words in bold refer to other A–Z entries.

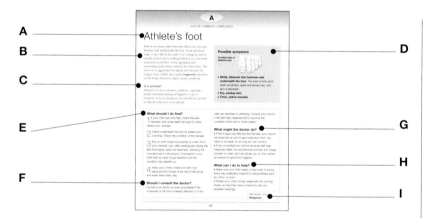

A — Heading
B —
C —
E —
F —
D —
G —
H —
I —

A Heading
Name by which the complaint is commonly known.

B Introduction
Gives a description of the complaint, explaining why it arises and how it is likely to develop.

C Is it serious?
States whether or not the complaint is serious, and the conditions under which it would become serious.

D Possible symptoms
Lists the symptoms that are likely to occur with the given complaint. Your child may have some or all of them; he may or may not develop them in the order given, although that is the most likely sequence of appearance.

E What should I do first?
Details what you should do if you suspect your child has a certain complaint. This may involve action to determine whether your child definitely has the complaint (taking his temperature, checking for a

rash); or may suggest home treatments that will provide immediate relief for your child while you contact the doctor (tepid sponging for fever, or calamine lotion for itchiness). If your child's case is an emergency, the section will say so and will suggest that you call an ambulance or go straight to the nearest casualty department.

F Should I consult the doctor?
This will tell you the circumstances under which you should seek medical assistance. There are four levels of immediacy.

1 Emergency
In a life-threatening situation, you will be told to call an ambulance or go straight to the nearest casualty department for help.

2 Consult your doctor immediately
This means call your doctor at once – even if it is the middle of the night or out of surgery hours – because your child needs medical attention as soon as possible. If the complaint is life-threatening and there is any risk

of a delay in the doctor's arrival, the entry will tell you to call an ambulance or go straight to the nearest casualty department.

3 Consult your doctor as soon as possible

This means call your doctor to make an appointment at the earliest time possible. If your child's symptoms develop out of surgery hours, don't worry, but do ring as soon as the surgery opens.

4 Consult your doctor for advice

Your child has no serious problem, but it may be one which worries him or you. Make an appointment to talk to your doctor about it whenever it is convenient.

G What might the doctor do?

The treatment most likely to be given to your child is outlined.

H What can I do to help?

Makes suggestions as to what a parent can do to assist the doctor in the treatment of the child, as well as home treatment and nursing tips for the complaint itself.

I See also box

A cross-referencing system to other articles within the A–Z. The parent may be cross-referred to another complaint because it could be the possible cause of the symptoms, or it may be of background interest to the complaint in question.

A–Z Index

AIDS

AIDS (ACQUIRED IMMUNE DEFICIENCY SYNDROME) is a progressively debilitating condition caused by the human immunodeficiency virus (HIV) that destroys the white blood cells in the body's immune system. In some cases HIV has been transferred via contaminated blood transfusions, but most HIV-infected children contract the virus from their mothers. However, not all HIV-positive mothers will transmit the virus to their babies, and there are also ways of reducing the risk before and around the time of delivery.

HIV infection produces few symptoms, but once the immune system is severely weakened, illnesses such as **pneumonia** develop unhindered. Most infected children will show symptoms before they are two years old, although some may not show any signs until they are more than five. Few children who are HIV-infected seem to make a full recovery and,

without a major medical breakthrough, the outlook for HIV-positive people in general is bleak. Death from AIDS will continue to occur in most infected children within a few years of the onset of symptoms.

Possible symptoms

▶ **Failure to thrive**.
▶ **Recurrent diarrhoea**.
▶ **Enlarged lymph nodes**.
▶ **Frequent infections**.
▶ **Attacks of pneumonia**.
▶ **Developmental delay**.

Should I consult the doctor?

If you suspect that your child has been infected with the HIV virus, you should seek your doctor's advice immediately. Children who are HIV-positive or who have developed AIDS require careful medical supervision.

What can be done?

▶ Your doctor will arrange counselling for you and your partner. With your consent, a blood test will be performed. Newborn babies of HIV-positive mothers can be difficult to diagnose because they do not show any symptoms of the virus, but their mothers' antibodies may be present in their blood for at least a year.

▶ Your doctor may prescribe drugs for your child to attack the virus and to slow the development and progress of the disease.

▶ Your doctor may give your child regular injections of gamma globulin and may prescribe antibiotics to help prevent or fight infections such as pneumonia.

▶ If you are HIV-positive, do not breastfeed your child as there is a small but definite risk that you might transmit the virus to your baby via your milk.

▶ If your child is HIV-infected, or has AIDS, you will be given counselling and advice on how to manage the illness.

For help and advice contact the Terrence Higgins Trust (see page 324).

Anaemia

ANAEMIA IS A DEBILITATING CONDITION that is due either to a reduction in the number of normal red cells in the blood or in the amount of haemoglobin, the oxygen-carrying pigment derived from iron that gives the red cells their colour. This reduction can be caused by inadequate production of red cells in the bone marrow, by lack of iron and other blood-forming substances, by diseases such as **leukaemia**, **sickle cell anaemia** and **thalassaemia**, by excess blood loss, or by infection.

Is it serious?

Anaemia is serious because it may be a symptom of an underlying disease and therefore all cases must be investigated.

Possible symptoms

▶ **Pale tongue and skin**, especially at the tips of the fingers, the lips and around the eyes.
▶ **Fatigue, lethargy and weakness.**
▶ **Shortness of breath** on exertion.
▶ **Dizziness.**
▶ **Raised pulse rate.**

What should I do first?

1 If your child seems listless and pale, and he is not eating well, check his eyes, mouth, fingertips and tongue for paleness.

2 Note whether your child is less active than his friends, if he is uncharacteristically breathless after a little exercise, or if he complains of **dizziness**.

Should I consult the doctor?

Consult your doctor immediately if you think your child is anaemic. Anaemia should always be investigated promptly and thoroughly by a doctor. You should never rely on home remedies.

What might the doctor do?

▶ Your doctor will first take blood samples and send them to a laboratory for analysis. If the diagnosis is confirmed, your child may have to go into hospital for a full investigation of the cause of the anaemia and possibly a blood transfusion if his condition is severe.

▶ If the anaemia is due to iron deficiency, your doctor will probably prescribe supplements of iron and may advise you to include more iron-rich foods in your child's diet. In addition, the cause of the iron deficiency should be tracked down by a paediatrician. Your child may need to attend a hospital clinic for tests.

What can I do to help?

Make sure that your child is eating a properly balanced diet as set out by your doctor or dietician. Iron-rich foods include liver, egg yolk, dark green leafy vegetables and nuts. Vitamin C helps in the absorption of iron, so give your child a glass of orange juice with his egg, for example.

SEE ALSO:
Dizziness 116
Leukaemia 174
**Sickle cell
  anaemia** 216
Thalassaemia 239

Appendicitis

APPENDICITIS OCCURS WHEN the appendix becomes partly or wholly blocked and a build-up of bacteria in the appendix causes an infection. The appendix becomes inflamed and swollen and may need to be removed surgically. An appendicectomy is a common emergency operation among children. However, appendicitis in babies under one year is rare.

Is it serious?

If appendicitis is diagnosed early, it is not a serious condition. However, if treatment is delayed for any reason, the build-up of pus in the blocked appendix can cause it to burst. This is known as peritonitis.

Possible symptoms

- **Abdominal pain**, starting around the navel, then moving down to the lower-right abdomen.
- **Slight temperature**, rarely above 38°C (100.4°F).
- **Loss of appetite**.
- **Vomiting**.
- **Diarrhoea or constipation**.

What should I do first?

1 If your child complains of an abdominal pain for more than a couple of hours, lay him flat on his back. Gently press his stomach a few centimetres to the right of, and just below, the navel. Pain on gentle pressure, and a sharp pain when you suddenly remove your hands, are signs of appendicitis. Consult your doctor immediately.

2 If your child is constipated and you suspect appendicitis, don't give him laxatives. They can cause an inflamed appendix to burst.

3 Don't give your child anything to eat or drink in case an appendicectomy, which is carried out under general anaesthetic, is necessary.

Should I consult the doctor?

Consult your doctor immediately. Any delay could spread the infection to the rest of the intestines.

What might the doctor do?

- Your doctor will examine your child's abdomen and ask you when the pain started and to describe any other symptoms. He will probably arrange for the transfer of your child to hospital to confirm the diagnosis and for surgical removal of the appendix, if necessary.

What can I do to help?

- Stay with your child at the hospital overnight; your presence should help speed his recovery.
- Encourage your child to rest and eat normally when he returns home from hospital, usually about five days after the operation. Your child should recover fully after two to three weeks.

SEE ALSO:
Constipation 92

Appetite, loss of

A SICK CHILD WILL NEARLY ALWAYS go off his food. Loss of appetite is a general sign of ill health and nearly always accompanies a fever. It is also a symptom of a problem in the stomach and intestines, such as **gastroenteritis**, or of a **sore throat** if the child finds swallowing painful. Minor disorders, such as **travel sickness**, will usually cause your child to lose his appetite, but this will be only temporary. You should not worry about loss of appetite being a symptom of an underlying problem if your child has simply missed a meal due to tiredness, or because you've had a battle of wills at mealtime. This is perfectly normal, and your child will make up for it in the following meals.

Is it serious?

If your child refuses to eat for 24 hours, and you can find no reason for the loss of appetite, this is a cause for concern.

What should I do first?

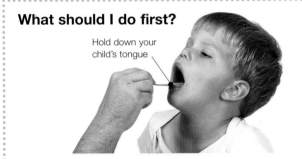

Hold down your child's tongue

1 If your child refuses food for a day, but he is taking plenty of fluids, check his temperature. Check to see if his tonsils are inflamed by gently holding down his tongue with the handle of a spoon, and ask him to say "aaah". He may be having difficulty in swallowing because of **tonsillitis**.

2 Check to see if your child is suffering from **earache**. An ear infection, such as **otitis media**, could be painful enough to put your child off his food.

3 Check for **appendicitis** by examining the lower right of the abdomen.

4 Check if there is any pain when your child passes urine. This could be a sign of a **urinary tract infection**.

5 If your child's temperature is normal, and there is no evidence of illness, although he still refuses food, get him to drink plenty of fluids.

Should I consult the doctor?

Consult your doctor if the loss of appetite persists, even without any other symptoms, for 24 hours.

What might the doctor do?

▶ Your doctor will examine your child to see if there is any physical reason why he should be off his food. If none can be found, your doctor will probably keep a check on your child's condition.
▶ Your health visitor can offer valuable advice and counselling.

What can I do to help?

Make sure your child gets plenty of nutrients by disguising them in drinks: for example, enrich a milkshake with wheatgerm and a banana.

SEE ALSO:
Appendicitis 54
Earache 122
Gastroenteritis 140
Otitis media 198
Sore throat 222
Tonsillitis 243
Travel sickness 248
Urinary tract infection 252

Arthritis

ARTHRITIS IS THE INFLAMMATION of a joint. This is usually accompanied by swelling, pain, stiffness and tenderness. Arthritis may be caused by an injury to a joint, or by an infection in the joint, when it is called septic arthritis. In rare cases, it may be caused by **rheumatic fever**, or by a malfunctioning of the body's defence mechanism which leads the antibodies to attack the body's own tissues, causing inflammation and a fluctuating temperature. This is called Still's disease or juvenile rheumatoid arthritis. Still's disease starts between the ages of two and five and affects mainly girls.

If your child is ill with an infectious disease such as **influenza** or **measles**, he may have arthritic pains in his joints. These will, however, disappear once the infection has passed.

Is it serious?
Arthritis is a serious disorder that can lead to permanent deformity.

Possible symptoms
- **Pain and swelling** in a joint or several joints.
- **Limping** if hip or knee joints are affected.
- **General aches** and pains all round the body.
- **A temperature** of 40°C (104°F) or higher, or a temperature that fluctuates from normal to 39°C (102.2°F).
- **Loss of appetite**.

What should I do first?

1 Check to see if your child has a temperature. If it is as high as 40°C (104°F), and there is pain in the joints, treat this as an emergency. This could be septic arthritis. If his temperature fluctuates from normal to as high as 39°C (102 2°F), and he seems unwell consult your doctor immediately. This could be Still's disease.

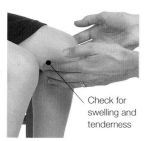

Check for swelling and tenderness

2 If you notice that your child is walking with a **limp**, check his joints for swelling and tenderness by pressing on and around them.

3 If your child has had an injury to a joint and he complains of aches and pains, check the joint for tenderness and swelling.

4 If the pain is felt by your child between the joints and not on the joint itself, this could be a **growing pain**. Check the calf and thigh muscles for tenderness.

5 Don't give your child any painkilling drugs until you have seen your doctor.

Should I consult the doctor?
Consult your doctor immediately if your child has a high, fluctuating temperature and a painful, swollen joint. Consult your doctor as soon as possible if you notice your child limping.

Continued from previous page

What might the doctor do?

▶ Your doctor will examine your child and ask about any other symptoms or illnesses your child may have had over previous months.

▶ If your doctor suspects arthritis, your child will probably be referred to a specialist for examination and blood tests to find a definite cause. Your child may have to stay in hospital to complete any necessary tests.

▶ If your child has septic arthritis, he will be given antibiotics intravenously to eradicate the infection in the joint.

▶ If your child has Still's disease, he may be prescribed paracetamol elixir and anti-inflammatory drugs. He will be taught a set of exercises to increase mobility in the affected joints.

What can I do to help?

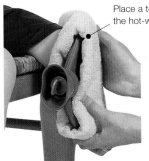

Place a towel around the hot-water bottle

▶ Wrap a hot-water bottle in a towel and rest it on the affected joint. Heat is sometimes soothing and can help to get the joint moving.

▶ Apply a cold compress to the joint if it is hot and swollen. Wrap a plastic bag filled with ice cubes in a piece of cloth and apply it directly to the joint.

▶ Make sure your child has plenty of rest and a protein-rich diet.

▶ Gently massage the joints. Sometimes this can relieve aches and pains.

▶ Take your child for regular 30-minute swimming sessions. Swimming in warm water is excellent exercise for arthritis sufferers. Check with your doctor before doing this.

Special exercises

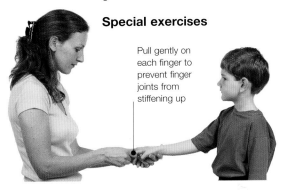

Pull gently on each finger to prevent finger joints from stiffening up

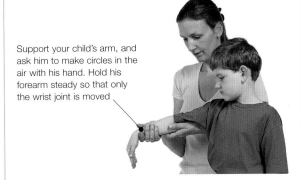

Support your child's arm, and ask him to make circles in the air with his hand. Hold his forearm steady so that only the wrist joint is moved

▶ Practise the special exercises at home with your child if the physiotherapist agrees.

SEE ALSO:
Growing pain 147
Influenza 167
Limp 176
Measles 177
Rheumatic fever 209

Asthma

ASTHMA IS AN ALLERGIC DISEASE that affects the air passages (*bronchi*). When the allergic reaction takes place, the bronchi constrict and become clogged with mucus, making breathing difficult. An asthma attack can be very frightening for a child because the feeling of suffocation can cause panic, making breathing even more difficult. The initial cause of the allergic reaction, the allergen, is usually airborne – pollen or house dust, for example. Once asthma is established, emotional stress and exercise can also bring on an attack.

Asthma does not usually begin until a child is about two years of age. The condition tends to run in families and is unfortunately usually accompanied by other allergic diseases, such as **eczema** or **hayfever**. However, most children get better as they get older.

Many babies under one year wheeze if they suffer from **bronchiolitis**, when their small air passages become inflamed. These babies are not necessarily suffering from asthma; as they grow older and their air passages start to widen, the wheezing will stop. Infection and not an allergic reaction is the usual cause of this wheezing.

Is it serious?

Asthma attacks can be frightening but, with medication and advice from your doctor, your child should suffer no serious complications.

Possible symptoms

▶ **Laboured breathing**: breathing out becomes difficult and the abdomen may be drawn inward with the effort of breathing in.
▶ **Sensation of suffocation**.
▶ **Wheezing**.
▶ **Persistent cough**.
▶ **Blueness around the lips (cyanosis)** because of lack of oxygen.

Area affected

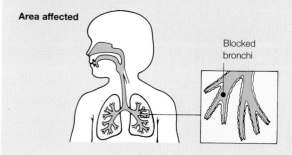

Blocked bronchi

What should I do first?

1 Consult your doctor immediately if your child is having an asthma attack.

2 If the attack occurs when your child is in bed, sit him up, propped up with pillows. Otherwise, have him sitting up straight on a chair and leaning forwards against a table or the back of another chair to take the weight off his chest; this allows his chest muscles to force air out more efficiently.

3 Stay calm; a show of anxiety would only make your child more fearful.

4 While you are waiting for the doctor, try to take your child's mind off the asthma attack. Sing to him, for example, to try to help him forget about the wheezing.

Should I consult the doctor?

Consult your doctor immediately if your child has an asthma attack.

Continued from previous page

What might the doctor do?

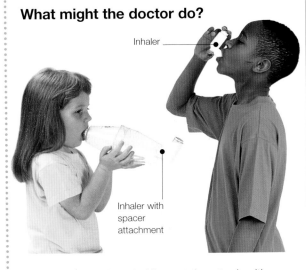

Inhaler

Inhaler with spacer attachment

▶ Your doctor will probably treat the attack with a bronchodilator drug, which is inhaled directly into the bronchi and gets right to the site of the restriction. A severe attack may require treatment in hospital where bigger doses of bronchodilator drugs may be given.

▶ If there is some evidence of a chest infection, antibiotics will be prescribed.

▶ Your doctor will measure your child's peak expiry flow rate (PEFR) to monitor his condition.

▶ Your doctor will discuss prevention of further attacks and may try to find the allergen. He will arrange for you to have a small supply of a bronchodilator drug, either in liquid form or as capsules for insertion into an inhaler or spacer. This should be given as soon as an attack begins. Your doctor will ask you to inform him if your child has a severe attack, or if an attack does not respond to two doses of the bronchodilator.

▶ Your doctor may prescribe a steroid drug if other simpler measures are not successful in preventing further attacks. A small dose of steroid may be inhaled by your child three or four times a day or,

if this is not effective, a larger dose will be given in tablet form.

▶ Your health visitor can help you monitor the severity and frequency of your child's attacks and give general advice about ongoing treatment.

What can I do to help?

▶ If your doctor failed to pinpoint the allergen, try to track it down yourself. Notice when the attacks occur and at what time of the day or year. Avoid obvious allergens, such as feather pillows, and keep the dust down in your house by vacuuming floors often.

▶ Many asthmatics are allergic to animals. If you have a pet, ask a friend to look after it for a while and see if your child's attacks are reduced.

▶ Make sure your child has the prescribed drugs nearby at all times in case of an attack. Inform his school about his asthma.

▶ Ask to be referred to a physiotherapist so that your child can learn breathing exercises to help him remain calm during an attack.

▶ Encourage your child to stand and sit up straight so that his lungs have more space. Don't let him become overweight as this will put an extra burden on his lungs.

▶ Moderate exercise can help his breathing, but too much can bring on an asthma attack. Swimming, however, can be especially helpful.

▶ Avoid smoking near your child.

▶ Use barrier covers for pillows and duvets and reduce soft furnishings if possible.

For help and advice contact the National Asthma Society (see page 324).

SEE ALSO:
Bronchiolitis 72
Eczema 124
Hayfever 152

Athlete's foot

THIS IS A FUNGAL INFECTION that affects the soft area between and underneath the toes. At an advanced stage, it also affects the nails. It is contagious and is usually picked up by walking barefoot in communal areas such as shower rooms, gymnasia and swimming pools, where infected feet have been. The infection is aggravated by sweaty feet because the fungus, *tinea*, which also causes **ringworm** elsewhere on the body, thrives in warm, moist conditions.

Is it serious?

Athlete's foot is a common condition, requiring simple treatment and good hygiene to cure it. However, as it is contagious, you should act quickly so that the infection is not spread.

Possible symptoms

Possible sites of blistered skin

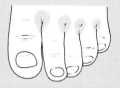

▶ **White, blistered skin between and underneath the toes**. The area is itchy and, when scratched, splits and leaves raw, red skin underneath.
▶ **Dry, peeling skin**.
▶ **Thick, yellow toenails**.

What should I do first?

1 If your child has itchy feet, check the area between and underneath the toes for white blisters and redness.

2 Check underneath the foot for blisters and cracking. Check the condition of the toenails.

3 Buy an anti-fungal foot powder or cream from your chemist, and, after washing and drying the feet thoroughly, apply the treatment, following the manufacturer's instructions. Emphasize to your child that he must not go barefoot until the condition has cleared up.

4 Keep your child's towel and bath mat separate from those of the rest of the family and wash them every day.

Should I consult the doctor?

Consult your doctor as soon as possible if the underside of the foot is already affected, or if the nails are distorted or yellowing. Consult your doctor if the self-help measures fail to improve the condition within two or three weeks.

What might the doctor do?

▶ If the fungus has affected the toenails, your doctor will prescribe an anti-fungal medication that may need to be taken for as long as nine months.
▶ If you consulted your doctor because self-help measures failed, he will prescribe another anti-fungal powder or cream and will advise you on the correct procedure for good foot hygiene.

What can I do to help?

▶ Make sure your child wears a clean pair of socks every day, preferably made from natural fibres such as cotton or wool.
▶ Rotate your child's shoes, especially his running shoes, so that they have a chance to dry out between wearings.

SEE ALSO:
Ringworm 210

Autism

AUTISM IS A DISABILITY THAT AFFECTS the way a child relates to people around him. It disrupts the development of social and communication skills, isolating those it affects from the rest of us. It occurs in varying degrees of severity (hence the description "autistic spectrum disorder") although all those affected have various impairments which affect social interaction, social communication and imagination. Many autistic children have accompanying learning disabilities. The spectrum of autistic disorders includes Asperger's syndrome, a condition that describes people who show the characteristics of autism, but are of average or above-average intelligence and have good communication skills.

Autism can be caused by a variety of conditions affecting brain development, which occur before, during and after birth. It cannot be diagnosed until it is realized that speech has not developed at the normal rate, if at all. By this time, you will probably have noticed that your child is withdrawn and spends hours in solitary play. He might adopt behaviour rituals, such as touching certain objects in sequence or rocking backwards and forwards. Disruption of

these behaviours may bring on severe temper tantrums. This behaviour reflects the child's need to surround himself with an environment that never varies. Some autistic children also have a heightened sensitivity to certain objects and sounds. With hindsight, parents may remember that their autistic child was not a cuddly baby, and seldom smiled.

Possible symptoms

▷ **Difficulty with verbal communication.**
▷ **Non-verbal communication difficulties.**
▷ **Difficulty with social relationships.**
▷ **Difficulty in the development of play and imagination.**
▷ **Resistance to change in routine.**

What can be done?

If you suspect that autism is present, it is essential that you take your child for a specialist diagnosis as early as possible – either to your doctor, Child Development Centre or Child and Family Guidance Centre. Early diagnosis is essential to ensure that families and carers have access to appropriate services and professional support. At present there is no cure for autism, but there are many different therapies and approaches that have been tried over the years with varying degrees of success. Specialized education and structured support can maximize a child's skills and minimize any

behaviour problems, enabling those who are affected by the condition to live their lives as independently as possible.

For help and advice contact the National Autistic Society (see page 324).

Balanitis

BALANITIS IS THE INFLAMMATION of the tip (*glans*) of the penis. It may be caused by **nappy rash**, by an allergic reaction to the soap powder in which your child's clothes are washed, or by a tight foreskin in boys aged three to five (**phimosis**). Up until then, the foreskin is normally tight.

Is it serious?

The condition is not serious, though it is important for your child's comfort that you treat the condition promptly. If balanitis is recurrent, your son may need to be circumcised.

Possible symptoms

- **Red, swollen tip** to the penis.
- **Discharge of pus** from the tip.
- **A foreskin that cannot be drawn back.**
- If your child is still in nappies, **a general inflammation around the buttocks and in the genital region**.

What should I do first?

1 If your child is over five, as soon as you notice any redness around the tip of the penis, carefully and gently try to draw back the foreskin. Don't force it. If the foreskin won't retract, leave it alone and consult your doctor as soon as possible.

2 If the foreskin will retract, wash and dry the penis thoroughly and apply an antiseptic ointment.

3 If the condition is part of nappy rash, change your child's nappies frequently, wash and dry the area thoroughly at every nappy change and liberally apply a barrier cream over the area covered by the nappy, including the penis.

Should I consult the doctor?

Consult your doctor as soon as possible if your child complains of pain, if you cannot retract the foreskin, or if home treatment fails to relieve the swelling within 48 hours.

What might the doctor do?

- Your doctor may prescribe an antibiotic cream to relieve the inflammation.

If the foreskin is tight, your doctor will keep a regular check on it; if the foreskin has failed to stretch by the time your son is six years old, the condition may need to be corrected surgically with circumcision. Your doctor will refer you to a paediatrician who will assess your child to see if he really needs to be circumcised.

What can I do to help?

- Always change your child's nappies frequently to prevent the recurrence of nappy rash.
- Teach your child good personal hygiene from an early age. Up until the age of five, regular bathing will keep the penis adequately cleaned. After this age, encourage your child to draw back the foreskin and wash the area every day.
- If an allergic reaction has caused balanitis, try changing your washing powder, and make sure that your child's clothing is thoroughly rinsed.

SEE ALSO:
Nappy rash 188
Phimosis 201

Bedwetting

CHILDREN MASTER BLADDER CONTROL at different ages. Just as they develop skills at different rates, so their ability to hold urine for long periods varies. However, although one in 10 normal boys still wets the bed at the age of five, most children become dry at night between the ages of three and four. A child should not be classified as a bedwetter while he is still training his bladder to last the 10–12 hours of night-time sleep.

A return to bedwetting once a child has gained bladder control is nearly always a sign of increased tension and anxiety. This often happens as a result of an important occasion, such as the arrival of a new baby in the house, or starting school. A few children may have a physical reason for their incontinence, such as a **urinary tract infection** or some abnormality of the urinary system. If bedwetting is accompanied by increased thirst and frequent urination during the day, these could be symptoms of **diabetes mellitus**.

Is it serious?

Although irritating for parents, bedwetting is not a serious problem.

What should I do first?

1 Put a rubber sheet on the bed and cover it with a small top sheet that can be easily washed and dried every day if necessary.

2 Examine your own behaviour. You may be the source of the problem. You may be pushing your child too hard or creating a tense atmosphere.

3 Make sure your child empties his bladder before going to bed; if he wishes, leave a potty in his room so that he doesn't have to go to the bathroom.

4 Check whether your child's urine has a fishy smell. This could indicate a urinary tract infection.

Should I consult the doctor?

Consult your doctor if both you and your child are becoming discouraged, or if you suspect that there may be some physical cause such as a urinary tract infection, which may cause frequent, painful urination. Your health visitor can give counselling.

What might the doctor do?

▶ Your doctor will examine your child and take a urine sample to exclude the possibility of a urinary tract infection or a malformation of the urinary tract.

▶ Your doctor may recommend that you fit a special pad on your child's bed which lets off an alarm when moistened. Your child can learn to react to the alarm and get up and go to the toilet. This is of use only if your child is over six years old and doesn't object.

▶ Your doctor or paediatrician may prescribe a medicine to reduce the urine produced overnight.

What can I do to help?

▶ Minimize the problem and make sure the rest of the household follows your lead. Don't scold your child and always make light of the subject, no matter how tiresome it becomes.

▶ Try giving your child a star for every dry night. He can place it on a calendar and watch his progress.

▶ Don't limit the amount of liquid you give your child before bedtime. This has no effect on his bedwetting.

▶ Don't try anything, such as the alarm pad, that your child objects to; it will only increase the tension.

▶ Avoid fizzy drinks at bedtime and drinks containing caffeine, which can cause excess urine production.

For help and advice contact ERIC (see page 324).

SEE ALSO:
Diabetes mellitus 111
Urinary tract infection 252

Birthmark

A BIRTHMARK IS A PATCH OF DISCOLORATION in the skin, caused by a collection of small blood vessels or pigment just under the surface. The birthmark, which may be flat or raised, may be present at birth or may appear in the first months of life.

Brown birthmarks are circular and may have hair growing out of them. They are called moles and are usually permanent and should not be interfered with by anyone but a specialist.

Storkbites are small, pink and spidery and appear on the back of the neck, the upper eyelids or the nose. They disappear within a few years.

A *Mongolian spot* looks like a blue bruise in the skin and is usually found among dark-skinned people. It occurs most often on the lower back or buttocks.

A *strawberry naevus* is a raised red mark with a bumpy surface which is sometimes shaped like a strawberry. It usually disappears by the time a child is five but, before it does, it enlarges alarmingly, growing darker or lighter, before gradually disappearing. It is most common in girls and can bleed spontaneously.

A *port-wine stain* looks exactly like its name – a red patch on the skin. It can appear over much of the face and forehead or the limbs, and it is usually quite large. This is the most distressing birthmark because it does not disappear, though it can fade to a paler pink. It is more common among blond children.

Is it serious?

A birthmark is almost always harmless and, apart from a port-wine stain, most will disappear by the age of five.

What should I do first?

1 The most important thing is not to rush at treatment because many birthmarks disappear spontaneously.

2 If a strawberry naevus bleeds, place a clean pad or handkerchief over the mark. It should stop bleeding after a minute or so.

Should I consult the doctor?

Consult your doctor for advice if you feel that the birthmark is disfiguring and that your child may suffer as a result in the future.

What might the doctor do?

If the birthmark is very unsightly, your doctor may refer you to a plastic surgeon. Birthmarks can be treated with a wide variety of modern techniques, including tattooing and laser therapy. If you decide against cosmetic surgery for any reason, your doctor may prescribe special camouflage make-up for your child.

What can I do to help?

❱ If the mark is unsightly and disturbs you and your child, use the camouflage make-up.

❱ Try not to show your child that you are anxious about the birthmark.

Bites

Most children love the company of animals but, because they are not always as gentle with them as they should be, bites do occur. The most common animal bites – from dogs and cats – leave puncture marks; humans leave teeth marks. Insect bites leave a weal resembling **hives** – a white centre on a red base. They are extremely itchy, but the pain and localized reaction fade within three to four hours.

The common flea, normally from a household pet, also bites to leave itchy weals.

Are they serious?
Animal, human and insect bites are rarely serious. If they are untreated, however, they could become infected and possibly serious.

What should I do first?
1 Reassure your child and calm him down. If he has been bitten by a dog or a horse, for example, it is important that he does not remain afraid of these animals throughout his childhood. Try to persuade him that it is an isolated incident.

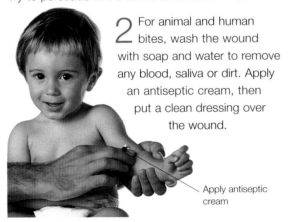

2 For animal and human bites, wash the wound with soap and water to remove any blood, saliva or dirt. Apply an antiseptic cream, then put a clean dressing over the wound.

Apply antiseptic cream

3 For insect bites, apply calamine lotion to relieve the irritation.

Should I consult the doctor?
Consult your doctor as soon as possible to check that an animal or human bite is not infected or deep enough to carry the risk of **tetanus**. Consult your doctor immediately if the wound is bleeding heavily or if, after 12 hours, the area looks red and swollen.

What might the doctor do?
◗ Your child may need to be immunized against tetanus infection.
◗ If the wound is infected, your doctor will probably prescribe antibiotics.

What can I do to help?
◗ You must emphasize to your child the need to treat animals carefully and not to tease them. In most cases, if a pet caused the injury, it will be an isolated incident and you should not need to get rid of the animal.
◗ If you are travelling abroad, be prepared for any problems by carrying a first-aid pack and updating tetanus boosters before you go.
◗ You will need to clean the carpet, curtains and furniture if you suspect that your child has been bitten by fleas. A special flea powder to dust furnishings is available from veterinary surgeons. Take your pet along to the vet for treatment too.
◗ If your child is being bitten by mosquitoes, apply an insect repellent to his skin or clothes, and put an incense stick in his room at night or spray the room with an insect repellent.

SEE ALSO:
Hives 163
Tetanus 238

Blepharitis

BLEPHARITIS IS AN INFLAMMATION of the skin around the edges of the eyelids. It usually affects both eyes. The inflammation can become worse if the area is infected: **styes** may occur. Blepharitis is often accompanied by dandruff and may be part of a condition known as seborrhoeic **eczema**.

Possible symptoms

▸ **Red, scaly eyelids**.
▸ **Discharge of pus** from the eyelid, which dries to look like dandruff clinging to the eyelashes.

Is it serious?

Even though the condition may initially be only a minor irritant, it should always be treated because it can recur.

What should I do first?

1 If you notice your child rubbing his eyelids, check to see if the area seems red and scaly, or if the eyelashes are matted together with pus.

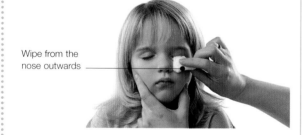

Wipe from the nose outwards

2 Don't use any patent creams or eye lotions. Wash away the discharge morning and night with warm boiled water, to which you have added a little salt or bicarbonate of soda. Use a clean cotton-wool swab for each eye and wipe gently from the nose outwards.

3 Check your child for **cradle cap** or **dandruff** on the scalp.

Should I consult the doctor?

Consult your doctor if the washing treatment doesn't clear the scaliness and redness within one week.

What might the doctor do?

▸ Your doctor may prescribe a soothing eye ointment to damp down the inflammation.
▸ If your child has seborrhoeic eczema, your doctor may prescribe special shampoos and scalp lotions.
▸ If there is an infection, such as a stye, your doctor may prescribe antibiotic ointment or eye drops to remove the pussy discharge.

What can I do to help?

▸ Pay particular attention to hygiene. If your child's eyelids have become infected, the infection can be easily spread to other members of the family, so wash your hands thoroughly before and after you administer the treatment.
▸ Discourage your child from touching his eyes.
▸ Apply a thin smear of Vaseline to your child's eyelids at night. The scales will then wash away easily in the morning.

SEE ALSO:
Cradle cap 100
Dandruff 107
Eczema 124
Stye 231

Blister

A BLISTER IS A FLUID-FILLED BUBBLE of skin that forms as a result of burns or friction, or as a result of exposure to extremes of temperature, which can cause **sunburn** or **frostbite**. Blisters vary in size, depending on the cause, and their purpose is to form a cushion to protect the new layer of skin growing underneath. The fluid is eventually reabsorbed by the body and the outer surface dries out and peels away, leaving the healed skin behind. If the blister is broken before healing has taken place, there is a risk of infection.

Is it serious?

A blister is not usually serious.

Possible symptoms

▶ **Raised surface of the skin**, filled with fluid, which may measure as much as several centimetres across.

What should I do first?

1 Don't prick a blister that has formed as a result of friction, burning or extremes of temperature: leave it intact.

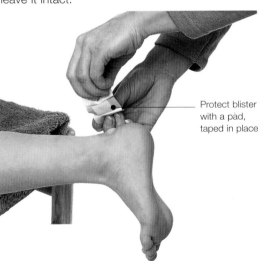

Protect blister with a pad, taped in place

2 Protect blisters where friction may cause them to burst. For example, if the blister is as a result of ill-fitting shoes or wearing shoes without socks, change your child's shoes for the time being, put two pairs of socks on your child, or use special sponge pads or corn plasters to protect the blister.

3 If the blister bursts, keep it clean and dry and cover it with a gauze dressing.

Should I consult the doctor?

Consult your doctor as soon as possible if the blister is large or the result of a scald or **sunburn**. Consult your doctor as soon as possible if the area becomes infected, that is, if the blister becomes pussy, if red streaks extend outwards from it, if the skin surrounding it becomes red, tender or swollen, or if your child complains of pain.

What might the doctor do?

▶ If the blister is large, it may require bursting. Your doctor will do this.
▶ If the blister has become infected, your doctor will prescribe antibiotics.

SEE ALSO:
Burn 76
Frostbite 139
Sunburn 232

Boil

A BOIL IS A LARGE, TENDER, RED LUMP that results when a hair follicle becomes infected with bacteria (*staphylococci*). (If the infection occurs further up the hair follicle, near to the skin's surface, this is called a pimple.) The pus-filled lump gradually comes to a white or yellow head and bursts after about two or three days, or it may heal on its own without bursting and slowly disappear. Because the hair follicles are so close together, the bacteria can infect a wide area, causing more boils to occur. This is most likely to happen on the face. The boils usually appear on areas where there are pressure points, such as where a collar rubs or on the buttocks.

Is it serious?

Although unsightly, a boil is not serious. However, it can be extremely painful, especially if it develops over a bony area such as the jaw or forehead where the skin is stretched tight.

Possible symptoms

▶ **Large, painful, red lump**.
▶ **Increasing tenderness and throbbing** as pus builds up inside the lump. After a day or two, the red lump forms a white or yellow pus-filled centre, which may or may not burst.

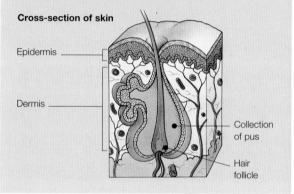

Cross-section of skin

Epidermis

Dermis

Collection of pus

Hair follicle

What should I do first?

1 If your child complains of throbbing pain, stop him from scratching or touching the area.

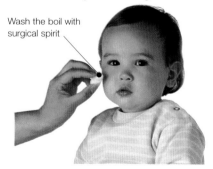

Wash the boil with surgical spirit

2 Wash the skin with surgical spirit or a solution of 5ml (one teaspoonful) of salt in a glass of warm water to prevent infection from spreading. Then put a sterile gauze dressing over the boil.

3 Do not try to squeeze the boil, even when it comes to a head. Squeezing will spread the infection to the surrounding area and make the outbreak much worse.

Should I consult the doctor?

Consult your doctor if boils are multiple or recurrent, or if the boil is causing your child a lot of pain because it is situated over a bony area or in an awkward place, such as the armpit. Consult your doctor as soon as possible if you notice red streaks spreading out from the centre of the boil. This may mean that the infection is spreading.

What might the doctor do?

▶ Your doctor will examine the boil and the surrounding area. If he can feel pus under the

Continued from previous page

skin, your doctor will probably lance the boil with a small scalpel and drain the pus, thus reducing pain immediately.

▶ If there is an infection and it has spread to the surrounding area, or if your child has had a number of boils over the previous months, your doctor may prescribe an anti-infective cream to treat the skin's surface, or antibiotic tablets to prevent the internal spread of the infection.

▶ If there are crops of boils, your doctor may prescribe a special antiseptic to put in your child's bath water.

▶ If the boils are recurrent, your doctor may arrange tests or refer you to a specialist (paediatrician or dermatologist) to find out the underlying cause.

What can I do to help?

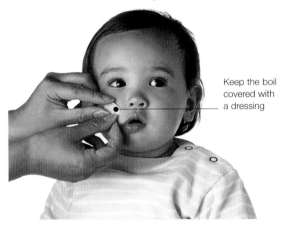

Keep the boil covered with a dressing

▶ Once the boil has burst, keep the area clean and covered with a dressing for a few days.

▶ Keep your child's towel and facecloth separate from those of the family.

▶ If the boil is in a place where clothing might rub against it, put a thick pad over the dressing to prevent any friction.

▶ If your child has a boil on the buttocks and is still in nappies, try to leave nappies off as much as possible. Change them frequently and use an antiseptic cream around the site of the boil.

Broken bone

CHILDREN'S BONES ARE LIKE YOUNG, bendy twigs on a tree; they do not snap as easily as the harder bones of an adult. A *greenstick fracture* is most common in children; the bone bends rather than breaks, and minimal damage occurs in the surrounding tissue. A *simple fracture* is where the bone breaks in one place but does not break the skin. In a *compound fracture*, the bone sticks through the skin and may damage the blood vessels and muscles. If the bone breaks through the skin or is exposed by a deep wound, this is known as an *open fracture*.

Is it serious?

A broken bone should always be treated promptly by a doctor for various reasons. The bone has to be set correctly, and any damage to surrounding organs or tissues has to be repaired. There is also a risk of infection if the break is an open fracture and the bone is exposed to the air.

Possible symptoms

- **Swelling** around the site of the injury.
- **Bruising** around the site of the injury.
- **Possible deformation** of the affected area.
- **Inability to move** the affected area normally or without pain.
- **Pain**.

Types of fracture

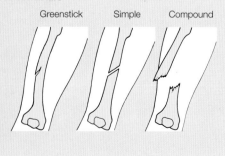

Greenstick   Simple   Compound

What should I do first?

1 Call an ambulance if the bone is curved or bent, or if the bone is sticking through the skin. Otherwise, take your child to the nearest hospital.

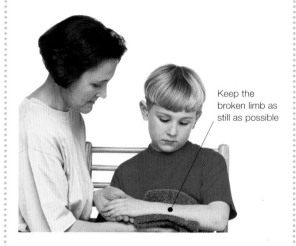

Keep the broken limb as still as possible

2 If the broken limb appears bent or curved, don't try to straighten it. Don't move your child unless you have to for his own safety. Any movement may increase internal damage and will cause more pain. If a bone has broken through the skin, or if there is a wound leading down to the fracture, drape a sterile dressing or gauze over the wound. Don't attempt any cleaning and don't touch the wound.

3 If there is no bone sticking through the skin, but your child cannot move the affected area without pain, immobilize the joints above and below the break to prevent worsening of the injury: for an arm, put it in a sling; for a leg, tie the knees and ankles together. Take your child to the nearest hospital if you can, but call an ambulance if the legs are affected because you will need a stretcher.

Continued from previous page

4 Don't give your child anything to eat and drink. He may need a general anaesthetic and this will be delayed if his stomach is not empty.

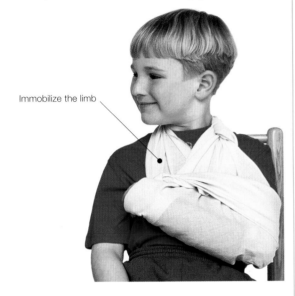

Immobilize the limb

5 Keep your child warm and as calm as possible while you get medical help. If possible, raise the affected part after immobilizing it.

Should I consult the doctor?

Call an ambulance if the limb is bent or curved, if the bone is sticking through the skin or if a leg is broken. Take your child to the nearest casualty department if you suspect your child has a broken bone.

What might the doctor do?

▶ The hospital doctor will X-ray your child to determine the extent of the damage. With a straightforward break, the bone will be immobilized by strapping with a tight bandage, or by setting it in a plaster-of-Paris cast.

▶ If the break is a compound fracture, the bones will be manipulated into position under a general anaesthetic before being immobilized in plaster.

▶ If there is an open wound with the broken bone, antibiotics will be given to prevent infection.

▶ If your child has a bad break in his leg, he may have to remain in hospital in traction. The damaged bone is pulled apart and held in the correct position for healing with a system of pulleys and weights.

What can I do to help?

▶ If your child has a plaster cast, make sure it stays dry and help your child to lead as normal a life as possible while the bone heals. Most broken bones in children heal within six to 10 weeks, depending on the severity of the fracture.

▶ If your child has to remain in hospital in traction, make his stay as entertaining as possible by bringing in his favourite games and toys, as well as new books and perhaps a personal stereo. Try to stay with him if you can.

Bronchiolitis

BRONCHIOLITIS IS AN INFLAMMATION of the smallest airways in the lungs (*bronchioles*). It is usually caused by a virus and occurs in babies under one year old. The condition may start as a **cough** or **common cold**. The virus causes the lining of the small airways to swell and to fill with mucus. This results in breathing difficulty and the baby will have to struggle for breath.

Is it serious?

Bronchiolitis is serious because the condition can cause severe breathing difficulties.

Possible symptoms

▶ **Rapid breathing** – over 50 breaths per minute.
▶ **Breathing difficulties**.
▶ **Raised temperature**.
▶ **Blueness** of the lips and tongue.
▶ **Drowsiness**.

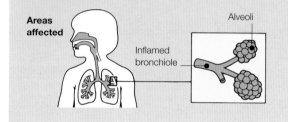

Areas affected

Alveoli

Inflamed bronchiole

What should I do first?

1 If your baby is distressed because of difficulty with breathing, and he starts to turn blue around the lips, treat this as an emergency. Consult your doctor immediately or take your child to the nearest hospital.

2 Try to soothe your baby; crying makes the breathing problem worse.

3 If you are breastfeeding, offer the breast frequently, or, if you are bottlefeeding, offer your baby frequent feeds to keep his fluid levels up.

4 Take your baby's temperature every six hours, and more often if he appears hot. If the temperature is over 38°C (100.4°F), give your baby paracetamol elixir to bring his temperature down.

Should I consult the doctor?

Consult your doctor immediately or take your baby to the nearest hospital if he has obvious breathing problems or if there is any sign of blueness around his lips and on his tongue. Consult your doctor immediately if you notice any deterioration in your baby's condition following a cold or cough.

What might the doctor do?

If your doctor is satisfied that your baby's infection is a mild one, he will advise you on nursing procedures so that you can look after your baby at home. However, most babies with this condition are usually admitted to hospital overnight for observation.

What can I do to help?

▶ If your baby is admitted to hospital, stay with him overnight. Your presence will reassure him.
▶ Try to keep your baby away from other children and adults who have coughs and colds.

SEE ALSO:
Common cold 90
Cough 98

Bronchitis

BRONCHITIS IS AN INFLAMMATION of the membranes that line the larger airways leading to the lungs. The condition may arise because a minor upper respiratory tract infection, such as a **common cold** or **sore throat**, reduces your child's resistance to infection. The infection, which may be viral or bacterial, causes the lining of the air passages to swell and mucus to build up, making breathing difficult. There is also a dry hacking **cough**, which, after one or two days, produces phlegm. If this is swallowed, the child may vomit it up.

Is it serious?

In children over a year old, bronchitis is not usually serious, but in rare cases wheezing and **vomiting** may be troublesome enough to require hospitalization.

Possible symptoms

▶ **Raised temperature**.

▶ **Dry hacking cough** that produces green or yellow phlegm.

▶ **Rapid breathing**, over 40 breaths per minute, with wheezing.

▶ **Breathing difficulties**.

▶ **Loss of appetite**.

▶ **Vomiting** with the cough.

▶ **Blueness of the lips and tongue**.

What should I do first?

1 If your child has recently had a cold, **sinusitis**, sore throat or an ear infection and his condition worsens, take his temperature to see if he has a **fever**. If your child has a fever, take his temperature every four hours. If it is as high as 38°C (100.4°F), lower it with tepid sponging (*see page 31*) or paracetamol elixir.

2 If your child is coughing persistently, check if there is any phlegm. If there is, encourage your child to cough it up. If he cannot understand how to do this, sit him on your lap leaning forwards and pat him gently on the back during the coughing attack.

Pat your child's back

3 Keep offering your child liquids; even if he won't eat, encourage him to take plenty of fluids to prevent the risk of **dehydration**.

4 Don't give him patent cough suppressants if there is phlegm, as this needs to be coughed up. However, your pharmacist may be able to recommend a soothing linctus to help soothe the throat.

5 Keep your child calm, quiet and warm.

Continued on next page

Continued from previous page

Should I consult the doctor?

Consult your doctor immediately or take your child to the nearest casualty department if your child is breathing with difficulty, drawing in his chest with every breath, or if there is any sign of blueness around his lips and on his tongue. This should be treated as an emergency. Consult your doctor as soon as possible if your child's upper respiratory tract infection gets worse.

What might the doctor do?

▶ If your child is in great distress because of breathing difficulties or vomiting, your doctor may admit him to hospital so that he can be given either oxygen to help with breathing or intravenous fluids to combat dehydration if your child has been vomiting as well.

▶ Your doctor will prescribe antibiotics if a bacterial infection is present. If your child's bronchitis is caused by a virus, your doctor will advise you on the nursing procedures for bronchitis because there will be no specific medication. Your doctor will show you how to help your child cough up the phlegm.

What can I do to help?

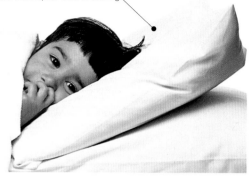

Prop your child up to ease breathing

▶ Prop your child up when he is sleeping so that he can breathe more easily.

▶ Keep your child as quiet as possible; running around and too much excitement may cause a coughing attack and vomiting.

Bruise

A BRUISE IS A PURPLISH-RED STAIN in the skin, usually resulting from a blow or a knock that ruptures the small blood vessels near the skin's surface. Children with fair skin show a bruise more readily than children with olive skin. It usually takes 10–14 days for a bruise to disappear completely; as it fades, it changes colour to maroon, and then to green or yellow as the blood pigments break down and are reabsorbed by the body.

Is it serious?

A bruise is rarely serious. If a bruise appears without reason, this may relate to uncommon but serious conditions such as **leukaemia** and **haemophilia**.

Possible symptoms

- **Purplish-red mark** on the skin which fades to maroon and then to green or yellow.
- **Tenderness** for a day or two.
- **Swelling** if the bruise is over the bone.

What should I do first?

1 A minor bruise needs no treatment at all, just a cuddle and reassurance if your child is upset.

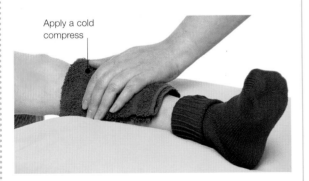

Apply a cold compress

2 If the bruise is large, apply a cold compress for half an hour or so. This will contain the bruising.

Should I consult the doctor?

Consult your doctor immediately if pain on the site of the bruise gets worse after 24 hours; an underlying bone could be broken. Consult your doctor immediately if a bruise appears spontaneously with no apparent cause.

What might the doctor do?

- Your doctor will examine your child to determine if there is a broken bone and refer you to a hospital casualty department for treatment if necessary.
- Your doctor will arrange blood tests or refer you to a specialist clinic if your child suffers from recurrent bruising or bruises that appear spontaneously to exclude anything serious.

SEE ALSO:
Broken bone 70
Haemophilia 150
Leukaemia 174

Burn

A BURN IS AN INJURY TO THE SKIN following exposure to heat from fires, hot liquids, chemicals, sun or electric current. The severity of a burn will depend on the situation and the cause. In a *superficial burn* there may be just a reddened patch of skin or a fluid-filled **blister**; in a *deep burn* layers of skin may actually be removed. Only small, superficial burns should be treated at home – no matter how minor a burn may seem to be, or how painless, there will always be some damage to the underlying tissue (in deep burns there may not always be pain because nerve endings have been damaged). All burns ooze a colourless liquid (plasma) and, if too much is lost, your child could go into a state of shock (*see page 299*).

Is it serious?

Apart from the most superficial burns, all burns should be treated seriously because of the possible scarring, risk of infection and shock. Electrical burns are serious because they may be deep but appear minor.

Possible symptoms

▶ **Raw, red areas**.
▶ **Fluid-filled blisters**.
▶ **Small blackened area** after an electric current has touched the skin.

What should I do first?
For small, superficial burns

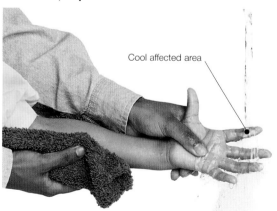

Cool affected area

1 Cool the affected area by placing it under cold running water for 10–15 minutes, or as long as your child can tolerate it, or apply ice cubes if only a small area is affected.

2 Cover the burn with a sterile dressing or a clean, ironed handkerchief; the dressing should extend beyond the injured area. Don't apply any creams or lotions, and certainly not butter or fat.

3 Give your child junior paracetamol tablets or elixir to relieve the pain.

4 Raise the affected part slightly so that blood flow to the area is slowed down. This will help to ease the pain.

For major, deep burns, or any electrical burn

1 If the burns were caused by liquids such as boiling water, oil or chemicals, put on a pair of rubber gloves or use a cloth or towel to prevent them from getting on to your skin, and remove your child's clothing. The clothes will continue to burn him until they are removed. However, do not remove any clothing that is sticking to the skin.

2 If your child has suffered an electric shock, first break his contact with the electricity by turning off the current or knocking him away with a non-conducting material, such as wood (*see page 304*).

Continued from previous page

3 Cool the affected area by running cold water over the skin for as long as your child can tolerate it. If the burns cover a large area, put your child into a cool bath.

4 Cover the affected area with a sterile dressing or any clean, non-fluffy material, such as an ironed handkerchief or pillowcase. Don't apply any creams or lotions, and certainly not butter or fat.

5 Lay your child down with his legs raised and supported and his head turned to one side. This prevents shock by keeping the essential blood supply in the vital organs. Wrap him in a clean sheet to reduce the risk of infection.

Raise your child's leg

6 Take your child to the nearest casualty department by ambulance or by car if someone else can drive you there.

Should I consult the doctor?

As only small, superficial burns should be treated at home, consult your doctor immediately or take your child to the nearest casualty department for all deep burns, burns on your child's face or any electric burn. Consult your doctor as soon as possible if a superficial burn does not heal in a week, or if the area becomes red and swollen and pus forms, indicating infection.

What might the doctor do?

▶ The hospital doctor will evaluate the burn and treat your child accordingly.

▶ If the burn has become infected, your doctor will cover the area with an antibiotic dressing. Your child may also be prescribed antibiotics to clear up the infection.

What can I do to help?

▶ Try to safeguard your child against hazards in the home by putting safety guards around the stove and fireplace and by fitting dummy plugs in unused electric sockets.

▶ Teach your child about the dangers of fire and burning as soon as he is old enough to understand.

▶ Check the labels when you buy clothing for your child to ensure that the fabric is non-flammable.

▶ Install a smoke alarm in your home.

SEE ALSO:
Blister 67
First aid 283

Catarrh

CATARRH IS AN EXCESS of mucus in the nose and throat. It may be the result of a **common cold**, it may occur with the onset of an infectious disease, such as **measles**, or it may be a symptom of **influenza**. With catarrh, the mucus is clear and runny, though it may become thick and yellow before the underlying condition clears up. One of the most dramatic forms of acute catarrh occurs in **hayfever** sufferers, when the allergic reaction of a runny nose is accompanied by itchy, tearful eyes and sneezing.

Chronic catarrh may be caused by **sinusitis**. The mucus from the infected sinuses runs down the back of the throat, causing the child to cough, particularly when lying down. Breathing becomes difficult, and, if a great deal of mucus is swallowed, this may lead to vomiting. Occasionally there may be catarrh with a middle-ear infection (**otitis media**), enlarged adenoids or nasal polyps.

Is it serious?

Catarrh that accompanies a minor illness is not serious. However, if your child suffers from chronic catarrh he will require treatment.

Possible symptoms

▶ **Nasal congestion**.
▶ **Runny nose** with a clear discharge.
▶ **Coughing**, especially at night.
▶ **Difficulty in feeding** in small babies.
▶ **Vomiting** if the mucus is swallowed.

What should I do first?

1 Encourage your child to blow his nose frequently. The catarrh will probably not need any more treatment than this.

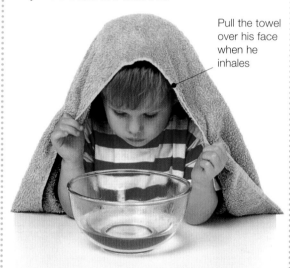

Pull the towel over his face when he inhales

2 If your child is having difficulty breathing, apply a menthol rub to his chest, or drops to his clothing or pillow at night. You can also encourage him, if he is old enough, to inhale the fumes from menthol crystals dissolved in hot water. Put the bowl on a safe work surface and cover both the bowl and your child's head with a towel so that he gets the full effect of the menthol. Menthol is also available in capsule and liquid forms.

3 If your child is coughing at night, prop him up with pillows so that the mucus doesn't drip down his throat.

4 Never use nose drops without your doctor's advice.

Continued from previous page

Should I consult the doctor?

Consult your doctor as soon as possible if the catarrh is making feeding difficult for your baby. Consult your doctor as soon as possible if you think the catarrh may be the result of an allergic reaction, such as hayfever, or if it persists for no apparent reason.

What might the doctor do?

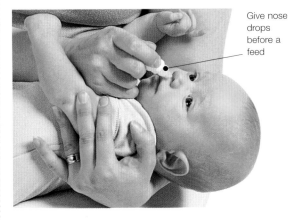

Give nose drops before a feed

▶ For a baby, your doctor may prescribe nose drops to relieve the congestion before a feed.

▶ If your doctor thinks the catarrh is caused by an allergy, he will probably give your child a series of tests to find the possible causes.

▶ If the catarrh is caused by chronic sinusitis or a middle ear infection (**otitis media**), antibiotics will be prescribed. If it is caused by enlarged adenoids or nasal polyps, surgical removal may be recommended by the doctor.

What can I do to help?

▶ Never try to clear your child's nose with a cotton-wool swab; this will only push the mucus further back up the nostrils.

▶ Unless your doctor recommends them, avoid using decongestant medicines, which can lead to a build-up of mucus; this is because they dry up the mucus so efficiently that the body makes more in order to compensate.

▶ Teach your child to blow his nose properly by clearing out one nostril at a time.

SEE ALSO:
Common cold 90
Hayfever 152
Influenza 167
Measles 177
Otitis media 198
Sinusitis 218

Cerebral palsy

CEREBRAL PALSY IS THE NAME GIVEN to disorders of the brain that occur early in life and result in a lack of full control of physical movement. In some children, the damage occurs in pregnancy; in others, during a difficult labour, when the baby may suffer from a lack of oxygen. Cerebral palsy may also result if a premature baby has severe breathing problems, with bleeding in the brain and lack of oxygen both contributing to the condition. Other less common problems that may damage the parts of the brain controlling movement, thus giving rise to cerebral palsy, are serious **head injury** and **meningitis**.

Because the more sophisticated voluntary control centres of the brain do not function in the first months of life, cerebral palsy may not be apparent at birth. After nine months it may show itself if the child is slow to sit up, is generally unsteady, or cannot grasp and hold an object. Cerebral palsy may affect only one side (for example, the right arm and leg), both legs with the arms hardly affected at all,

or all four limbs and the trunk. Walking is delayed but usually possible. If the limbs tend to be stiff and fixed in certain postures, the child is technically termed "spastic". If he is prone to frequent, purposeless, writhing movements, he is said to be "athetoid".

Cerebral palsy is not a progressive disease which steadily gets worse. Nor is it uncommon for children with cerebral palsy to have normal intelligence and normal social capabilities.

Possible symptoms

▶ **Delayed sitting**.
▶ **Delayed walking**.
▶ **Stiffness** in arms and legs.
▶ **Persistent abnormal postures**.

What can be done?

The treatment for cerebral palsy consists of trying to develop the child's physical, mental and social capabilities to the full. Therefore it is important that the child is fully assessed by a specialist and a physiotherapist so that he can be given treatment at an early age. Stretching exercises will prevent fixed deformity of the limbs; orthopaedic appliances such as calipers, and in some cases surgery, can improve mobility; and treatment, such as speech therapy, can compensate for the physical disability.

Where there is no mental handicap, the outlook for the child is extremely good. Children adjust quite well to severe lack of motor function as long as their intellectual capacity is good and they can make themselves understood. The reaction of the family is of great importance. Parents must guard against feeling sorry for the child. If there are other children in the family, the child must be treated, as far as possible, in the same way as they are, although this may be hard for parents. As with all disabled children, the emphasis should be on what the child can do rather than on what he cannot.

For help and advice contact Scope (formerly the Spastics Society), (see page 324).

SEE ALSO:
Head injury 154
Meningitis 178

Chapping

CHAPS ARE SMALL CRACKS IN THE SKIN that can be painful if they are deep. In nearly all cases, chapping is preceded by drying out of the skin due to its exposure to cold air or to hot, dry air. Chapping is therefore most common in exposed parts of the body such as on the lips, fingers, hands and ears.

Is it serious?
Chapping is not serious.

Possible symptoms

▶ **Small cracks in the skin**, most commonly on the lips, fingers, hands and ears.
▶ **Bleeding** if the cracks are deep.

What should I do first?

1 Keep your child's skin well moisturized with a gentle cream.

2 Keep your child warm in cold weather, particularly his hands and ears.

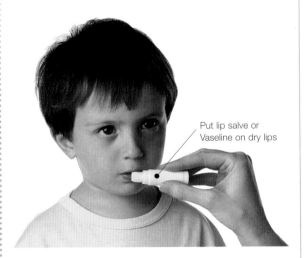

Put lip salve or Vaseline on dry lips

3 If your child has dry lips, put lip salve or Vaseline on regularly throughout the day.

4 If the chap cracks, place a piece of surgical tape or adhesive tape over it, where possible, for about 12 hours, to stop it drying out and cracking even more.

Should I consult the doctor?
Consult your doctor as soon as possible if the chaps fail to heal or become infected, that is, if they are red, tender and pus-filled.

What might the doctor do?
▶ Your doctor will give you general advice on how to stop your child's skin from drying to the point of cracking and he may prescribe an emollient cream to keep the skin moist.
▶ If there is an infection, your doctor will prescribe a course of antibiotics.

What can I do to help?
▶ Don't wash your child with soap too often during cold weather. Soap defats the skin and makes it rough. An emollient cream or baby lotion can be used instead of soap to clean the skin.

SEE ALSO:
Chilblains 83

Chickenpox

CHICKENPOX IS A COMMON, infectious, childhood disease. It has an incubation period of between 14 and 21 days and causes only mild symptoms. Some sufferers may have a headache and a fever, though the majority give no indication of illness at all except for the characteristic itchy chickenpox spots. The spots cover most parts of the body and can even appear in the mouth, anus, vagina or ears. They appear in crops every three to four days and quickly develop tiny **blisters** that leave a scab. Your child is infectious until the scabs have dropped off. The spots may leave shallow scars when they heal if the child scratches too vigorously.

Is it serious?

Chickenpox is not serious. However, in rare cases, the chickenpox virus may cause **encephalitis** or be complicated by **Reye's syndrome**.

Possible symptoms

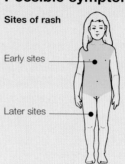

Sites of rash

Early sites

Later sites

▶ **Small blisters** appearing in new batches every three to four days, usually starting on the trunk, then spreading to the face, arms and legs, and eventually scabbing over.
▶ **Intense itchiness**.
▶ **Headache and fever**.

What should I do first?

1 Damp down the itchiness by applying calamine lotion to the rash, or by giving your child warm baths in which you have dissolved a handful of bicarbonate of soda.

2 As far as possible, keep your child away from other children; don't send him to school or nursery until the scabs have all dropped off.

Should I consult the doctor?

Consult your doctor as soon as possible to confirm that your child has chickenpox. Consult your doctor as soon as possible if any of the spots develops a redness with swelling, which indicates infection, or if the child is unable to stop scratching the spots. Consult your doctor immediately if your child is

feverish or complains of neckache when the spots have scabbed over and he should be feeling better.

What might the doctor do?

▶ Your doctor will prescribe an anti-infective cream if any of the spots is infected.
▶ If itchiness is causing your child sleepless nights, your doctor may prescribe a sedative.

What can I do to help?

▶ If your child is still in nappies, change them frequently and leave them off whenever possible to allow the spots to scab over.
▶ Cut your child's fingernails short and discourage him from scratching.

SEE ALSO:
Blister 67
Encephalitis 126
Itching 170
Reye's syndrome 208

Chilblains

CHILBLAINS ARE AREAS OF RED, ITCHY SKIN that are the result of a hypersensitivity to cold. When the skin of a cold-sensitive child is exposed to cold and damp, the blood vessels beneath the skin close up to conserve heat, causing the skin to become numb and pale. When the blood vessels dilate again with warmth, the skin becomes red and itchy. Chilblains usually appear on the ankles, hands and feet and on the backs of the legs.

Are they serious?
Chilblains are not serious, but they are irritating.

Possible symptoms

▶ **Pale, numb skin**, particularly on the hands and feet.

Common sites

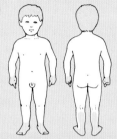

▶ **Red, swollen and itchy skin** when the affected area warms up.

What should I do first?

1 If your child has been out in the cold without sufficient warm clothing and then complains of itchiness, dust the skin with talcum powder or cornflour to ease the irritation.

Dust affected area with talc

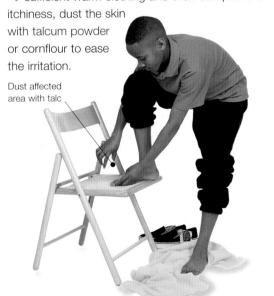

2 Stop your child from breaking the skin of the affected areas by covering them with clothing or putting mittens or gloves on your child.

Should I consult the doctor?
Consult your doctor as soon as possible if the chilblains give your child a great deal of discomfort.

What might the doctor do?
Your doctor may prescribe a vasodilator cream to improve circulation.

What can I do to help?
▶ Keep all the susceptible parts on your child's body covered up and warm in damp and cold weather.
▶ Put thermal insoles in your child's shoes to keep his feet warm.

SEE ALSO:
Itching 170

Choking

CHOKING OCCURS WHEN A FOREIGN BODY becomes lodged in the throat and either blocks the airway or causes muscular spasms. If, despite the obstruction, there is still enough air getting through to the lungs, your child will be able to cough the object back up into his mouth.

Is it serious?

If your child is coughing and gasping for breath, or turning red then blue in the face, this is an emergency (*see page 294*). If the airway is totally blocked, your child will lose consciousness and stop breathing; if this happens, call for medical help and give mouth-to-mouth ventilation.

Possible symptoms

▶ **Coughing**.
▶ **Grasping the throat**.
▶ **Redness, followed by blueness in the face** – blood vessels in the neck and face may stand out.

What should I do first?

1 With a baby, lay him along your forearm, with his head lower than his chest and his chin supported between your fingers. Give up to five sharp slaps on the middle of his back with your other hand. With an older child, bend him forward with his head lower than his chest. Give up to five firm back slaps between his shoulders.

2 If the foreign body is coughed into the throat and you can see it, try to hook it out with a finger. Do not feel blindly down the throat, and be very careful not to push the object further down the throat. Hold your baby or child steady with your other hand to prevent him from re-inhaling the object.

3 If you cannot hook out the object, give your baby alternate back slaps and chest thrusts, or your child back slaps, chest thrusts and abdominal thrusts (*see page 294*). Check your child's mouth to see if the obstruction has cleared.

Should I consult the doctor?

If the obstruction has not cleared and your baby or child turns blue or loses consciousness, call for an ambulance immediately and inform the operator of his condition. Continue giving your baby alternate back slaps and chest thrusts, or your child back slaps, chest and abdominal thrusts while you are waiting for medical help to arrive. If your child loses consciousness, lay him in the recovery position (*see page 287*) until help arrives. Stay with him and, if he stops breathing, start giving mouth-to-mouth ventilation (*see page 288*).

What might the doctor do?

The ambulance attendant or the doctor will try to revive your child, if necessary, and remove the foreign body if it is still lodged in the throat.

What can I do to help?

▶ Make sure your child understands that he must not put any small toys in his mouth because of the risk of choking. Toys small enough to be swallowed should not be given to children under three years of age.
▶ Never leave a small child unattended when he is eating in case he chokes.
▶ Never give peanuts or other small foods to a child under three years of age.

Coeliac disease

COELIAC DISEASE, OR GLUTEN SENSITIVITY, is the result of an allergic reaction in the lining of the small intestine when the intestine comes into contact with gluten. (Gluten is a protein found in cereals and grains and is therefore difficult to avoid in a normal diet.) The lining of the intestine becomes smooth, preventing nutrients from being properly absorbed and metabolized. The child fails to thrive because valuable proteins, calories, vitamins and minerals pass out of his body in the stools. Symptoms of coeliac disease normally appear within a few weeks of cereals being introduced into the diet. Because of the dietary deficiencies, the child may appear unhappy and irritable.

If left undiagnosed and untreated by a change of diet, coeliac disease leads to a distended abdomen (because of wind), and to stick-like limbs. The buttocks in particular become flat, wasted and saggy.

Is it serious?

Coeliac disease is serious if undetected because it could permanently stunt your child's growth.

Possible symptoms

▶ **Frequent, bulky, pale, foul-smelling stools**, which are difficult to flush away because they are so full of fat.
▶ **Loss of appetite**.
▶ **Failure to thrive**.
▶ **Distended stomach** because of wind.
▶ **Stick-like limbs**.
▶ **Irritability and lethargy**.
▶ **Saggy, flat buttocks**.

What should I do first?

1 If your baby has recently been weaned on to cereals, and his stools become foul-smelling and frequent, try to flush the motions down the lavatory to see if they float.

2 Don't put your child on to a gluten-free diet without medical advice. You may be unnecessarily reducing your child's protein intake and causing problems by restricting the diet without medical supervision.

Should I consult the doctor?

Consult your doctor as soon as possible if your child is not gaining weight and his bowel motions are frequent and foul-smelling. Your health visitor can advise you on whether your child's growth rate is normal and can arrange tests for coeliac disease.

What might the doctor do?

▶ To check for coeliac disease, your doctor will arrange blood and faeces tests for your child. If these indicate the likelihood of coeliac disease, your child will probably be admitted to hospital for a biopsy (removal under anaesthetic of a tiny piece of the intestine for testing).
▶ Once the diagnosis has been confirmed, your child will need to eat a gluten-free diet for life. Your doctor will refer you to a dietician for advice about the kinds of foods your child should have. The reaction once the diet is begun is startling. Within days there is an improvement in mood, an increase in appetite and a return to normal bowel motions.

Continued on next page

Continued from previous page

What can I do to help?

❱ The best way to approach the special diet is to make gluten-free dishes for all the family so that your child does not feel different. Special gluten-free flours are available, and some cereals – for example, maize, rice and buckwheat – don't contain gluten. There are also a number of cookery books on the market with gluten-free recipes.

Foods to avoid	**Foods to eat**
	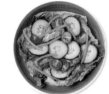
Non-dairy ice cream	**Vegetable salad**
Wholemeal bread	**Rice and prawns**

❱ Familiarize yourself, with the help of the hospital dietician, with foods to be avoided: non-dairy ice cream, muesli, cocoa powder and mustard, for example, all contain gluten.

❱ If buying prepared dishes, check the labels to make sure they don't include ingredients containing gluten.

❱ As your child gets older, you will have to emphasize the need to be wary of all foods that you haven't prepared yourself or checked for gluten. School lunches, party foods and restaurants will present problems, but with planning you should be able to prevent your child from feeling abnormal.

For help and advice contact the Coeliac Society (see page 324).

SEE ALSO:
Diarrhoea 112

Cold sores

COLD SORES ARE tiny **blisters** that form around the nostrils and lips and elsewhere on the face. The blisters break open and weep before they crust over and disappear. Cold sores are caused by a virus (*Herpes simplex*) that lives permanently in the nerve endings of some adults and children. A rise in skin temperature – perhaps caused by a cold, or by going out in the sun – activates the virus. The first attack may take the form of painful **mouth ulcers**. Subsequent attacks, which tend to occur most often when children are run down, take the form of blisters.

Are they serious?

Cold sores are not serious unless they occur near the eye, where they may cause an ulcer to form on the front of the eyeball.

Possible symptoms

Common site

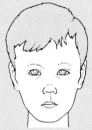

▶ **Raised red area**, usually around the nostrils and lips, which tingles and feels itchy. Tiny blisters then form around the spot.
▶ **Weeping blisters**, which then crust over.

What should I do first?

1 Apply anti-viral cream (acyclovir), which is available over the counter, during the tingle phase before blisters appear to reduce the length and severity of the attack. Once blisters have formed, stop your child from touching the area. Keep his hands clean.

2 Apply surgical spirit to the cold sores to dry them up, or smear a soothing cream such as Vaseline on to them to keep them moist while the virus runs its course. One or the other treatment may give your child some relief.

Should I consult the doctor?

Consult your doctor as soon as possible if a cold sore is near your child's eye. Consult your doctor as soon as possible if the cold sores become redder and develop pussy centres. They will have become infected with bacteria. Ask your doctor's advice if your child suffers from recurrent cold sores.

What might the doctor do?

▶ If the cold sores are infected, your doctor will prescribe an antibiotic ointment that lubricates the area and treats the infection.
▶ Your doctor may prescribe an anti-viral cream to spread over the affected area regularly to contain the attack.

What can I do to help?

▶ Make sure that your child uses his own clean towel and facecloth.
▶ Don't let your child kiss other children. The virus can be transmitted this way.
▶ If your child tends to develop cold sores after exposure to sunlight, smear a sunblock on his lips or nose when he plays out in the sun.

SEE ALSO:
Blister 67
Mouth ulcers 182
Sunburn 232

Colic

COLIC, AS APPLIED TO A BABY under four months of age, describes a crying spell, during which the baby's face becomes very red and both legs are drawn up to his stomach as if he is in great pain. This crying spell usually comes in the early evening; during the rest of the day the baby is generally contented. The crying can reach screaming pitch and last from one to three hours. It doesn't usually stop as a result of the proven methods of soothing. Colic is so common that it is regarded by paediatricians as normal, but for parents it can be difficult to endure. The cause of the apparent spasmodic pain is not known. It is often at its worst at three months of age but goes by four months.

Is it serious?

The fact that your baby is contented during the rest of the day means that this crying bout is not related to a serious physical problem. Colicky babies are usually healthy and thriving.

Possible symptoms

▶ **Your baby cannot settle** in the early evening and cries no matter what you do to calm him.
▶ **He becomes red-faced** and draws his legs up into his stomach as if in pain.
▶ **He may wake from a short sleep** with a startled cry.

What should I do first?

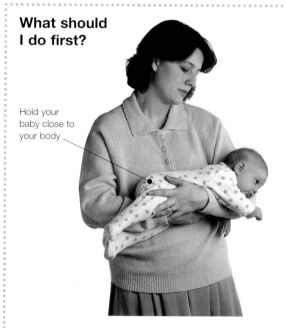

Hold your baby close to your body

1 Try all the methods of soothing your baby that you know work at other times of the day. This may mean you are constantly offering the breast or bottle, changing nappies, burping, nursing and rocking, walking with the baby held over your shoulder, putting the baby in a sling against your body, playing music to give a constant background noise, or walking him in a pram.

Continued from previous page

2 Lay him on his tummy over a hot-water bottle wrapped in a towel.

3 Try using a pacifier: your baby may need to suck all the time.

4 Don't use any patent medicines without your doctor's advice.

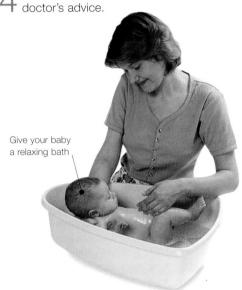

Give your baby
a relaxing bath

5 Bathe your baby at this difficult time of the day. A warm bath relaxes most babies and this will pass the time when the crying seems worst.

Should I consult the doctor?

Consult your doctor as soon as possible if you find you cannot cope with the nightly crying sessions.

What might the doctor do?

▌ Your doctor will reassure you that your baby is healthy. He may discuss the use of dicyclomine, which relaxes the intestine and does relieve colic symptoms in older babies. It is not usually given to babies under six months.

▌ If you are being driven to breaking point, ask your doctor to refer you to someone who can help you develop strategies to cope. For instance, your health visitor may be able to fill this role.

What can I do to help?

▌ Make sure you look after yourself. Sleep during the day, if you can, when the baby sleeps. You will be better able to cope with the evenings.

▌ Invite good friends in to share that time of the evening; a relaxed atmosphere may calm both you and your baby.

▌ Talk to other parents who have had colicky babies. Once you realize you are not alone and that colic does pass, you may find it easier to bear.

▌ Consult your health visitor for valuable advice and support on coping with colic.

SEE ALSO:
Crying 102

Common cold

THE COMMON COLD IS CAUSED BY A VIRUS that enters the body through the nasal passages and throat and causes inflammation of the mucous membranes lining these passages. The body's defences take around 10 days to fight off the virus.

Is it serious?
A common cold is not serious but, because it lowers the body's resistance, complications such as **bronchitis** and **pneumonia** have been known to arise. A cold should be regarded more seriously in a baby because minor cold symptoms, such as a blocked nose, can cause him to have feeding problems.

Possible symptoms
- **Sneezing**.
- **Runny or blocked nose**.
- **Raised temperature**.
- **Coughing**.
- **Sore throat**.
- **Aching muscles**.
- **Irritability**.
- **Catarrh**.

What should I do first?
1 Take your child's temperature. If it is high, 38°C (100.4°F) or more, and it does not subside within four to five hours, put him to bed and bring his temperature down (*see page 31*).

2 Check your child's nasal discharge. Yellow discharge can indicate a secondary infection, while clear mucus could signify **hayfever**.

3 Don't give your child any patent medicines without your doctor's advice.

Should I consult the doctor?
Consult your doctor immediately if you think your child has developed a secondary infection. If your baby is having trouble sleeping at night or feeding, consult your doctor or health visitor.

What might the doctor do?
▶ Your doctor will treat a secondary infection.
▶ Your doctor may prescribe nose drops to ease feeding. Use them as directed, as over-use can damage the lining of the nose.
▶ Your doctor may prescribe a cough suppressant or an expectorant to ease a bad cough.

What can I do to help?
▶ Ease your baby's breathing by placing a pillow under the cot mattress to raise his head.
▶ Give your child plenty to drink.
▶ Make nose-blowing easier by blowing one nostril at a time.
▶ If possible, create a humid atmosphere in your child's bedroom so that the raw lining of his nose does not become dry.
▶ Smear Vaseline on to your child's nose and upper lip if constant blowing has made them sore.
▶ Capsules of camphor sprinkled on to clothing or bedding will ease your child's breathing at night.
▶ A hot bedtime drink of freshly squeezed lemon juice and water will ease your child's sore throat and clear his nasal passages.

SEE ALSO:
Bronchiolitis 72
Catarrh 78
Cough 98
Croup 101
Fever 134
Hayfever 152
Pneumonia 202
Sore throat 222

Conjunctivitis

CONJUNCTIVITIS IS AN INFLAMMATION of the conjunctiva, which is the membrane covering the eyeball and the inside of the eyelid. The inflammation may be caused by a viral or bacterial infection, or by injury from a **foreign body** or chemicals, or it may be the result of an allergic reaction. The eyes become red and weepy, and they can be painful or extremely itchy, and may be irritated by bright light. If caused by an infection, the condition, which may affect one or both of the eyes, is contagious.

Is it serious?

Although conjunctivitis is not a serious eye infection, it should always be treated by a doctor.

Possible symptoms

▶ **Weepy, red eyes** that feel sore or itchy.
▶ **Intolerance of bright light**.
▶ **Discharge of pus** causing eyelashes to stick together after a night's sleep.

Cross-section of the eye

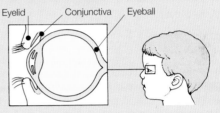

Eyelid   Conjunctiva   Eyeball

What should I do first?

1 Check to see if there is a foreign body in the eye; if possible, remove it (*see page 130*).

2 As a temporary measure, before consulting your doctor, bathe each eye, whether both are affected or not, with a solution of 5ml (one teaspoonful) of salt dissolved in a glass of warm, previously boiled, water. Using a new ball of cotton wool for each eye, soak it in the solution, then wipe from the inner corner of the eye outwards.

3 To prevent the spread of infection, encourage your child to keep his hands clean and not to rub his eyes.

Should I consult the doctor?

Consult your doctor as soon as possible if you suspect conjunctivitis.

What might the doctor do?

▶ If the condition is caused by an infection, your doctor will prescribe antibiotic eye drops or ointment to clear it. If the infection does not respond to treatment within a few days, your doctor may refer you to an eye specialist.
▶ If the irritation is caused by an allergy, such as **hayfever**, your doctor will prescribe anti-inflammatory eye drops and antihistamine medication.
▶ If there is a foreign body in your child's eye, your doctor will remove it.

What can I do to help?

▶ Make your child understand that it is easy to spread the infection with his hands. Encourage him to keep his hands clean and to use a separate facecloth and towel.
▶ If your child suffers from hayfever, try to keep him away from freshly mown lawns during the worst hayfever months.

SEE ALSO:
Eye, foreign body in,
  130
Hayfever 152

Constipation

A CHILD WHO IS CONSTIPATED passes hard, pebble-like stools and this may cause discomfort or actual pain when the stools are passed. Constipation is a word that is used to describe the consistency of stools and not the regularity or frequency of bowel movements. During babyhood, constipation is unlikely for either breastfed or bottlefed babies. When they start on solid food, however, they can suffer from constipation if their diet doesn't contain enough fresh fruit and vegetables and liquids. By the age of two or three, constipation may become a problem for a different reason: some parents are so obsessed with the importance of "regularity" during the period when their child is learning bowel control that the child reacts by holding back the stools as a weapon in a battle of wills.

As a guiding rule, if your child is perfectly happy and healthy and shows no signs of discomfort when going to the toilet, and if his stools are not as hard as pebbles, he is not constipated. Furthermore, if your child's stools are hard and dry during a period when, because of illness, he is feverish or has been vomiting, this is not true constipation. The body compensates for loss of fluid from vomiting or fever by absorbing water from the stools, and bowel activity should return to normal when the illness has passed.

If your child involuntarily soils his underpants when he was previously toilet-trained, he may be developing **encopresis**, which is the passage of formed stools in inappropriate places. Constipation is often, but not always, associated with this condition.

Is it serious?

Occasional constipation is not serious and can be avoided by means of a diet rich in fibre. Chronic constipation can be a serious matter because it can cause problems in later life. Blood in the stools may indicate an underlying disorder and should always be cause for concern.

Possible symptoms

▶ **Hard, pebble-like stools**.
▶ **Pain** in the lower abdomen.
▶ **Blood** on nappy or underpants.

What should I do first?

1 If your child strains when passing stools and complains of pain, check the consistency of what she has passed.

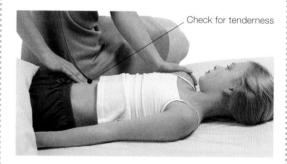

Check for tenderness

2 If she complains of stomach pain, check the right side of her abdomen below her navel (*see page 54*) for possible **appendicitis**.

Should I consult the doctor?

Consult your doctor as soon as possible if your child complains of pain when moving her bowels. Consult your doctor immediately if you notice red blood on her nappy or underpants; the passing of a large, dry stool may have injured her anal passage. This is called an anal fissure and your child may be reluctant to pass any more stools for fear of the pain caused by this tiny crack. Consult your doctor immediately if you suspect appendicitis.

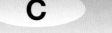

Continued from previous page

What might the doctor do?

❱ Your doctor may prescribe a very mild laxative, specially formulated for babies and children, which is safe to give your child for short periods. He will also give you advice about your child's diet.

❱ If your doctor suspects an anal fissure, he will examine your child's rectum, and if there is a fissure he may prescribe a stool-softening laxative or advise you of other methods to alleviate constipation.

❱ Your health visitor can provide helpful dietary advice and general counselling.

What can I do to help?

❱ Never use laxatives unless your doctor advises it. Laxatives encourage a lazy bowel.

❱ Don't leave your child sitting on his potty for long periods of time. He may get the impression that if he doesn't perform he will lose your approval.

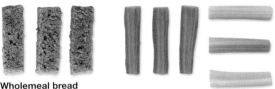

Wholemeal bread

Fresh vegetables

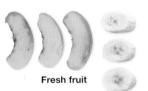

Fresh fruit

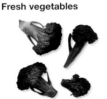

❱ Include as many natural, unprocessed foods as possible in your child's diet, with some dietary fibre in the form of whole grains – such as brown rice and wholemeal bread – and fresh fruit and vegetables. It is not a good idea just to scatter bran over your child's meals; this can deplete certain minerals in the diet. A few stewed prunes or dried figs, however, can produce a soft stool within 24 hours.

❱ If your child has been prescribed a laxative, follow the manufacturer's instructions precisely.

❱ Make sure your child is getting plenty to drink.

❱ Don't rush your school-age child when he goes to the toilet. If the pace is hectic in the morning, make sure he has time to go to the toilet without the anxiety of having to rush off to school. Many children prefer to go to the toilet at home because they find the school facilities lack privacy.

SEE ALSO:
Appendicitis 54
Encopresis 127

Convulsion

A CONVULSION IS A FIT OR SEIZURE that occurs when the brain reacts abnormally. During the convulsion, your child loses consciousness, becomes rigid for some seconds while holding his breath, then rhythmically bends and straightens his arms and legs for some minutes. Your child may cry out at the beginning of the seizure; he may urinate and he may defecate. When the convulsion is over, your child will be in a confused state and he may want to sleep.

The most common cause of convulsions is a raised temperature that accompanies a viral infection such as **influenza**. This type of convulsion is known as a febrile convulsion and generally occurs between the ages of six months and six years. The tendency to suffer from febrile convulsions runs in families. Convulsions may also be caused by **meningitis**, **encephalitis** and, rarely, by chemical abnormalities of the blood, such as a low level of glucose in diabetics. Sometimes no specific cause is found. **Epilepsy** is another cause of convulsions.

Is it serious?

Though dramatic and frightening, a convulsion is not life-threatening but it should be treated seriously.

Possible symptoms

▶ **Sudden rise in temperature**.
▶ **Crying out** and loss of consciousness.
▶ **Rigid phase** with the breath held.
▶ **Rhythmic jerking** of the limbs.
▶ **Urination and/or defecation**.
▶ **Confusion and drowsiness**.

What should I do first?

1 As soon as your child loses consciousness, remove any furniture or other solid objects from the area so that he does not injure himself when he has a seizure. With a baby or young child, put him face down over your knee to ensure that his tongue does not fall backwards and obstruct the airway.

2 Don't leave your child alone for a moment.

3 Don't try to stop him from jerking his limbs; you may injure him.

4 Don't try to force anything into his mouth and never try to force the teeth apart if they are clenched.

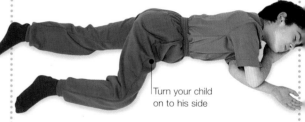
Turn your child on to his side

5 As soon as the violent movements have ceased, turn your child on to his side so that he does not inhale saliva and so that his tongue cannot fall to the back of his throat and obstruct his airway.

Should I consult the doctor?

Consult your doctor immediately as soon as the convulsion has passed. If there is someone with you, ask him to call the doctor while you stay with your child. If the doctor hasn't arrived within 15 minutes, or if the convulsion hasn't passed, take your child to the nearest hospital. Any fit

Continued from previous page

that continues for 20 minutes should be stopped with an anti-convulsant drug.

What might the doctor do?

❱ If the convulsion is continuing, your doctor will give your child an anti-convulsant drug, usually administered rectally.

❱ Your doctor may admit your child to hospital immediately so that tests can be carried out to exclude any serious cause of convulsions, such as meningitis.

❱ With an older child, your doctor will refer him to hospital if the cause of the convulsion is not clear. Tests will be carried out, and the paediatrician will advise whether or not anti-convulsant drug treatment is needed in the event of your child contracting another infectious fever.

❱ Your doctor will give you advice on how to avoid a rapid rise in temperature in the future.

What can I do to help?

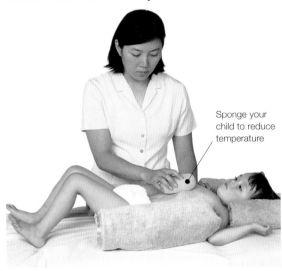

Sponge your child to reduce temperature

❱ Once the convulsion is over, if your child is feverish and has a high temperature, remove her clothing and cool her skin by tepid sponging (*see page 31*). Cover her with a light sheet when she sleeps.

❱ Don't give her any patent medicines without your doctor's advice.

❱ Stay calm.

SEE ALSO:
Encephalitis 126
Epilepsy 128
Fever 134
Influenza 167
Meningitis 178

Cot death

SUDDEN INFANT DEATH SYNDROME (SIDS), or cot death, is the sudden and often unexplained death of a seemingly healthy baby. There is no single known cause of cot death, although research has shown that some deaths are the result of an abnormality in the breathing and heart rate. Current areas of research include the development of a baby's temperature-control mechanism and respiratory system in the first six months, and the recent discovery that an inherited enzyme deficiency may be responsible for around one per cent of cases. Studies connecting SIDS with flame-retardant chemicals in cot mattresses have, so far, proven inconclusive.

The death of an infant from SIDS is a highly distressing experience. Severe grief can be compounded by intense feelings of guilt and misplaced blame, and family relationships can suffer as a result. Parents of cot-death infants may have to discuss the incident with the police and be prepared for a post-mortem examination of the baby. Your doctor, paediatrician and health visitor should provide valuable support and counselling in this situation, and talking to other parents who have experienced a cot death, or to a professional organization, can provide great comfort.

Possible symptoms

▶ **Common cold-like symptom** of stuffy nose.
▶ **Inexplicable weight loss**.

What can I do to help?

While the causes of cot death are not clear, there are ways in which you can significantly reduce the risks.

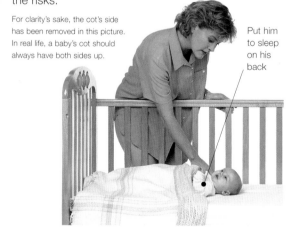

For clarity's sake, the cot's side has been removed in this picture. In real life, a baby's cot should always have both sides up.

Put him to sleep on his back

▶ Always put your baby to sleep ON HIS BACK, NEVER ON HIS FRONT. Babies who sleep on their backs are at less risk of cot death. This position also helps control your baby's body temperature (*see below*). Older babies are able to turn over during the night. Place an older baby on his back in the cot and then allow him to find his own position. In babies over six months, the risk of cot death is greatly reduced.

▶ Place your baby's feet at the foot of the cot so that he can't slip beneath his bedclothes.

▶ Make sure your baby has enough blankets – a sheet and no more than three blankets is quite sufficient in a room temperature of 18°C (65°F). Use less blankets if the room temperature is higher – no more than one sheet and blanket on a warm night of 24°C (75°F), (*see chart, page 97*).

▶ Don't wrap your baby too warmly in too many nightclothes or bedclothes, especially during winter, or put him to bed in a room that is too hot. Use a thermostatically controlled heater in your baby's room so that temperatures do not rise too high or drop too low.

Continued from previous page

What bedding to use according to the temperature

Temperature	What to use
15°C (60°F)	A sheet and four blankets.
18°C (65°F)	A sheet and three blankets.
21°C (70°F)	A sheet and two blankets.
24°C (75°F)	A sheet and one blanket.
27°C (80°F)	A sheet only.

❱ Be careful not to swaddle or tuck your baby in as this will prevent him from throwing off his bedclothes if he gets too hot. Baby nests, sheepskins, duvets and cot bumpers all prevent heat loss and should not be used for young babies. Cover her with a cotton sheet and cellular blankets according to room temperature (*see chart, above*).

❱ Avoid smoking during pregnancy and after your child is born. The risk of SIDS in babies born to smokers is twice that for babies born to non-smokers, and with every 10 cigarettes a day the risk increases threefold. Avoid taking your baby into smoky environments.

❱ Don't increase the amount of bedding when your baby is unwell.

❱ Whenever possible, breastfeed rather than bottle-feed your baby.

❱ Avoid taking unnecessary drugs during pregnancy.

❱ If you think your baby is unwell, don't hesitate to contact your doctor. If he has a fever, don't increase the wrapping, but reduce it so he can lose heat. After a minor illness, keep a closer eye than usual on your baby for several days until the symptoms have completely disappeared.

For help and advice contact the Foundation for the Study of Infant Death (see page 324).

Cough

A COUGH IS EITHER A SYMPTOM of an illness or the body's way of reacting to an irritant in the throat or air passages. A cough may bring up phlegm from the chest and clear mucus from the air passages, for example, during an attack of **asthma** or **whooping cough** (this is known as a productive cough). A dry cough, which produces no phlegm, serves no useful purpose and its cause is not always obvious. The irritation provoking the cough may be mucus from chronically infected sinuses or nasal discharge from a common cold, both of which dribble down and tickle the back of the throat. A dry cough may also be the body's way of bringing up a foreign body stuck in the windpipe. Coughing may be caused by "passive smoking". If adults around your child smoke a lot, the smoke may irritate your child's throat and cause a cough. Children may also adopt a cough as an attention-seeking device, when it becomes a **tic** or mannerism.

Is it serious?
A cough is not usually serious, although it can be irritating. However, a cough which causes breathing difficulties, such that your child turns blue around the lips and gasps for breath, is serious and should be treated as an emergency.

What should I do first?

1 If your child is coughing up phlegm, sit him in your lap leaning slightly forwards while you pat him gently on the back to help him bring up the phlegm.

2 Don't give your child cough-suppressant medicines for a cough that produces phlegm. The risk of infection increases if the phlegm is not coughed up.

3 If you think that your child has a foreign body in his throat, try to remove it (*see page 294*).

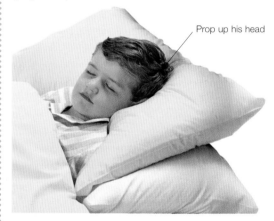

Prop up his head

4 If your child is coughing at night, prop up his head and shoulders with pillows. This will stop mucus or nasal discharge from dribbling down the throat.

5 To soothe your child's throat, give him a hot lemon drink sweetened with honey.

Continued from previous page

Should I consult the doctor?

Consult your doctor as soon as possible if your child's cough doesn't get better after three or four days, if your child is not getting any sleep at night or if you cannot remove the foreign body from your child's throat. Consult your doctor immediately if your baby develops a hacking cough or if your child's coughing is accompanied by rapid, laboured or wheezy breathing. This could be a sign of croup or asthma.

What might the doctor do?

▶ If your child's cough is part of an infection such as **otitis media**, **tonsillitis** or croup, your doctor may prescribe antibiotics to clear up that infection.

▶ If your child is suffering from a viral infection, your doctor will advise you on how to relieve the symptoms and also on how to help your child to cough up the phlegm.

▶ If the cough is part of an asthmatic condition, your doctor may prescribe bronchodilator drugs that help to widen the air passages.

▶ Your doctor may prescribe nose drops to administer sparingly to your child before he goes to bed. These drops ease congestion and prevent mucus from dribbling down the back of your child's throat.

▶ Your doctor may prescribe a cough medicine: either a cough suppressant (to reduce irritation and soothe the throat) or an expectorant (to encourage the coughing up of phlegm).

What can I do to help?

▶ Keeping your child quiet and warm may help to prevent any minor infection from spreading into the lungs and causing a more serious condition such as bronchitis.

▶ Don't let your child run around too much during the day. Breathlessness can bring on a coughing fit.

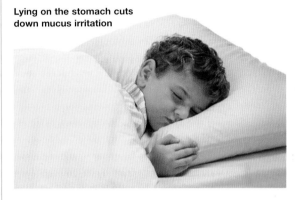

Lying on the stomach cuts down mucus irritation

▶ If your child is over 18 months old, encourage him to lie on his stomach or his side at night so that mucus will not dribble into his throat.

▶ Keep the air in your child's room moist by leaving a window open. Don't overheat the room.

▶ Don't smoke at home and don't take your child into smoky atmospheres.

SEE ALSO:
Asthma 58
Bronchiolitis 72
Croup 101
Otitis media 198
Tic 242
Tonsillitis 243
Whooping cough 261

Cradle cap

CRADLE CAP IS A THICK, YELLOW encrustation on the scalp. It occurs mainly in babies, though children up to the age of three can have cradle cap. The yellow scales appear in small patches or can cover the entire scalp. Cradle cap is not due to poor hygiene. Babies who suffer from it probably just have greasier scalps.

Is it serious?
Cradle cap may appear unsightly, but it is quite harmless unless it is accompanied by red, scaly areas elsewhere on your baby's body, in which case your baby may have seborrhoeic **eczema**.

Possible symptoms

▶ **Thick, yellowish scales** over part or all of the scalp.

What should I do first?

1 Do not try to remove the scales with your fingers. If they won't brush out, they must be loosened first.

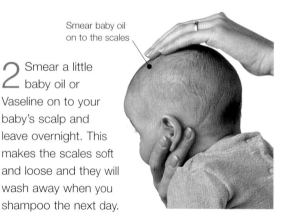

Smear baby oil on to the scales

2 Smear a little baby oil or Vaseline on to your baby's scalp and leave overnight. This makes the scales soft and loose and they will wash away when you shampoo the next day.

3 Do not use anti-dandruff shampoos without consulting your doctor.

Should I consult the doctor?
Consult your doctor if you are worried about the condition or if your baby has any red, scaly areas elsewhere on his body.

What might the doctor do?
Your doctor or health visitor will prescribe a special shampoo to prevent the scales from forming and give you general advice on brushing and other home treatments that help prevent cradle cap.

What can I do to help?
▶ You can prevent scales from building up by brushing through your baby's hair daily, even if there is very little of it, with a soft-bristled brush.
▶ Never rub the scalp very hard when washing your child's hair. Shampoos remove dirt within seconds, so you only need to bring the shampoo to a lather and then rinse it off thoroughly.
▶ If the cradle cap becomes quite hard and thick, you may have to continue with the baby oil or Vaseline treatment over a 10-day period to loosen all the encrustations.

SEE ALSO:
Dandruff 107
Eczema 124

Croup

CROUP IS THE NAME GIVEN to the sound made when air is breathed in through a constricted windpipe, past inflamed vocal cords. It usually occurs only in young children, who are susceptible because their air passages (bronchi) are narrow and become blocked with mucus when inflamed – most commonly because of a virus such as a **common cold**, or an infection such as **bronchitis**. In rare cases, croup can be caused by an inhaled foreign body. In older children the condition is less serious and is known as **laryngitis**.

The first attack of croup can come on quickly, usually at night, and it may last a couple of hours. Your child will have a croaking cough and laboured breathing.

Is it serious?

If your child has a severe attack of croup, he could develop breathing difficulties. This should be treated as an emergency.

Possible symptoms

▶ **Croaking cough.**
▶ **Laboured breathing** when the lower chest caves in at every inhalation.
▶ **Wheezing.**
▶ **Face colour becoming grey or blue.**

What should I do first?

1 Stay calm and try to calm your child so that he won't panic and make his breathing more difficult.

2 Your child's air passages will be soothed by moist air. If the air outside is cool and damp, take him to the window and get him to take a deep breath of air, or take him into the bathroom and turn on the hot taps to build up a steamy atmosphere.

3 Prop your child up in bed with pillows or hold him on your lap. It will be easier for him to breathe if he is sitting up.

Should I consult the doctor?

Consult your doctor immediately if your child's skin turns grey or blue and he has to fight for breath. Consult your doctor as soon as possible to tell him that your child has had an attack of croup.

What might the doctor do?

▶ In a serious attack your doctor will give your child oxygen to help his breathing.

▶ If necessary, your doctor will prescribe antibiotics to eradicate any underlying infection.
▶ You will be given advice on what to do should there be another attack.
▶ If the attack is caused by an inhaled foreign body, your doctor will remove the foreign body.

What can I do to help?

In future attacks, stay with your child and follow your doctor's instructions.

SEE ALSO:
Bronchiolitis 72
Common cold 90
Laryngitis 173
Nose, foreign body in 191

Crying

ALL BABIES CRY, BUT SOME CRY much more often than others. Crying is a baby's means of communicating, and you will soon come to recognize whether the crying is a symptom of an illness or not. By the age of about six weeks, your baby will be passing part of his waking hours by taking in his surroundings and making gurgling noises instead of just crying, feeding and sleeping. By six months, babies spend most of their waking time playing and communicating in all sorts of ways. A baby who cries rather than plays by the age of six months may be an anxious child, or cutting teeth, or one who is easily bored. In a minority of cases, the baby may cry because he has some sort of physical illness. Most healthy babies stop crying as soon as they are fed, cuddled and made comfortable. If there are certain times of the day (especially in the evening) when nothing stops the crying, your baby could be suffering from **colic**, which is a common cause of crying in babies. A toddler will usually cry only for obvious reasons of illness or injury or as a show of temper.

Is it serious?

Crying is not normally serious. Persistent crying can, however, cause problems if you become angry, resentful and overtired. A persistently crying baby is a common cause of child abuse.

What should I do first?

1 Pick your baby up and cuddle him, or give him a pacifier if he finds sucking calming.

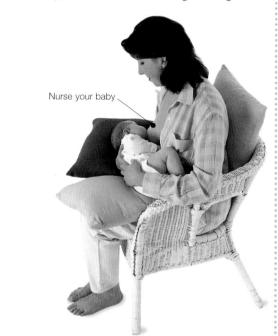

Nurse your baby

2 Feed him or, if you have fed him recently, give him a spoonful of cooled, boiled water.

3 Change your baby's nappy and make sure that he isn't too hot or too cold in the clothes he is wearing.

Should I consult the doctor?

Consult your doctor as soon as possible if the crying seems to be following a different pattern from usual, and there are symptoms of illness such as **diarrhoea**, **fever** or **vomiting**. Consult your doctor as soon as possible if you are exhausted by your active baby and you think you might lash out in anger.

Continued from previous page

What might the doctor do?

Your doctor or health visitor will question you about the extent of your baby's crying. He will examine your baby for any symptoms of illness. If your baby is healthy, your doctor will probably reassure you that there is nothing to be anxious about.

Should I consult the doctor?

▌ You must think of ways to help yourself if you have a particularly demanding baby. Rest whenever you can and take turns with your partner if your baby is difficult at night and seems to need little sleep.

▌ Stay calm yourself; try not to resent your baby's need to be close to you.

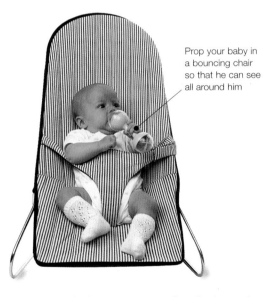

Prop your baby in a bouncing chair so that he can see all around him

▌ Keep your baby near to you when he is awake. Prop him up in a bouncing chair so that he can watch you at work. Carrying him around in a sling may also give him comfort and reassurance.

▌ Always go to your crying baby. Parental apathy and lack of response can inhibit a child's attachment to others in later life. There is no such thing as spoiling a baby.

For help and advice contact CRYSIS (see page 324), a support telephone-advice line for parents of crying babies.

SEE ALSO:
Colic 88
Diarrhoea 112
Fever 134
Sleeplessness 219
Teething 234
Vomiting 257

Cuts and grazes

SMALL CUTS AND GRAZES CAN BE treated at home, and should be cleaned up and possibly dressed to prevent germs entering and causing infection. The best dressing for a cut or graze is a piece of sterile gauze held in place with adhesive tape so that the air can get to the wound. Plasters can be used to dress a cut and prevent it from becoming infected.

Are they serious?

Few cuts and grazes are serious enough to need medical attention. However, if a cut is particularly deep, there is a risk of **tetanus** or another infection developing. In some cases, stitches may be necessary and, if there is a great deal of blood loss, shock might follow (*see page 293*). In all of these incidences, it is advisable to seek medical help immediately. If there is more than just gravel or dirt embedded in the wound, do not remove it as you may cause further damage and bleeding. Place a piece of gauze over it to minimize the risk of infection, and bandage (*see page 292*). Take your child to hospital.

What should I do first?
If the wound is large and bleeding

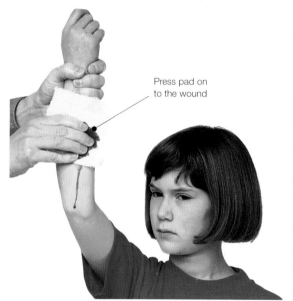

Press pad on to the wound

1 Use a clean pad or handkerchief, or the palm of your hand, to press firmly on the wound to compress the ends of the damaged blood vessels. At the same time, raise your child's arm above the level of her heart.

2 Help your child lie down with her head low. You can put a thin pad under her head for comfort. Keep the injured area raised and keep pressing on the wound for up to 10 minutes.

3 Cover the wound with a clean, non-fluffy dressing that is larger than the wound itself, still keeping the injured area raised above the heart. Secure the dressing in place with a bandage, tied firmly, but not so tightly as to cut off the blood supply (*see page 302*). If any blood comes through the bandage, secure another dressing with a second bandage firmly on top. If necessary, support the wounded area in a sling (*see page 301*). Call for an ambulance immediately.

Continued from previous page

If the wound is a small cut or graze

1 Sit your child down and gently wash the cut or graze with soap and water using a gauze pad, making sure you remove all dirt or gravel. If this causes a little fresh bleeding, press the wound with a clean pad.

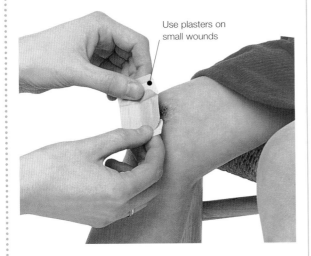

Use plasters on small wounds

2 Dress the wound with a plaster that has a pad large enough to cover the wound. Do not cover cuts with cotton wool: fluffy materials stick to a wound and delay healing.

Should I consult the doctor?

Consult your doctor immediately or take your child to the nearest casualty department if the wound is large, if bleeding persists after 10 minutes of pressure, if the wound is very deep and bloody, if the wound is on the face, if the wound is gaping, if there is dirt or a foreign body in the wound that you can't get out, if the wound is deep but has only a small puncture hole in the skin, or if your child was playing in an area where horses are kept and the wound has been contaminated by dirt or gravel. Consult your doctor as soon as possible if, after a day or two, you notice red streaks extending from the wound as this could be a sign of infection.

What might the doctor do?

▶ The doctor will clean the wound and stitch it, if necessary, under a local anaesthetic; any wound on the face will be stitched to minimize scarring.

▶ If the bleeding doesn't stop, a blood vessel may have been lacerated; this will be tied off by the doctor under anaesthetic.

▶ If there is a deep wound or a wound contaminated with dirt, the doctor will ask you when your child last had a tetanus booster. If there is any doubt, your child will be given a tetanus injection.

▶ If there is any sign of infection, the doctor will cover the area with an antibiotic dressing and he may also prescribe antibiotics to be taken by mouth to eradicate the infection.

What can I do to help?

▶ Change the dressing daily. Your doctor may advise you to leave the dressing off at night as wounds heal more quickly if exposed to the air.

▶ When you change the dressing check for any redness extending from the wound. If you notice any, contact your doctor as soon as possible.

▶ A graze tends to cover a larger area, and it may need to be protected against rubbing. Use a dry gauze strip and hold it in place with surgical tape. Don't apply any adhesive dressing directly to the wound as it will be very painful to remove.

▶ Put a handful of salt in your child's bath water to clean the skin and deter infection.

Cystic fibrosis

CYSTIC FIBROSIS IS A RARE DISEASE that is present at birth and inherited from both parents. If the mother and father are healthy, but each carries one defective gene for cystic fibrosis, each child conceived has a 25 per cent chance of inheriting two defective genes and being born with the disease.

Cystic fibrosis causes several glands in the body to be defective, particularly the glands in the lining of the bronchial tubes. Instead of producing the normal thin mucus, the bronchial glands produce a thick, sticky phlegm, which creates blockages in the air passages, and this, in turn, leads to lung infections. When small parts of the lungs collapse, **pneumonia** results. This is a common and recurrent infection in cystic fibrosis sufferers.

In the intestines of a child with cystic fibrosis, the pancreas fails to produce certain enzymes that are vital to digestion. These enzymes break down food so that it can be absorbed easily by the body. When these enzymes are missing, food is poorly digested, which leads to diarrhoea and foul-smelling stools. Because the body does not absorb many of the nutrients that are essential to good health, the child with cystic fibrosis tends to be small, underweight and fails to thrive. Furthermore, the bouts of diarrhoea may alternate with constipation, which can actually block the intestine.

Possible symptoms

▶ **Recurrent chest infections** with a cough and some breathing difficulty.
▶ **Diarrhoea, alternating with constipation.**
▶ **Greasy and foul-smelling bowel motions.**
▶ **Failure to thrive.**
▶ **Swollen abdomen and wasted limbs.**

What can be done?

There is no cure for cystic fibrosis, but early detection of the condition lessens the chance of permanent damage to the lungs. Simple tests on the blood or stools of a newborn baby can be carried out, but the definitive test for cystic fibrosis is a sweat test because there is an increased salt level in the sweat of sufferers. This will be done on all brothers and sisters of a child with cystic fibrosis, or if a baby has recurrent bouts of pneumonia or fails to thrive. The tests are carried out when the baby is about three months of age.

A child with cystic fibrosis has to have a special low-fat diet, with vitamin supplements and enzyme replacements, which can be taken by mouth. Physiotherapy and breathing exercises must be given daily to loosen and drain mucus from the lungs. Exposure to moist air and a cold steam vaporizer can also help the lungs. Respiratory infections are treated with antibiotics; sometimes a spray form is used for speedy inhalation. Other treatments include inhaling enzymes to help dissolve lung secretions, or a heart-lung transplantation. Parents with an affected child who are planning a further pregnancy are offered genetic counselling.

For help and advice contact the Cystic Fibrosis Trust (see page 324).

Dandruff

DEAD CELLS ARE SHED CONSTANTLY from the surface of the skin. However, on the scalp they tend to become trapped and build up because of the hair. This build-up of cells is known as dandruff. It is not a disease, nor is it infectious or contagious; it is simply a variation of the normal. The amount of dandruff seen on the scalp varies from person to person according to how rapidly the skin cells are being shed and how greasy the scalp is. If the scalp is irritated, for example, by vigorous rubbing or by a medicated shampoo, more dead cells will be shed. If dandruff-like flakes appear on your child's eyelashes, this may be part of seborrhoeic **eczema** known as **blepharitis**.

Is it serious?

Dandruff is never serious; it can, however, be embarrassing, particularly as your child gets older. Although dandruff cannot be prevented if your child's scalp is greasy, it can be controlled.

Possible symptoms

▶ **Flakes of white skin** that are present on the scalp and can be easily wiped away with a finger.
▶ **White flakes** that appear on your child's shoulders after hair brushing.

What should I do first?

1 If you notice white flakes on your child's scalp, try to wipe them off with your fingers. If they move easily, this is dandruff. If not, don't pick at them; it could be an infestation of **lice**.

2 Wash your child's hair every other day using a baby shampoo.

3 Don't rub the scalp hard thinking that this will get rid of the dandruff. It will make it worse by stimulating the scalp.

Should I consult the doctor?

Consult your doctor as soon as possible if home treatment fails to clear up the white flakes.

What might the doctor do?

Your doctor will reassure you, and advise you how best to cope with the dandruff.

What can I do to help?

Don't use anti-dandruff shampoos more than once every two weeks. Avoid those containing selenium; this can irritate a child's scalp. Wash your child's hair with baby shampoo at other times.

SEE ALSO:
Blepharitis 66
Eczema 124
Lice 175

Deafness

DEAFNESS, EITHER PARTIAL OR TOTAL, may be the result of a congenital defect – that is, a defect already present at birth – or of an illness during a baby's first six weeks. There is normally some residual hearing so, with early diagnosis, hearing aids will help to develop speech, as will the stimulation of touch and vision. More often, a child may suffer hearing loss as a result of an ear infection, such as **glue ear** or **otitis media**, or a build-up of **wax in the ears**. The problem for parents is how to recognize whether their child is deaf or not. It is not easy to spot deafness in a newborn baby: all babies make gurgling noises up to the age of nine months or older, and loud noises don't seem to disturb very young babies.

However, after about four to six months, a deaf baby won't chatter the way a normal baby does because he hasn't been stimulated by his own or other people's voices.

Is it serious?

If a baby cannot hear properly, learning to talk can be a much more difficult task. Much of a child's language should have been learned before he starts to talk. Therefore, the longer a child is unable to hear, the greater will be the resulting delay in communicating. Even partial deafness will interfere with speech development.

What should I do first?

Test your child's hearing by making a fairly loud noise when your child's head is turned away from you to see if he turns around. Make sure he doesn't see you. If he responds, make the sounds gradually fainter and note the level at which he ceases to hear. Your health visitor can arrange hearing tests if you are concerned.

Should I consult the doctor?

Consult your doctor as soon as possible if you suspect a hearing problem. Consult your doctor immediately if your child has had an ear infection and you detect some hearing loss.

What might the doctor do?

▶ Your doctor will perform routine hearing tests on your child. If a hearing difficulty is diagnosed, your doctor will refer your child to an ear, nose and throat specialist for tests to determine the extent of the deafness. In a few cases, a hearing aid will be fitted. A baby can be fitted with a hearing aid from a very

early age (before six months). Your child may have aids fitted to both ears even if the hearing difficulty is only in one ear. You will be given advice on how to talk to your child.

▶ If the deafness is the result of repeated attacks of otitis media, surgery may be necessary to insert tubes to drain the fluid causing the deafness.

What can I do to help?

▶ Don't be concerned if your child remains silent for several months after hearing aids are fitted. It may take time for him to develop speech from the words that he is able to hear.

▶ Communicate with your child as clearly as you can. Make sure everyone else talks to him clearly, too. Never resort to shouting to make yourself clear.

▶ If your child is at school, ask the teacher if he can sit near the front of the class so that his school work does not suffer as a result of his disability.

SEE ALSO:
Glue ear 145
Otitis media 198
Wax in ears 260

Dehydration

THE BODY NEEDS ADEQUATE SUPPLIES of water to carry the essential minerals through the system to maintain body chemistry and to get rid of waste from the body. If your child loses water by **vomiting**, **diarrhoea** or **fever** and doesn't take in enough to replace the lost fluid, dehydration will result. Diarrhoea in babies can cause dehydration to develop rapidly as the intestines are not given enough time to absorb water. So, while a loose bowel motion is nothing to worry about, diarrhoea lasting six hours, especially if it is accompanied by vomiting, can cause dehydration in a baby or child. Dehydration will be compounded if your baby or child has a fever and is losing fluid through sweating. The body chemistry will be upset, essential nutrients will be lost and the volume of blood circulating through the body will be dangerously lowered.

Is it serious?

Dehydration is extremely serious and should be treated as an emergency. If dehydration is advanced, this can lead to brain damage and even death.

Possible symptoms

▶ **Dry mouth and lips**.
▶ **Lethargy**.

Affected areas

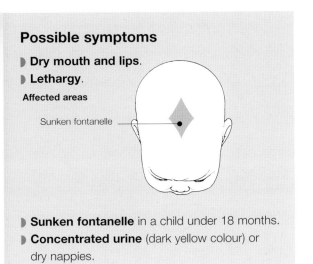

Sunken fontanelle

▶ **Sunken fontanelle** in a child under 18 months.
▶ **Concentrated urine** (dark yellow colour) or dry nappies.

What should I do first?

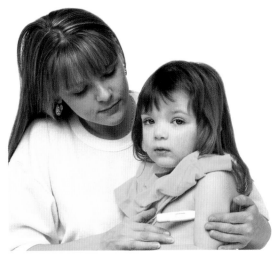

1 If your baby or child has diarrhoea or is vomiting, check her temperature for a fever. If she has, try to reduce it with tepid sponging.

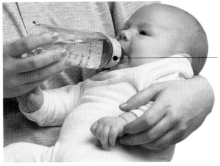

Bottlefeed with cooled, boiled water

2 If your bottlefed baby is not yet weaned, stop all milk feeds and give her only cooled, boiled water off a spoon or from a bottle or cup for six hours. Continue breastfeeding your baby. If the diarrhoea or vomiting hasn't stopped after six hours, consult your doctor immediately.

Continued on next page

Continued from previous page

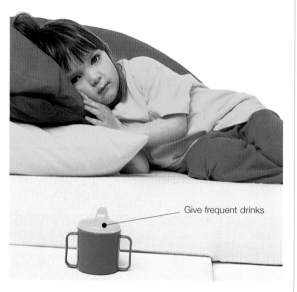

Give frequent drinks

3 Encourage your child to take small amounts of fluids frequently – every ten minutes or so. Don't give your child milk or undiluted fruit juices.

4 Buy a rehydration solution from a pharmacy and make it up with water according to the directions on the package. The solution contains salts and glucose in the correct proportions – follow the directions carefully because the solution must not be too weak or too strong, and make it just before using. The glucose supplies energy and the salts, though only in small quantities, are vital, as salt loss can add to the problems of dehydration.

5 Never give your child patent medicines for vomiting or diarrhoea, unless you are given a prescription by your doctor.

Should I consult the doctor?

Consult your doctor immediately if your baby or child has had diarrhoea for a period of more than six hours and has other signs of illness, such as a fever and vomiting.

What might the doctor do?

⦿ Your doctor may prescribe a powder to add to your child's drinks. This replaces the essential minerals that have been lost as a result of diarrhoea or vomiting. In severe cases, your child may be admitted to hospital and given essential fluids by intravenous drip.

⦿ In rare instances, your doctor may advise you to change your baby's formula milk feed to one that contains no sugars as your baby may be allergic to the sugar in the milk (lactose).

What can I do to help?

⦿ Check the colour of your child's urine. Clear, regular urine indicates that the body fluid levels are returning to normal.

⦿ When the illness has passed, you can reintroduce milk feeds gradually. Dilute your baby's normal formula milk feed with three times the usual amount of boiled water. Gradually reduce the water in the feed to the normal amount over the next two or three days.

⦿ If you are weaning your child on to solid foods, remember to keep his fluid intake up. Breast and formula milk have a high percentage of water and, when they are replaced by solid foods, your child's fluid levels may be reduced without you realizing it.

Diabetes mellitus

THERE ARE TWO FORMS OF DIABETES: one affects children and young adults, and one comes on in middle age. Both are due to a lack, or relative lack, of insulin in the body. Insulin is the hormone responsible for the normal metabolism of glucose in the body. We take in glucose in our diet mainly in the form of carbohydrates. Insulin is produced by the pancreas and promotes the absorption of glucose from the blood into the cells of the body and into the liver for storage. If the body is short of insulin, glucose collects in the blood and the body cells are deprived of their energy source. To make up for this deficiency, the body starts to break down fats and proteins to replace the lost energy. This means of energy production leads to weight loss and results in the production of poisonous waste substances, such as acetone and ketones.

Diabetes can start quite suddenly, for no known reason, though the disease may be inherited. Because the excess glucose spills over into the urine, the first symptom in a child is the frequent passing of large amounts of urine every hour; and because of the loss of body fluid, your child will be very thirsty. He may also start to wet the bed.

Possible symptoms

▶ **Large amounts of urine** passed every hour, possibly leading to bedwetting.
▶ **Increased thirst**.
▶ **Weight loss**.
▶ **Irritability and listlessness**.
▶ **Smell of pear drops on the breath**, signifying presence of acetone.
▶ **Reduced resistance to infection**.

What can be done?

The diagnosis is confirmed by blood tests that show an inappropriately high blood level of glucose. Your child will be prescribed a regime of insulin injections – the digestive juices destroy insulin taken by mouth – and you and your child will be taught how to administer them. Many children over the age of five confidently give themselves injections, under parental supervision. Insulin injections must be given daily and often twice a day to keep blood glucose levels to normal limits.

Your child will also need a special diet to keep the glucose steady in the blood throughout the day. No meals should be missed.

The hospital will provide you with special equipment to use at home to test the urine for sugar every day. The result will help you to adjust the dose of insulin to keep glucose levels normal in your child. You may also be shown how to measure the blood glucose level by using a drop of blood from a finger. It is advisable for your child to wear a bracelet or medallion engraved with details of his condition in case problems occur when you are not with him. As diabetic children are extremely prone to infectious illnesses, consult your doctor as soon as your child gets any infection; infection can affect your child's insulin requirements.

For help and advice contact the British Diabetic Association (see page 324).

Diarrhoea

Consult your doctor immediately if your child has loose, watery bowel motions for more than six hours and has any other signs of illness.

Accompanying symptoms	Common causes
Your child has no symptoms except looser stools than normal, and seems perfectly well and contented in himself.	He has possibly eaten too much of a food high in dietary fibre (such as prunes). Unless the stools are very watery or frequent, this is not true diarrhoea and you have no need to worry.
Your child has a sudden attack of diarrhoea and vomiting, with a slight fever.	He possibly has "gastric" 'flu, *page 140*, or a bowel infection such as **Food poisoning**, *page 137*.
Your child has no symptoms other than the diarrhoea, but he is anxious about something: for example, school.	Stress can cause bouts of diarrhoea in older children. If this happens often, consult your doctor.
Your child has other symptoms, such as a cough, for example, for which your doctor has already given him medicine.	Many medicines cause diarrhoea. Tell your doctor, but don't stop giving the medicine.
Your child has abdominal pain around his navel and to the lower right side of his groin.	**CONSULT YOUR DOCTOR IMMEDIATELY** Your child may have **Appendicitis**, *page 54*.
Your baby has severe abdominal cramps, is vomiting and his bowel motions are filled with blood and mucus resembling redcurrant jelly.	**CONSULT YOUR DOCTOR IMMEDIATELY** Your baby may have a bowel blockage known as **Intussusception,** *page 169*.
Your child soils his underpants involuntarily, even though he is toilet-trained.	This is not true diarrhoea, but possibly a condition called **Encopresis**, *page 127*.
Your child fails to thrive and his stools are pale, bulky and foul-smelling and float when you try to flush them down the toilet.	He could have **Coeliac disease**, *page 85*.

Diarrhoea *continued from previous page*

DIARRHOEA IS THE FREQUENT PASSAGE of loose, watery stools. It is a sign of an irritation of the intestines in which the intestines contract more than normal, hurrying food along. Consequently there is not sufficient time for water from foodstuffs to be absorbed into the body and this can result in profound water loss or **dehydration**, especially in babies.

Babies on a milk diet pass liquid motions many times a day. This is perfectly normal. Once a baby begins to take solid foods, bowel motions become firmer and more regular. Loose, frequent stools can result when a baby or child eats too much of a certain food that is rich in dietary fibre, such as fruit, or they may be a symptom of an infection. Infection in the intestines is commonly caused by viruses or bacteria. Food may have been contaminated with bacteria (**food poisoning**) or an infection from contaminated stools may have been spread to the mouth by unwashed hands. The infection need not be in the intestines;

diarrhoea can also be the symptom of a non-intestinal infection, such as **otitis media** or **influenza**, when the diarrhoea may be accompanied by a **fever**.

Ironically, stools similar to those of diarrhoea may be caused by **constipation**. If an older child soils himself, this may be because constipation has resulted in a blockage but the liquid stools still manage to escape past it. This involuntary soiling is known as **encopresis**.

Is it serious?
Diarrhoea in a baby is always serious because of the dangers of dehydration. Diarrhoea accompanied by **vomiting** in a young child is also serious for the same reason, especially if it is accompanied by fever and sweating. Diarrhoea in which the stools are greasy and foul-smelling can be a symptom of a more serious long-term condition such as **coeliac disease** or **cystic fibrosis**, in which there is a failure by the body to absorb the nutrients in food.

What should I do first?

1 If your baby is under one year old and has had diarrhoea for six hours with other signs of illness, consult your doctor immediately.

2 Don't give an older child any food or milk but give frequent drinks of rehydration solution, which you can buy as a powder at the chemist's.

3 Check your child's temperature to see if he has a fever. Reduce any fever with tepid sponging (*see page 31*).

4 Check the chart opposite to find a possible cause of your child's diarrhoea.

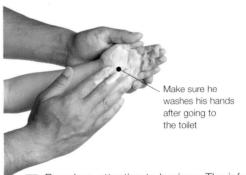

Make sure he washes his hands after going to the toilet

5 Pay close attention to hygiene. The infection could spread throughout the family if your child doesn't wash his hands after going to the toilet or if you don't wash yours after changing his nappies, if he wears them.

Continued on next page

Continued from previous page

Should I consult the doctor?

Consult your doctor immediately or take your baby to the nearest hospital if he has had diarrhoea for more than six hours with other signs of illness, such as a fever. Consult your doctor immediately if your child has diarrhoea with fever and vomiting, if he still has diarrhoea after 12 hours, or if the stools are greasy or contain mucus or blood.

What might the doctor do?

▶ After diagnosing the cause of the diarrhoea, your doctor will treat the illness accordingly.

▶ Your doctor may prescribe a powder to be added to all your child's drinks. This contains glucose and essential salts that will have been lost. Your doctor will recommend bed-rest and a liquid diet until any fever has passed. As a rough guide, your child should drink at least 200ml (7fl oz) of liquid per kilogram (2.2lb) of his body weight in 24 hours while he has diarrhoea. For a bottlefed baby, your doctor will probably suggest that you replace milk feeds with glucose and salt solutions, and then slowly reintroduce the milk. If your baby is breastfed, you will be advised to continue breastfeeding.

▶ If your baby is seriously ill, your doctor may admit him to hospital so that he can be given fluids intravenously.

What can I do to help?

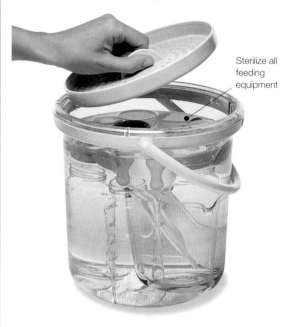

Sterilize all feeding equipment

▶ Be meticulous about hygiene. Wash your hands before preparing food and after changing your baby's nappies. If your baby is under six months, sterilize all feeding equipment.

▶ Advise anyone with diarrhoea to stay away from your baby.

▶ When the diarrhoea has cleared up, introduce bland foods to your baby's diet such as yogurt, bananas, rice and soups.

Diphtheria

DIPHTHERIA IS A SERIOUS BACTERIAL INFECTION that is very contagious. It produces symptoms like those of **tonsillitis** – a **sore throat**, accompanied by a **cough**, which sounds like **croup**. If diphtheria is not treated promptly, the infection may cause **pneumonia** to develop and heart failure due to paralysis of the cardiac muscle. Muscles of the limbs may weaken and become paralysed, too. A fine web of grey membrane forms over the tonsils, and may make breathing difficult if the windpipe is affected. However, a child can be rendered immune from the infection in the first year of life with a series of injections. This immunization programme has virtually eradicated the disease.

Is it serious?
Diphtheria is always serious as it is both life-threatening and contagious.

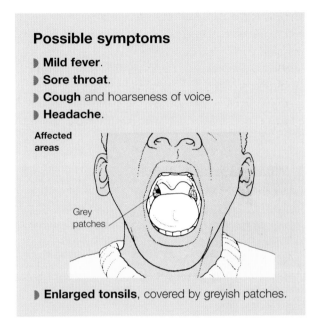

Possible symptoms

▶ **Mild fever.**

▶ **Sore throat.**

▶ **Cough** and hoarseness of voice.

▶ **Headache.**

Affected areas

Grey patches

▶ **Enlarged tonsils**, covered by greyish patches.

What should I do first?
1 Diphtheria rarely occurs spontaneously; there are nearly always several cases in the community, so you should be on the alert if you hear of any outbreaks and your child has not been immunized.

2 Check to see if your child's tonsils are swollen and coated with greyish patches.

Should I consult the doctor?
Consult your doctor immediately or take your child to the nearest hospital if you suspect diphtheria.

What might the doctor do?
Your doctor will admit your child to hospital immediately. Your child will then be given powerful antibiotic drugs and, if there are breathing difficulties, a tracheotomy will be performed to keep the airways open. This is a surgical procedure to insert a tube into the windpipe, bypassing the blockage in the throat.

What can I do to help?
▶ You will need to help medical staff to trace all known contacts of your child so that they can be checked for immunity.

▶ Your child will need a full course of immunization injections as the disease itself does not give complete immunity.

SEE ALSO:
Cough 98
Croup 101
Pneumonia 202
Sore throat 222
Tonsillitis 243

Dizziness

DIZZINESS DESCRIBES A FEELING of unsteadiness and spinning about. When a child is out of breath, he may feel a bit dizzy because there is a less-than-normal supply of oxygen reaching his brain. Your child may also feel dizzy if he is suffering from **anaemia**. A bang on the head that results in loss of consciousness or a **convulsion** may be preceded by dizziness. Under normal circumstances, dizziness should pass within a few minutes.

Is it serious?

Momentary dizziness is not serious but, if dizzy spells last longer than 12 hours, they may be caused by anaemia.

What should I do first?

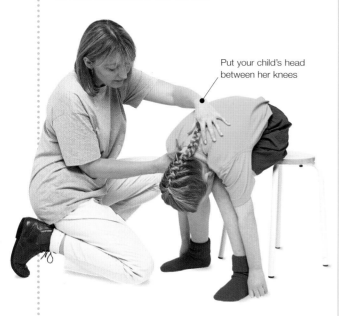

Put your child's head between her knees

Should I consult the doctor?

Consult your doctor immediately if your child experiences dizzy spells over a 12-hour period but has no other symptoms. Consult your doctor as soon as possible if your child is always complaining of dizziness after strenuous activity; this may be a sign of anaemia.

What might the doctor do?

After examining your child, your doctor will determine the cause of the dizziness. If the dizziness is a symptom of a more serious disorder, such as anaemia, your doctor will treat this accordingly.

1 Sit your child down and put her head between her knees to increase the flow of blood, and therefore oxygen, to her brain. Tell her to take a few deep breaths.

2 Keep her quiet and calm, still sitting, if that is what she wants.

3 Note how long your child says that the dizzy feeling lasts.

SEE ALSO:
Anaemia 53
Convulsion 94
Head injury 154

Down's syndrome

DOWN'S SYNDROME IS THE MOST common chromosomal abnormality. Children with Down's syndrome have 47 chromosomes instead of the normal 46 in each cell. The extra chromosome, chromosome 21, usually comes from the mother's egg.

The incidence of Down's syndrome babies rises sharply with maternal age, but various forms of screening in pregnancy can identify the condition in the fetus and a termination can be performed if the parents wish. Chorionic villus sampling or scans of the fetal neck can be carried out between nine and 13 weeks into the pregnancy. At around 14–20 weeks, an amniocentesis test is usually offered to pregnant women of 37 or over. Blood tests (known as a triple test) can also be carried out at this stage.

Children with Down's syndrome share obvious physical characteristics, such as a wide-bridged nose and upward-slanting eyes. The hands are short and broad, with a deep crease running across the middle of the palm, and there may be a large gap between the first and second toes. Down's children may suffer some degree of learning difficulty, and around 50 per cent have a heart defect; a smaller number are born with blocked intestines.

Possible symptoms

▶ **Small, upward-slanting eyes**, **nose with a wide bridge**, **short, broad hands** with a deep crease across the palm, **gap between first and second toes**.
▶ **Some degree of learning difficulty**.
▶ **Even-tempered and affectionate nature**.

What can be done?

The degree of learning difficulty varies widely in children with Down's syndrome, and some children are within the normal intelligence range. Modern theories reject the idea that all children with Down's syndrome should be educated in special institutions. The education of a child with Down's syndrome must be determined by the specific learning difficulty of the child, but children with Down's syndrome are usually educated in mainstream schools. As with all children, the emphasis should be on what the child can do rather than on what he cannot.

Almost all children with Down's syndrome will learn to walk and talk, and many will learn to read and write. They will need extra help to fulfil their potential, but with this help many will go on to lead semi-independent lives.

For help and advice contact the Down's Syndrome Association (see page 324).

Drowsiness

DROWSINESS IN A NORMALLY ALERT CHILD can be a symptom of a **fever,** hypothermia (when the body temperature falls below normal) or **dehydration**. It can also occur before or after a **convulsion,** or as a result of medication, such as antihistamines.

Is it serious?

If a child is drowsy but contented, is feeding well and has a normal temperature, there is no cause for alarm – your child is probably just feeling a little sleepy. If, however, a child becomes drowsy while recovering from an infectious disease such as **measles** or **chickenpox,** and he complains of headache and neck pain, this could be an indication of **encephalitis, meningitis** or **Reye's syndrome,** all of which are serious conditions and should be treated immediately.

What should I do first?

1 Check your child's temperature. If it is over 38°C (100.4°F) he has a fever; if it is under 35°C (95°F) he will be suffering from hypothermia.

2 If drowsiness is accompanied by vomiting and diarrhoea, keep up your child's fluid intake to prevent the risk of dehydration.

3 Check to see if your child has received a blow to his head.

4 Check if your child is suffering from a headache, or has neckache.

5 Smell your child's breath and check the liquor cabinet – he may have drunk alcohol. Check the medicine cabinet for sleep-inducing drugs.

6 If your child has had a convulsion, leave him to rest after the fit has passed.

Should I consult the doctor?

Consult your doctor immediately if your child's temperature is over 38°C (100.4°F) or below 35°C (95°F) and he is difficult to rouse. Consult your doctor immediately if he has a headache or neckache, if he has just had measles, chickenpox or mumps, or after a first fit.

What might the doctor do?

After examining your child, your doctor will determine the cause of the drowsiness, and will treat your child accordingly.

SEE ALSO:
Chickenpox 82
Convulsion 94
Dehydration 109
Encephalitis 126
Fever 134
Measles 177
Meningitis 178
Mumps 184
Reye's syndrome 208

Dysentery

DYSENTERY IS THE INFLAMMATION of the lining of the large bowel and causes the symptoms of **diarrhoea** and **fever**. The bacterium (*Shigella bacillus*) is passed out with the faeces and, if the hands are not washed after going to the toilet, they will become contaminated. The bacterium will then be passed on by contact. Dysentery is rare in countries where sanitary conditions are good.

Is it serious?

Dysentery is especially serious in children because of the risk of **dehydration**.

Possible symptoms

- **Griping abdominal pain**.
- **Loose, frequent motions**, every half-hour or so, which may contain mucus, blood or pus.
- **Fever**.
- **Nausea**.
- **Lethargy and weakness**.
- **Vomiting**.

What should I do first?

1 If you are living or travelling in an area of poor sanitation and your child has frequent loose stools, check the stools for any blood, mucus or pus. If you notice any, consult a doctor immediately.

2 Check your child's temperature to see if he has a fever.

3 Give your child frequent drinks in order to keep his fluid levels up.

Should I consult the doctor?

Consult a doctor at once if you notice mucus, blood or pus in your child's loose bowel motions. Consult a doctor as soon as possible if your child's bowel motions are still loose after 12 hours, or if his urine is infrequent and concentrated (dark yellow colour).

What might the doctor do?

- The doctor will treat your child for dehydration and send a sample of your child's faeces to a laboratory for investigation.
- If your child has a severe case of dysentery, he might be admitted to hospital and put on an

intravenous drip to counteract the dehydration. In many places, public health authorities must be notified of any cases of dysentery, and not only will your child's stools be tested but those of the whole family as well. The child will not be allowed to return to school until the stools are free of the bacterium.

What can I do to help?

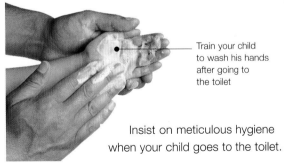

Train your child to wash his hands after going to the toilet

Insist on meticulous hygiene when your child goes to the toilet.

SEE ALSO:
Dehydration 109
Diarrhoea 112
Fever 134

Dyslexia

DYSLEXIA IS A SPECIFIC learning disorder concerning reading and writing. Dyslexic children have problems interpreting visual symbols. Although their hearing and vision are normal and they have the manual dexterity needed to form letters, they may have difficulty in perceiving letters or words in their proper order, or they may confuse certain letters, such as b and d, and p and q. Dyslexic children may misread words which have a similar overall configuration, they may disregard punctuation and read monotonously, and quite often they produce incorrect spellings that nevertheless reflect the sound of words (for example, lite for light) or that transpose letters (lihgt for light).

Dyslexic children are of average or above-average intelligence, though many of them appear clumsy. If the problem is not diagnosed and handled properly, the frustration with learning can lead to behavioural problems and unnecessary emotional strain.

Possible symptoms

▶ Written words that have the **letters misplaced**.
▶ **Poor reading ability**.
▶ **Difficulty in visualizing words**, even those just seen.

What can be done?

Dyslexia need not be educationally disabling. Provided the problem is detected early on, and the child has the correct tuition from educational psychologists and teachers (this can be done within a normal school), he should be able to overcome reading problems and reach the standards required for examinations. Dyslexic children are helped if emphasis is given to their non-verbal skills and activities.

The artistic and creative side of their development should be stressed so that they never become insecure and develop behavioural problems to mask feelings of inadequacy.

Parents and teachers must persist if they believe a child has been wrongly assessed as being of low intelligence or as having some problem with sight or hearing. Dyslexic children need to be encouraged and have their confidence boosted.

For help and advice contact the British Dyslexia Association (see page 324).

Ear, foreign body in

THE MOST COMMON FOREIGN BODIES to become stuck in a child's ear are inevitably small objects, like beads, which may be pushed in by the child himself or by a playmate. Very rarely, a small insect may fly into the ear and be trapped there.

Is it serious?

Any foreign body in the ear that cannot easily be removed should be regarded as serious because it may cause an infection of the external ear canal, **otitis externa**, or damage the eardrum.

What should I do first?

1 If the object is small and soft, try to remove it with a pair of tweezers. If you cannot grasp it without poking around in the ear, leave it and consult your doctor immediately.

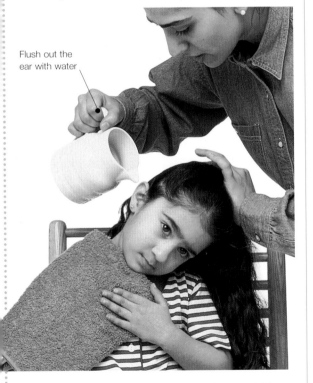

Flush out the ear with water

2 If the foreign body is an insect, sit your child on a chair with the affected ear uppermost and gently pour warm water into the ear. The insect should float out.

Should I consult the doctor?

Consult your doctor immediately if the object cannot be removed, or if your child complains of pain and tenderness in her ear.

What might the doctor do?

After examining your child's external ear canal, your doctor will remove the object and will treat any damage to the skin, or any infection that may have been caused by the foreign body.

What can I do to help?

Don't let a child under four play with small objects which he could put in her nose, or mouth, thus risking choking.

SEE ALSO:
Otitis externa 196

Earache

THERE ARE A NUMBER OF CAUSES of earache. The most common cause is an infection of the middle ear, called **otitis media**. This is especially true in children under six because the tube that runs from the throat to the ear – the Eustachian tube – is relatively short, and so infections of the nose and throat can be easily spread to the middle-ear cavity. A baby may not be able to isolate the site of the pain, and will scratch and rub the side of his face if the pain is severe. A child may complain of earache if he is suffering from **toothache**, **tonsillitis** or **mumps**, when the glands in his neck are swollen, or if he has been out in a cold wind without protective headgear. Earache with intense pain will result from an infection of the outer ear (**otitis externa**) if, for example, a foreign body has been poked into the ear by the child or if a **boil** has developed.

Is it serious?

Earache plus loss of hearing is serious. If the condition is not diagnosed and treated, it could cause permanent damage to the middle ear, resulting in a loss of hearing that will affect your child's speech development and learning ability.

Possible symptoms

▶ **Pain** in the area around the ear.
▶ **A temperature** of over 38°C (100.4°F).
▶ **Discharge** of pus from the ear.
▶ **Deafness**.
▶ **Inflammation** of the tonsils.
▶ **Pain** when the ear is touched.
▶ **Swollen glands**.
▶ **Rubbing and pulling** of the ear in the case of a young child.

Cross-section of the ear

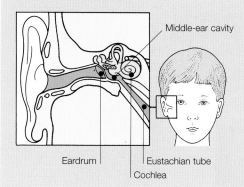

Middle-ear cavity

Eardrum

Eustachian tube

Cochlea

What should I do first?

1 Take your child's temperature to see if he has developed a fever.

2 Check to see whether there is any discharge coming from the ear.

3 Check whether your child's hearing is diminished. To do this, call his name quietly when his head is averted. See if he turns around.

4 Examine the back of your child's throat to see if the tonsils are abnormally enlarged or red (*see page 243*). This could indicate tonsillitis.

5 Check to see if there is any inflammation in the outer-ear cavity; such inflammation could be caused by a boil. Do not put anything into the ear, not even a cotton-wool swab.

6 Never use eardrops, or put anything into your child's ear, unless your doctor advises it.

Continued from previous page

Should I consult the doctor?

Consult your doctor as soon as possible if your child complains of earache; most earache is caused by infection. Consult your doctor immediately if your child is in pain with a high fever, and especially if you notice a discharge from the ear. Consult your doctor immediately if your child is too young to tell you he's in pain but is crying, generally off-colour and possibly pulling or rubbing one of his ears.

What might the doctor do?

Your doctor will examine your child to determine the cause of the earache. If it is caused by a bacterial infection, your doctor will probably prescribe a course of antibiotics.

What can I do to help?

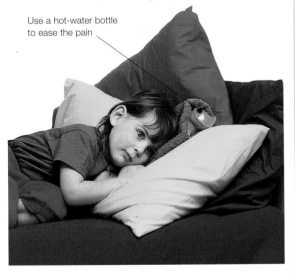

Use a hot-water bottle to ease the pain

▶ Place a hot-water bottle, covered by a towel, next to your child's ear to relieve pain, as long as the source of the earache is not a boil.

▶ Prevent water from entering the ear during bathing until the infection has cleared up.

SEE ALSO:
Boil 68
Ear, foreign body in, 121
Mumps 184
Otitis externa 196
Otitis media 198
Tonsillitis 243
Toothache 245

Eczema

ECZEMA IS AN ALLERGIC SKIN CONDITION that produces an extremely itchy, dry, scaly, red rash on the face, neck and hands, and in the creases of the limbs. The most common form of eczema in children is atopic eczema, which usually develops when a baby is about two to three months old, or at around four to five months, when solid foods are introduced. Certain foods, most commonly dairy products, eggs and wheat, and skin irritants such as pet fur, wool or washing powders, are among the main causes. An attack of eczema can also be triggered by stress or an emotional upset. It is common for eczema to be followed by other allergic complaints such as **hayfever** and penicillin sensitivity. It is also quite common for a child with eczema to suffer from **asthma**. Although most children grow out of eczema by the age of three, the associated allergic conditions may remain.

Another form of eczema, known as seborrhoeic eczema, occurs where the sebaceous glands are numerous. This is most commonly found on the scalps of young babies (**cradle cap**), on the eyelashes and eyelids (**blepharitis**), in the external ear canal (**otitis externa**) and in the greasy areas around the nostrils, ears and groin. This seborrhoeic eczema is not as itchy a condition as atopic eczema and it responds well to treatment.

Is it serious?
Eczema is not serious, although it can be very irritating for an affected child.

Possible symptoms

▶ **Dry, red, scaly skin** which is extremely itchy. The rash usually starts off as minute pearly blisters beneath the skin's surface.
▶ **Sleeplessness** if the itchiness is very bad.

Affected areas

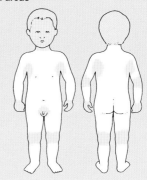

What should I do first?

1 If your child is scratching, inspect his neck and scalp, his face, his hands and the creases of his elbows, knees and groin for any rash.

2 Keep his fingernails short to minimize the possibility of breaking the skin. If the skin becomes broken, put mittens on his hands to prevent infection.

3 If you've just started weaning your breastfed child and he develops eczema, consult your doctor or health visitor for advice.

4 Apply an emollient such as aqueous cream to ease irritation and soothe the skin. Don't apply any astringent lotions.

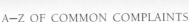

Continued from previous page

Should I consult the doctor?

Consult your doctor as soon as possible if you suspect eczema.

What might the doctor do?

▶ Your doctor will question you on your family's medical history, particularly whether anyone has ever suffered from eczema-related conditions, such as asthma or hayfever.

▶ He will ask you about any changes in your child's diet, whether you have recently changed washing powders, whether you have just brought a pet into the house, and whether your child wears natural or synthetic fibres.

▶ Your doctor may advise you to avoid foods such as dairy products, eggs and wheat, which may have caused the reaction.

▶ If you have just started weaning your baby from the breast or bottle, your doctor may recommend that you avoid dairy products and continue breastfeeding or formula milk, or recommend soya milk instead.

▶ Your doctor may prescribe an anti-inflammatory (steroid) skin cream to reduce redness, scaliness and itchiness. These creams should be used sparingly. Your doctor may also recommend emollient creams or ointments.

▶ Your doctor may prescribe anti-histamine medication to help your child sleep if the itching is keeping him awake at night.

▶ If your child's skin has become infected through scratching, your doctor may prescribe antibiotics.

▶ He will advise you to add bath oil to your child's bath water and to stop using soap as this can be an irritant. The oil will help to keep your child's skin supple and moisturized.

What can I do to help?

▶ Use an emollient cream whenever your child washes. This will keep his skin soft, prevent it from drying out and damp down the itchiness.

▶ Underplay the condition in front of your child. Your anxiety can make the condition worse.

▶ Keep your child's fingernails as short as possible and put gloves or mittens on his hands at night so that scratching doesn't cause the skin to break and become infected.

▶ Make sure all your child's clothes, and anything that comes next to his skin, are rinsed thoroughly to remove all traces of powders and conditioners.

▶ You may need to consider giving your family pet away if the reaction is found to be caused by pet fur.

▶ Dress your child with cotton next to his skin at all times to reduce irritation.

▶ Don't eliminate any foods from your child's diet without your doctor's supervision.

▶ Remove as many irritants from your child's environment as possible. For example, feather and down pillows can be a source of irritation.

For help and advice contact the National Eczema Society (see page 324) for advice and support.

Encephalitis

ENCEPHALITIS IS AN INFLAMMATION of the brain. The most common causes in children are viral infections like **chickenpox** or **mumps**. The major symptoms of encephalitis are fever, headache, pain when the neck is stretched and intolerance of bright light. Very rarely, encephalitis occurs as a severe reaction to the **whooping cough** vaccine. If your child is irritable, with a fever, and especially if he has a **convulsion**, this could be the first sign of sensitivity.

Is it serious?
Encephalitis is always a serious condition and in babies it can be fatal.

Possible symptoms
▶ **Fever**.
▶ **Severe headache**.
▶ **Pain** when the neck is stretched.
▶ **Intolerance of bright light**.
▶ **Loss of appetite** and perhaps **vomiting**.
▶ **Drowsiness**.
▶ **Listlessness**.
▶ **Confusion** and, in later stages, **convulsion** and **coma**.

What should I do first?

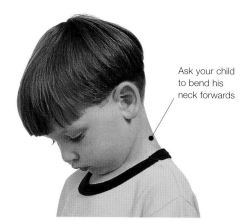

Ask your child to bend his neck forwards

If your child is recovering from an infectious disease and seems unwell, with a fever, ask him to bend his neck forward so that his chin touches his chest. See if this causes him pain.

Should I consult the doctor?
Consult your doctor immediately if you suspect that your child may have encephalitis.

What might the doctor do?
▶ Your child will be admitted to hospital where diagnostic tests will be carried out to determine the severity of the disease. These will include a lumbar puncture in which spinal fluid is drawn off under anaesthetic for examination.
▶ The hospital staff will treat the accompanying symptoms of encephalitis and your child should be better in a couple of weeks.

What can I do to help?
▶ Once your child has been discharged from hospital, keep him comfortable and well-fed.
▶ If there has been any weakness or stiffness of your child's muscles, you may have to do exercises with him to help him regain control over them. You will be advised how to do this by a hospital physiotherapist.

Encopresis

IF A CHILD FREQUENTLY PASSES solid stools in his pants or in inappropriate places after he has bowel control, he has encopresis. In a child of four or five, uncontrollable bowel motions should be regarded as a symptom of a problem rather than of slow development. The most common cause of encopresis is chronic **constipation**. The problem often starts as the result of some emotional disturbance in the child's life, such as the arrival of a new baby. Occasionally, children persist in soiling their pants from infancy onwards. This soiling may be a reaction against over-fussy toilet training.

Is it serious?
Encopresis is not a serious problem.

Possible symptoms
▶ **Involuntary bowel motions** after the child has been toilet-trained.
▶ **Chronic constipation**.

What should I do first?
1 Try to determine whether your child is constipated. Ask him how long ago he last went to the toilet.

2 Check whether your child is affected by stress caused by a new baby, moving house or starting school.

Should I consult the doctor?
Consult your doctor as soon as possible if you think your child has chronic constipation. If you can find no reason for the involuntary soiling, your doctor may be the best person to discover a possible cause of tension.

What might the doctor do?
▶ If your child is constipated, your doctor will prescribe a mild laxative, specially formulated for babies and children, which is safe for short-term use.
▶ Your doctor or health visitor will advise you on how to reduce the constipation in the future.
▶ If there is some emotional reason for the encopresis, your doctor will assess the situation after discussion with you and your child. If further investigation is needed, your doctor or health visitor may refer you and your child to a psychotherapist.

What can I do to help?
▶ Make sure your child has a diet rich in dietary fibre and liquids.
▶ Don't punish your child or show disgust if he soils his pants; this will make the condition worse.
▶ Watch for signs of poor school performance. Your child may become a target of scorn because of the odour if he soils himself at school. Provide him with spare underpants.

SEE ALSO:
Constipation 92
Diarrhoea 112

Epilepsy

EPILEPSY IS A DISORDER THAT CAUSES periodic seizures, and these occur when the normal electrical impulses in the brain are disturbed. There are two main forms of epileptic seizure. The *grand mal* form involves recurring attacks of convulsions. These involve a loss of consciousness and a stiff phase lasting a minute or less, followed by a series of rhythmic jerks of the limbs, clenching of the teeth (when your child might bite his tongue), involuntary urination and frothing at the mouth. The child then usually lapses into sleep.

The *petit mal* form of epilepsy has no convulsions. There is only a second or two of unconsciousness – rather like daydreaming – when the child's eyes glaze over; the child appears not to see or hear anything. This form of epilepsy is often not recognized and not diagnosed as epilepsy. Although the scale of the problem is different from the *grand mal* convulsions, frequent *petit mal* seizures can interfere with a child's life, particularly with school performance and certain physical activities, such as riding a bicycle. There is not usually any mental disability associated with either form of epilepsy, which is a condition that tends to run in families.

About three to five per cent of children under the age of six have an occasional convulsion, but nearly all of these are harmless febrile convulsions, when the electrical disturbance in the brain is caused by a high temperature preceding or during an infectious illness.

Is it serious?
Epilepsy is not a life-threatening disorder. Most children grow out of the *petit mal* form of epilepsy by late adolescence. However, children who suffer from grand mal epilepsy may need special consideration throughout their lives, even though the condition is controlled by drugs. They will need supervision during activities such as swimming and cycling.

Possible symptoms
Grand mal
▶ **Loss of consciousness**.
▶ **Clenching of teeth**.
▶ **Stiffness**, followed by a rhythmic jerking of the limbs.
▶ **Involuntary urination**.
▶ **Frothing** at the mouth.

Petit mal
▶ **Daydream-like state**, lasting one or two seconds, from which the child cannot be roused.

What should I do first?
During a *grand mal* seizure:

1 Protect your child from injury by moving any furniture or other solid objects out of his way during a seizure. Loosen the clothing around his neck and chest. Stay with your child until the seizure has finished.

2 Don't try to hold your child's teeth apart if they are clenched, or put anything in his mouth. Any injury to his tongue will occur at the beginning of the attack, therefore there is nothing you can do until the attack is over.

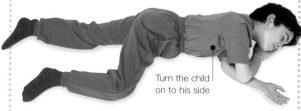

Turn the child on to his side

3 As soon as your child stops moving violently, turn him gently on to his side so that he cannot choke on his tongue or on saliva.

Continued from previous page

4 Watch exactly what happens during your child's seizure – your account will help your doctor to make a diagnosis.

During a *petit mal* seizure:

1 Guide your child to safety if he is in the street or near a stairway, for example.

2 Stay with your child until the seizure has completely passed.

Should I consult the doctor?

Consult your doctor as soon as the convulsion has passed, whether you think it is a *grand mal* seizure or a febrile convulsion. Consult your doctor as soon as possible if you think your child has *petit mal* seizures.

What might the doctor do?

If your child has a convulsion, your doctor will examine him and question you about the attack in order to determine what form of seizure your child has suffered from.

If your child has recurrent convulsions, he will be referred to hospital for laboratory examinations. These may include blood tests for glucose and calcium, an EEG (electroencephalogram), and possibly a brain scan to find out if an abnormal area of the brain is causing the seizures. During the scan the child is stimulated, for example, with strobe lights, so that any abnormal behaviour in the brain can be picked up with the scanning equipment. Some of these tests are also used to diagnose *petit mal* seizures.

The hospital paediatrician will prescribe anti-convulsant drugs to be taken daily to reduce the frequency of both *petit mal* and *grand mal* seizures. There are no drugs to cure the condition.

Your child's condition will be reviewed periodically by the paediatrician. If there are no seizures for a year or two, the doctor may decide to phase out the drugs.

What can I do to help?

It can be a shock to realize that your child has epilepsy. Both you and your child will need to get your confidence back. You can do this through your doctor, who can advise you how to cope with the seizures.

Make a note of the frequency of your child's *petit mal* seizures so that you can tell your doctor.

Watch your child carefully and report any mental or personality differences which may be the result of the drugs. It is important that your child's medication is given in the proper amounts so as not to cause any undesirable side effects.

Treat your child as normally as possible. Tell his friends and teachers about the condition so that they will not be frightened and shocked if your child has a convulsion in their presence.

Have a bracelet or medallion engraved with information about your child's epilepsy in case of an attack when you are not there and make sure your child wears it all the time.

If your child is prescribed anti-convulsant drugs, do not stop them without medical advice. To do so could cause a severe, prolonged convulsion after a few days.

Teach your child to recognize the signs of an on-coming attack. Some sufferers from epilepsy experience strange sensations, such as unpleasant smells, distorted vision or an odd feeling in the stomach, just before a convulsion. This is known as an "aura" and, if your child is old enough to identify these sensations as warning signs, he may be able to avoid having an accident.

For help and advice contact the Epilepsy Support Group (see page 324)

SEE ALSO:
Convulsion 94

Eye, foreign body in

IF A FOREIGN BODY such as a speck of dust or grit enters your child's eye, the eye will water and your child will be loath to open it. If you can see something moving loosely over the white part of the eye, you can try to remove it. If, however, the foreign body is embedded in the eyeball or is on the coloured part of the eye (the iris), don't touch it.

Is it serious?

Small specks of dust or grit are not serious as they are washed out naturally by the tears, but, if your child's eyeball is scratched, if an object has pierced it or there is a cut on the eyeball or eyelid, this is serious and should be treated as an emergency.

Possible symptoms

▶ **Watery eye**.
▶ **Reluctance** to open eye.
▶ **Pain and irritation**.
▶ **A visible embedded object**.

What should I do first?

Look closely to see whether the foreign body is moving or is embedded in the eye. Encourage your child to blink; this may dislodge the foreign body, as may tears if your child has been crying because of the pain and irritation.

If the foreign body is embedded in the eye

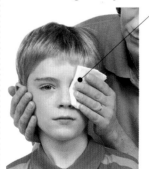

Keep eye closed

Do not attempt any first aid. Keep your child's eye closed by putting a pad or clean handkerchief over the eyelid and taping it in place. Go straight to the nearest casualty department.

If the foreign body is not embedded in the eye

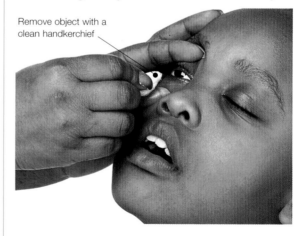

Remove object with a clean handkerchief

1 Ask your child to look upwards and gently pull down the eyelid to see if the object is there. If it is, remove it with the corner of a clean handkerchief or a cotton-wool swab.

2 To expose the area beneath the top lid, lay a matchstick or a cotton-wool swab along the middle of the top lid. Take hold of the eyelashes and

Continued from previous page

pull them back over the matchstick or swab. Remove the object with a handkerchief or cotton-wool swab. If your child won't co-operate, you will need someone to help you. You may have to restrain your child bodily if he resists.

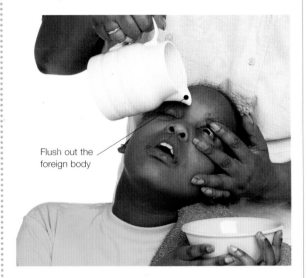

Flush out the foreign body

3 If these methods don't work, try to flush the foreign body out by pouring a glass or jug of water, to which you have added a pinch of salt, across the open eye.

Should I consult the doctor?

Go immediately to the nearest casualty department if the eyeball is scratched or if a foreign body has pierced the eye. Consult your doctor immediately if you have failed to remove a floating foreign body from your child's eye within one hour. Consult your doctor as soon as possible if your child still complains of pain an hour or two after you have removed the object.

What might the doctor do?

❱ The hospital doctor will remove an embedded foreign body from your child's eye after putting drops of a local anaesthetic into the eye.

❱ If the eyeball is scratched, the doctor will prescribe antibiotic drops to guard against infection and may bandage the eye to keep it closed for about 24 hours.

❱ If you went to your doctor because your child's eye was still sore, your doctor will examine the eye and remove any foreign object that he finds.

What can I do to help?

After the removal of a foreign body, the pain should subside in an hour or so. If it does not, consult your doctor as soon as possible.

SEE ALSO:
Eye, injury to 132

Eye, injury to

INJURIES TO THE EYE should be treated promptly because they could have long-term consequences for your child's sight. If your child receives a blow to the eye, the eye socket will probably protect the eye itself, but the surrounding area will swell and **bruise** as the tiny blood vessels beneath the skin break.

If a chemical substance is accidentally splashed into the eye, this should be treated as an emergency. Soap in the eye may cause your child to make a lot of fuss but

it will do no damage. If a toy or other sharp implement penetrates the eyeball or makes a **cut** near the eye, or on the eyelid, this should be treated as an emergency.

Is it serious?

A black eye looks bad but it is rarely serious. However, if a chemical substance or a sharp object injures your child's eye, this is serious and should be treated as an emergency.

What should I do first?

1 If your child receives a blow to his eye, place a cold compress over the eye for half an hour to limit the extent of the bruising.

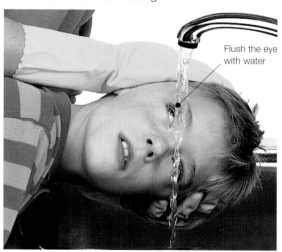

Flush the eye with water

2 If your child's eye is injured by a chemical substance, try to flush the chemical out with water immediately, before consulting your doctor or going to the nearest casualty department. If you can, carry your child to a sink or basin and hold his head under the cold tap with the injured eye lowermost so that no chemical can run into the unaffected eye or down on to his face. Hold the eye

open and let the water run in from the inner corner. Do this for 15 minutes. Alternatively, lay your child on the ground with his head turned to one side so that the injured eye is lowermost and pour cold water from a jug, bowl or bucket into the eye. Apply a pad or clean handkerchief, held in place with tape, to the eyelid to keep it closed.

3 If there are chemical particles sticking to the eyeball, don't attempt to remove them. Apply a pad or clean handkerchief, held in place with tape, to the eyelid to keep it closed, and take your child to the nearest casualty department.

4 If the injury is caused by a sharp implement, cover the injured eye with a pad or clean handkerchief, tape in place and go at once to the nearest casualty department.

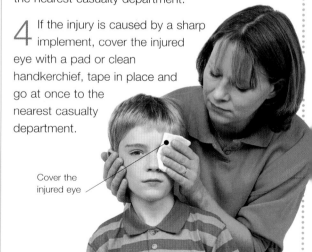

Cover the injured eye

Continued from previous page

5 If there is blood coming from the wound, hold a pad firmly against the cut to stem the blood flow, and then take your child to the nearest casualty department.

Should I consult the doctor?

Consult your doctor immediately or go to the nearest casualty department after flushing the chemicals from your child's eye. Go to the nearest casualty department immediately if your child suffers any other injury to his eye other than a black eye or minor cut.

What might the doctor do?

▶ How the doctor in the casualty department will treat the eye depends on the cause of the injury. If the problem was caused by a chemical substance, take the bottle containing the chemical with you; otherwise note what caused the damage and tell the doctor at the hospital.

▶ If your child's eyelid was cut, the doctor will stitch the cut to reduce scarring.

Fever

A fever is a temperature of 37.7°C (100°F) or over. Consult your doctor if your baby's temperature remains high despite tepid sponging (*see page 31*).

Consult your doctor immediately if your child's temperature is as high as 40°C (104°F).

Accompanying symptoms	Common causes
Your child has a cough and a runny nose.	He possibly has a **Common cold**, *page 90*.
Your child has a cough, sore throat and aches and pains.	He possibly has **Influenza**, *page 167*.
Your child has a sore throat and is experiencing difficulty in swallowing.	He may have **Tonsillitis**, *page 243*. If his voice is hoarse, he may have **Laryngitis**, *page 173*. If his neck glands are swollen, he may have **Glandular fever**, *page 143*.
Your child has a rash of itchy, red spots starting on the trunk.	He may have **Chickenpox**, *page 82*.
Your child passes urine frequently and, if he is old enough, complains of a burning sensation.	He may have a **Urinary tract infection**, *page 252*.
Your child had a runny nose and sore eyes and now has a brownish-red rash.	He possibly has **Measles**, *page 177*.
The sides of your child's face and the area under his chin are swollen.	He possibly has **Mumps**, *page 184*.
Your child has earache or, if he is too young to tell you, he cries and tugs at his ear.	He possibly has a middle-ear infection, **Otitis media**, *page 198*.
Your child has diarrhoea.	He could have "gastric" 'flu, *page 140*, or **Food poisoning**, *page 137*.
Your baby or child is breathing rapidly and with great difficulty.	**CONSULT YOUR DOCTOR IMMEDIATELY** Your child may have **Bronchitis**, *page 73* **Bronchiolitis**, *page 72*, **Pneumonia**, *page 202* or **Croup**, *page 101*.
Your child cannot bend his neck without pain and turns away from bright light.	**CONSULT YOUR DOCTOR IMMEDIATELY** Your child may have **Meningitis**, page 178.

Fever *continued from previous page*

THE RANGE OF NORMAL BODY temperature is 36–37°C (96.8–98.6°F). Anything over 37.7°C (100°F) is a fever, although the height a temperature reaches is not necessarily an accurate reflection of the seriousness of the sickness. A fever is not in itself an illness, but rather a symptom of one (*see page 134*). Apart from any illness, your child's temperature will reflect the time of day and activity level: after a very strenuous game of football, for example, the temperature could temporarily be over 38°C (100.4°F).

Is it serious?

A temperature of over 37.7°C (100°F) is always serious in a baby under six months old. If the temperature remains high, there is also a slight risk of a **convulsion** occurring.

What should I do first?

1 If you suspect that your child has a fever, take her temperature (*see page 30*), then check it again 20 minutes later. Note down each reading.

2 Put your child to bed and remove most of her clothing, even if the room is cool. A child with a fever need only be covered by a light sheet.

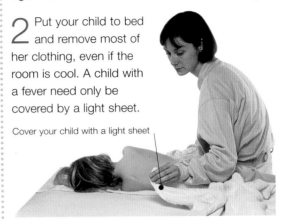

Cover your child with a light sheet

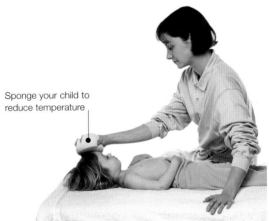

Sponge your child to reduce temperature

3 Lower a temperature of over 40°C (104°F) by sponging your child all over with tepid water (*see page 31*). Check the temperature every five minutes and stop tepid sponging when the temperature drops to 38°C (100.4°F). Never sponge your child with cold water as this causes the blood vessels to constrict, preventing heat loss and therefore increasing the temperature.

Continued on next page

Continued from previous page

4 Give paracetamol elixir only if other methods of reducing the fever (*see above*) have failed. Never give aspirin to a child under 12 years, particularly if he has the symptoms of **chickenpox** or **influenza**, as this has been linked to the development of **Reye's syndrome**.

5 Encourage your child to drink small amounts of fluid at regular intervals.

Should I consult the doctor?

Consult your doctor immediately if your child is under six months old. Consult your doctor immediately if your child has a **convulsion**, if he has had a convulsion in the past, or if febrile convulsions run in the family. Consult your doctor as soon as possible if the fever lasts for more than 24 hours, or if you are worried about any of the accompanying symptoms.

What might the doctor do?

The course of treatment will depend on the underlying cause of the fever. If the cause is bacterial infection, antibiotics will probably be prescribed. If the cause is an ailment like chickenpox, or a **common cold**, then most likely no medication will be given, just advice on how to make your child comfortable.

What can I do to help?

❯ Change the sheets on your child's bed frequently and cover him with a sheet only.

❯ Place a cold compress or a wet facecloth on your child's forehead.

❯ Don't wake your child to take his temperature. Sleep is more important.

Food poisoning

FOOD POISONING IS A FORM of **gastroenteritis** caused by eating food that is contaminated with poisons, usually bacteria. Within three to 24 hours, depending on the poison, the symptoms of abdominal cramps, **fever**, **vomiting** and **diarrhoea** occur with unpleasant ferocity. If the food was contaminated with bacteria, they release their own poisons, known as toxins, which have a direct effect on the lining of the bowel, causing inflammation. There are many types of bacterium that cause food poisoning, but the most common are *salmonella*, *shigella*, *staphylococcii* and *E. coli*, which is the bacterium most commonly responsible for food poisoning among babies, usually in bottlefed babies. Of the non-bacterial types of food poisoning, symptoms can arise from eating chemicals, insecticides or certain plants.

Is it serious?
In a baby, this condition is serious because the symptoms can rapidly lead to **dehydration**.

Possible symptoms

- **Abdominal cramps**.
- **Fever**.
- **Vomiting**.
- **Frequent, loose stools** that may contain blood, pus or mucus.
- **Muscular weakness and chills**.
- **Loss of appetite**.

What should I do first?

1 If your child is vomiting and has diarrhoea, check his temperature to see if he has a fever.

2 Check your child's stools for the presence of mucus or blood.

3 Put your child to bed and stop all foods, but keep up his fluid levels by offering frequent small drinks of rehydration solution (available in powder form from the chemist).

4 Try to determine what your child could have eaten to cause the symptoms.

Should I consult the doctor?

Consult your doctor immediately or take your baby to the nearest casualty department if vomiting and diarrhoea continue for more than six hours and you cannot bring them under control with a fluids-only diet. Consult your doctor immediately if your child's condition has not improved within 24 hours or if you suspect that your child has drunk an insecticide or eaten a poisonous plant. If your doctor is delayed in such cases, take your child to the nearest casualty department, taking the suspected poison with you.

What might the doctor do?

In the majority of cases there is no special treatment for food poisoning except to replace the fluid and

Continued on next page

Continued from previous page

salts that have been lost through diarrhoea and vomiting. Your doctor will probably prescribe a powder containing glucose and essential salts to be added to all your child's drinks and to replace all milk feeds in a bottlefed baby. If your baby or child is in danger of dehydration, your doctor will admit him to hospital to be given fluids intravenously. If the vomiting is very severe, your doctor may give your child an injection of an anti-emetic drug to stop the vomiting.

What can I do to help?

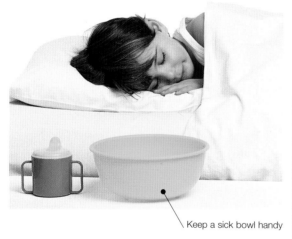
Keep a sick bowl handy

▶ Place a bowl next to your child's bed for her to be sick into, so that she doesn't have to run to the toilet.
▶ Keep her cool and refreshed with an icepack or a damp facecloth if she has a fever.
▶ Help your child to rinse her mouth out with water after she has been sick.
▶ Be meticulous about hygiene. Food poisoning is infectious; make your child wash her hands after going to the toilet. Wash your hands after changing nappies.
▶ To prevent food poisoning, refrigerate all cooked food and, if you reheat it, do so thoroughly. Salmonella thrives in warmed food but is killed by high temperatures.

▶ If your child refuses to drink enough fluids, or doesn't like the taste of the special powder, give her cubes of melon to suck.
▶ Defrost foods well before cooking, particularly poultry and pork, and make sure they are thoroughly cooked.
▶ Reintroduce foods that are easily digested, such as soups, yogurt, jellies and non-fatty foods, as soon as your child asks for something to eat. The effects of the illness usually pass within a week.
▶ Follow your doctor's instructions for reintroducing milk feeds for a bottlefed baby.
▶ Check back over what your child has eaten in the previous 24 hours. Throw out any cooked meats, fish, dairy products or pastries that you suspect may have caused the illness.

SEE ALSO:
Dehydration 109
Diarrhoea 112
Fever 134
Gastroenteritis 140
Vomiting 257

Frostbite

FROSTBITE OCCURS AFTER EXPOSURE to extreme cold, when the blood flow to the exposed area stops and the affected area of skin becomes frozen. Typically the skin first becomes red, then shiny and then a dull, greyish colour. Occasionally blisters may form. The fingers, toes, nose and ears are the parts of the body most often affected.

Is it serious?

Frostbite is serious and should be treated as an emergency, but there is a first-aid routine (*see below*) that you should carry out immediately. If treated quickly, frostbite has no lasting effect, but severe cases can lead to gangrene and eventually amputation of the affected part.

Possible symptoms

▶ **Hard, red, cold skin**, usually on the hands, toes, nose or ears, which becomes shiny then a dull, grey colour.
▶ **Tiny blisters** on the affected area.
▶ **Numbness** in the affected area.

What should I do first?

1 Get your child out of the cold immediately. If you can, get someone else to call for medical help. If you are on your own, don't stop to call a doctor until you have followed the first-aid procedure.

2 Do not apply direct heat or rub the affected part. If the fingers or toes are frostbitten, immerse them in warm water and keep adding warm water so that the temperature remains constantly warm. If you have no access to warm water, keep the affected part warm by putting your child's hands or feet under your armpits, or by holding his face against your body.

3 Wrap your child in blankets and give him hot drinks. Feed the drinks to him yourself if his hands are affected. Don't let your child walk on a frostbitten foot.

4 When the affected part becomes pink, stop warming, wrap in gauze, cotton wool or any soft, warm fabric that you have to hand and go at once to the nearest casualty department.

5 While you are travelling to the hospital, keep the affected part level with your child's chest to encourage blood flow. For example, raise his feet or put his hands across his chest.

Should I consult the doctor?

Take your child to the nearest casualty department as soon as you have restored pinkness to the affected skin.

What might the doctor do?

The doctor will check that circulation has returned to the frostbitten area. Drugs to improve blood circulation may be necessary if the blood flow has not returned to normal.

What can I do to help?

Always wrap your child up warmly in cold weather.

Gastroenteritis

GASTROENTERITIS IS AN INFLAMMATION of the stomach and intestines. The symptoms include **vomiting**, nausea, **diarrhoea**, abdominal cramps and loss of appetite. The most common cause of gastroenteritis in children is the *rotavirus*, which can be inhaled and tends to spread easily through a community. It may also be caused by direct infection of the intestines with bacteria, usually from contaminated food, when it is known as **food poisoning**, or by a parasite, when the condition is sometimes known as **dysentery**. Gastroenteritis may also be a symptom of another infection, such as **influenza**, when the infecting bacteria may spread to the bowel via the bloodstream. When vomiting and diarrhoea accompany 'flu symptoms, this is often referred to as "gastric 'flu".

Gastroenteritis in babies is most common in bottlefed babies and is usually the result of poor sterilization of feeding equipment.

Is it serious?

Gastroenteritis is very serious in children, especially babies, because the symptoms of vomiting and diarrhoea can rapidly lead to **dehydration**.

Possible symptoms

▶ **Vomiting**.

▶ **Nausea**.

▶ **Diarrhoea**.

▶ **Abdominal cramps**.

▶ **Loss of appetite**.

▶ **Raised temperature**.

What should I do first?

1 Stop all foods and milk and give your child only water in small amounts every 15 minutes.

2 Put your child to bed with a bowl by the bed in case he vomits.

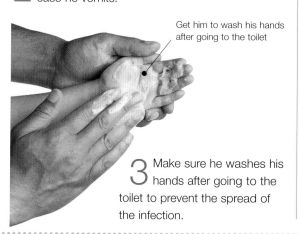

Get him to wash his hands after going to the toilet

3 Make sure he washes his hands after going to the toilet to prevent the spread of the infection.

Should I consult the doctor?

Consult your doctor immediately if your child has diarrhoea and vomiting for more than six hours and you cannot bring them under control with a fluids-only diet.

What might the doctor do?

▶ Your doctor will probably prescribe a powder to be added to all your child's drinks. This contains the glucose and essential minerals that have been lost through vomiting and diarrhoea. To avoid dehydration, your child should be given 200ml (7½fl oz) of water for every kilogram (2.2lb) of his body weight in the first 24 hours of diarrhoea and vomiting.

▶ Your doctor will recommend bed-rest and a liquid diet until the vomiting and diarrhoea have subsided.

▶ For a bottlefed baby, your doctor may recommend

Continued from previous page

that you replace all milk feeds with the glucose solution and he will then provide you with a regime for reintroducing the formula feeds.

▶ If your baby is seriously ill, your doctor may admit him to hospital so that he can be given fluids intravenously to counteract dehydration.

What can I do to help?

▶ If your child is admitted to hospital, try to stay with him. Most hospital authorities now encourage parents to do this.

▶ Be meticulous about hygiene. Sterilize all feeding equipment if your baby is bottlefed. Wash your hands before preparing any food for your child and after changing nappies.

▶ Avoid giving your child acidic drinks such as orange and grapefruit juice. They may irritate the stomach further.

▶ Reintroduce foods slowly when your child seems interested, starting with bland, easily digested foods such as jellies, yogurt, soups and non-fatty foods.

▶ If your child refuses to drink enough fluids, or doesn't like the taste of the special powder, give him cubes of melon or watermelon to suck.

SEE ALSO:
Appetite, loss of 55
Dehydration 109
Diarrhoea 112
Dysentery 119
Food poisoning 137
Influenza 167
Vomiting 257

German measles

GERMAN MEASLES, OR RUBELLA, is a mild, infectious disease that is caused by a virus. It is contagious and has an incubation period of 14 to 21 days. The rash usually starts behind the ears before spreading to the forehead and the rest of the body. It looks more like a large patch of redness than a series of spots. The rash lasts about two to three days and is rarely accompanied by serious symptoms, just a mild fever and enlarged glands at the back of the neck. The main danger with German measles is not to your infected child but to any pregnant woman who may contract the disease from your child. Rubella can cause birth defects such as blindness and deafness.

Is it serious?

This is not a serious childhood illness. However, you should keep your child in isolation for five days after the rash appears. Like other childhood infectious diseases, rubella carries a slight risk of **encephalitis**.

Possible symptoms

▶ **Slightly raised temperature**.

▶ **Tiny pink or red spots**, starting behind the ears and spreading to the forehead, then the rest of the body.

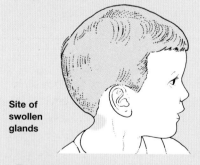

Site of swollen glands

▶ **Enlarged, swollen glands** at the back of the neck.

What should I do first?

1 Make sure that anyone who might be pregnant and has been in contact with your child is informed of your child's infection.

2 Keep your child away from school and from public places.

3 If your child's temperature rises above 38°C (100.4°F), give him paracetamol elixir.

4 If your child is feeling unwell, put him to bed.

Should I consult the doctor?

Consult your doctor by telephone to confirm that your child has German measles. Consult your doctor immediately if your child complains of a stiff neck or a headache.

What might the doctor do?

There is no treatment for German measles, but your doctor will advise you to alert any women you know who might be pregnant, if you haven't already done so.

What can I do to help?

Make sure that your child is vaccinated against the disease.

SEE ALSO:
Encephalitis 126
Rash 206

Glandular fever

GLANDULAR FEVER, OR INFECTIOUS mononucleosis, is a viral infection that starts in much the same way as **influenza**, with a runny nose, **sore throat**, aches, pains and tiredness. In a small number of cases, the infection begins with a rash similar to that of **German measles**. It is a fairly common disease affecting mostly teenagers and young adults; children can also contract it, but they tend to be less severely affected by the disease. In common with other viral infections, there is no known cure for glandular fever; it has to run its course – usually, for about a month. As part of the body's reaction to the infection, the glands become swollen and the spleen may become enlarged. This does not in itself give rise to unpleasant symptoms, and the spleen, which is part of the lymphatic-gland system, returns to normal once the infection has gone.

Is it serious?

Although debilitating, glandular fever is not usually serious but, as so many of its symptoms are similar to those of other illnesses, you should consult your doctor for a diagnosis.

Possible symptoms

▶ **Runny nose**.
▶ **Sore throat**.
▶ **Aches and pain**.

Affected glands

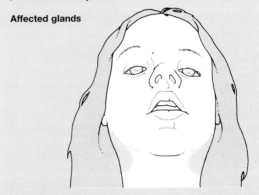

▶ **Swollen glands**, most commonly in the neck, accompanied by a fever.
▶ **Depression and lethargy**.
▶ **Rash** which starts behind the ears, spreading to the forehead.

What should I do first?

1 While many of the early symptoms of glandular fever are similar to those of other ailments, be alerted if the neck glands are swollen and there is a **fever**. Check your child's temperature regularly if his glands are swollen. If his temperature remains high, give him a dose of paracetamol elixir.

2 Keep your child isolated until you have a definite diagnosis. The virus is infectious and is passed on by intimate contact, such as kissing.

Should I consult the doctor?

Consult your doctor immediately if you suspect your child is not just suffering from influenza or a **common cold**.

What might the doctor do?

Your doctor will take a blood sample for analysis. Glandular fever can be diagnosed with certainty only by finding antibodies in the blood. You will be advised to keep your child indoors and to make sure he has plenty of rest; no further treatment is required.

Continued on next page

Continued from previous page

What can I do to help?

▶ Your child may feel well enough to return to school after two or three weeks, but he should avoid over-exertion or strenuous exercise for at least another month or so.

▶ If your child wants to stay in bed, let him. If he doesn't, keep him indoors at least until the fever subsides.

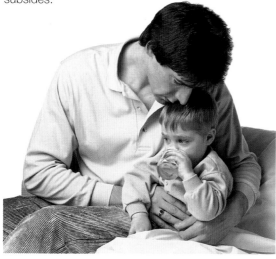

▶ If your child has a temperature, offer him plenty of fluids to prevent **dehydration**.

▶ Glandular fever is debilitating and it may be six months before your child is completely fit and his old self again.

▶ Keep him entertained and cheerful. The length of time the disease takes to run its course can lead to boredom and depression. So, although your child needs plenty of rest, keep him busy in quiet ways with books, puzzles and television.

▶ The virus may reappear during the two years after the first attack of glandular fever, so watch for a recurrence of the symptoms and consult your doctor if you are at all worried.

SEE ALSO:
Common cold 90
Dehydration 109
Fever 134
German measles 142
Influenza 167
Sore throat 222

Glue ear

GLUE EAR IS THE NON-MEDICAL TERM for a condition that results when the Eustachian tube and middle ear fill with fluid, often as a result of infection. The Eustachian tube, which runs from the throat to the ear, produces large quantities of fluid as a response to chronic infections such as **sinusitis**, enlarged adenoids, **tonsillitis** or, most commonly, **otitis media**. If the tube in either ear is blocked by inflammation, the fluid cannot drain and becomes glue-like, impeding the efficient vibration of sound, causing loss of hearing.

Is it serious?

Although painless, glue ear should be treated seriously because it can lead to deafness and eventually permanent loss of hearing in the affected ear. If undetected, it can cause problems with speech development and learning.

Possible symptoms

▶ **A feeling of fullness** in the ear.
▶ **Partial loss of hearing** or deafness in one or both of the ears.

What should I do first?

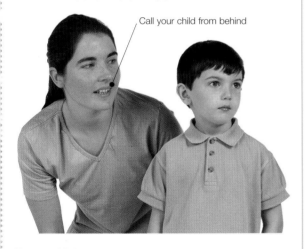
Call your child from behind

If your child seems inattentive and has recently had some upper respiratory tract infection, such as otitis media or a **common cold**, do a hearing test. Call quietly when the head is averted and see if there is a response. Even if your child can hear you, the hearing may be impaired in such a way that the child cannot tell where you are calling from.

Should I consult the doctor?

Consult your doctor as soon as possible if you suspect that your child's hearing has deteriorated in any way over time.

What might the doctor do?

▶ Your doctor will examine your child's ears with a special instrument (an otoscope), and treat the glue ear according to the severity of the blockage.
▶ In mild cases, your doctor will prescribe antibiotics to clear up the infection, and he may also prescribe vasoconstrictor drugs, which promote drainage by reducing swelling in the Eustachian tubes.

Continued on next page

Continued from previous page

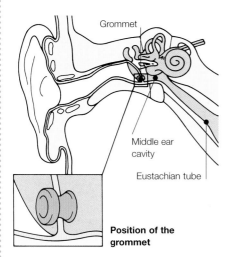

Grommet

Middle ear
cavity

Eustachian tube

**Position of the
grommet**

▶ In severe and recurrent cases, your child will probably be referred to an ear, nose and throat specialist and may be admitted to hospital to have the fluid drained off under a general anaesthetic. At the same time, the specialist may insert grommets in the affected ear. These are tiny plastic tubes that allow mucus to drain away, thus preventing further build-up of the sticky secretions. The grommets either fall out after several months when the ears are healthy again, or can be removed by the specialist. If glue ear is a result of repeated infections or enlarged adenoids, the underlying problem will also be treated to prevent recurrences.

What can I do to help?

▶ If your child has had grommets inserted, he should wait until two weeks after the operation to go swimming and should not dive. Some ear, nose and throat specialists advise against swimming altogether when grommets are in place.

▶ Try to keep the ear as dry as possible at all times.

SEE ALSO:
Common cold 90
Deafness 108
Otitis media 198
Sinusitis 217
Tonsillitis 243

Growing pain

A GROWING PAIN IS A DULL, VAGUE ACHE in a limb; it does not last long and the child can usually be distracted from it. One in six children of school age suffers from some kind of growing pain. Such pains can occur when your child is going through a growth spurt; the muscles and bones grow at slightly different rates, leading to an aching soreness that is worse in the evening. They can also occur after strenuous activity. It is important to distinguish a growing pain from joint pain. A growing pain is felt between the joints of a limb; joint pain is specific to the joint area. In a child, a joint pain can also be a symptom of **rheumatic fever** or **arthritis**.

Is it serious?
A growing pain is not serious, but any pain in the joint may be, particularly if it is accompanied by a fever. This could be septic arthritis.

Possible symptoms

▶ **Aches and pains** in the arms or legs, most often in the legs.
▶ **Disturbed sleep** if the pain is severe.
▶ **Painful muscles** after strenuous activity.

What should I do first?

1 Check your child's joints for swelling and tenderness by pressing on and around them. If there is neither, check the muscles in the same way.

2 Watch carefully to see if your child limps when he walks.

3 Ask your child when the pain started and how long it lasts.

Should I consult the doctor?
Consult your doctor as soon as possible if the pain is sited over a joint and is accompanied by a fever, or if it lasts longer than 24 hours.

What might the doctor do?
After excluding other possible causes of the pain, your doctor will reassure you and your child that there is no cause for concern.

What can I do to help?
▶ Show sympathetic interest in the pain – this may be sufficient to relax your child.

▶ Give your child a warm bath or a hot-water bottle: these can be soothing if your child is having difficulty sleeping.
▶ Gently massage the affected muscles as this will help relax any tension.

SEE ALSO:
Arthritis 56
Limp 176
Rheumatic fever 209

Growth hormone deficiency

THE GROWTH HORMONE, as its name implies, ensures that development of physical stature proceeds normally. In a very small percentage of children, the pituitary gland in the brain, which produces the growth hormone, fails to produce enough and this leads to stunted growth. Very occasionally the deficiency is caused by a tumour in the pituitary gland. Deficiency of growth hormone is often picked up at regular childhood check-ups when your child's weight and height are plotted on a graph to check that he is within the range of the average for his age. If your child is small for his age, a variety of laboratory tests can be performed to give a full clinical evaluation. Generally the tests involve a stay in hospital so that a full profile of the hormonal activity in your child's body can be compiled by a specialist in hormones – an endocrinologist. A series of blood samples is used to assess the rise of growth hormone in the body in response to a stimulus, such as exercise or a test drug. In a normal child, this kind of stimulus would cause the pituitary gland to produce and release the growth hormone.

Possible symptoms

▶ **Exceptionally short stature.**
▶ **Slow rate of growth.**

What can be done?

The treatment for growth hormone deficiency is sophisticated, and replacement therapy is easily controlled, giving good results. The hormone may be given by intra-muscular injections two or three times a week. The maximum growth response occurs during the first year of the treatment: the rate at which your child grows may be twice that expected for his chronological age as he makes up for lost time. The treatment usually continues until your child reaches adolescence. In the rare cases where the deficiency is caused by a pituitary tumour, the tumour will be removed surgically or with radiotherapy.

Gum boil (dental abscess)

A GUM BOIL, OR DENTAL ABSCESS, is a pus-filled cavity that develops at the root of a decayed tooth. In a primary tooth, a gum boil can damage the underlying permanent tooth if it is left untreated. Gum boils are nearly always very painful as they are in such a confined area and the pain does not always respond to painkillers.

Is it serious?

A gum boil should be treated seriously as it causes great discomfort and can result in a lost tooth.

Possible symptoms

- **Red, inflamed lump** on one side of the tooth in the gum.
- **Throbbing pain**.
- **Tenderness and swelling** on the affected side of the face.
- **Swollen neck glands**.
- **Pain** below the ear on the affected side.

What should I do first?

1 Examine the gum around the tooth and, if you notice a red lump, gently feel it with your fingertip. It will be soft and spongy because of the underlying collection of pus.

2 Give your child doses of paracetamol elixir to try to relieve the pain. Do not use local anaesthetics such as oil of cloves. These can damage the gum margin, leading to more dental problems.

3 Rinse your child's mouth with a weak salt-water solution to speed the bursting of the boil and to wash away any pus that has seeped out.

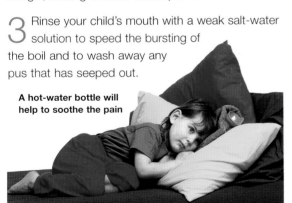

A hot-water bottle will help to soothe the pain

4 Apply a covered hot-water bottle to your child's cheek to soothe the pain.

Should I consult the doctor?

Consult your *dentist* immediately or take your child to the nearest casualty department.

What might the doctor do?

- The dentist or doctor will drain the pus by either opening the gum or removing the tooth if there is no possibility of saving it. Both procedures will be done under an anaesthetic.
- Your dentist or doctor will prescribe a course of antibiotics to eradicate the infection. Your child may also be prescribed a mouth wash to be used three or four times a day until the wound has healed.

What can I do to help?

- Maintain regular tooth brushing in order to minimize tooth decay.
- Take your child to the dentist regularly from the age of three.
- Cut down on sweets and sugary foods in your child's diet.

SEE ALSO:
Earache 122
Toothache 245

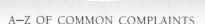
Haemophilia

HAEMOPHILIA IS AN INHERITED DISEASE of the blood, caused by a faulty gene. It is carried by some females, in whom the disease does not show. A carrier female may pass it on to her daughter, who then becomes a carrier herself, or to her son, who will be a haemophiliac.

Haemophiliacs lack a substance called *antihaemophilic globulin* (*AHG*), commonly known as Factor VIII, which is essential for the blood to clot. A haemophiliac therefore bleeds profusely from even small wounds, and the blood flow does not stop. Normally, a trivial knock produces a little bleeding into the tissues, which results in a bruise; in a haemophiliac, it produces deep bruising, swelling and pain for several days.

Possible symptoms

- **Profuse and prolonged bleeding** from any open wound.
- **Heavy bruising, pain and swelling** after even a light knock.
- **Stiff joints or muscles** due to internal bleeding.

What can be done?

Most haemophiliac families are aware that the disorder exists. Boys in such families should be tested after birth to see if haemophilia is present. Women in such families are advised to consult their doctor and a genetic counsellor before conceiving to assess the risks involved. During pregnancy, amniocentesis – a process in which amniotic fluid is drawn off from the fetus through a needle – can determine the sex of the baby. If it is a boy, and the mother is a carrier of the haemophiliac gene, a termination of the pregnancy will be offered. Haemophilia can also be diagnosed early during pregnancy by chorionic villus sampling.

In unsuspected cases, the symptoms tend to show themselves when the baby boy is several months old and is becoming more active, learning to crawl and walk.

The main treatment for haemophilia is replacement of the missing AHG by intravenous injection, as soon as possible after bruising, swelling or injury, or before dental and surgical procedures. In the case of injury, this injection may have to be repeated daily until the bleeding or swelling has ceased. Many older boys can insert the needle themselves, with the help of the parent or telephone supervision by a doctor.

You should be swift to apply the correct first-aid techniques if your child is injured. Bleeding must be staunched at once with firm pressure and the affected part raised to reduce blood flow. Keep your child very still while waiting for medical assistance.

A haemophiliac should wear a disc that states he has the disease, his blood group, and what to do in the case of an emergency.

The doctor or nurse may also pass on advice on how to protect your son against injury. For example, your child should sleep on a low bed, be careful on slippery floors and avoid playing with hazardous toys that may lead to physical injury.

For help and advice contact the Haemophilia Society (see page 324).

Hair loss

CHILDREN RARELY LOSE their hair. However, in newborn babies, the first fluffy hair is often lost just after birth and the second growth may be slow, so your baby will appear to be bald for several months. Babies also lose hair through friction. Simply by the pressure of their heads on the cot sheet, they may have large bald patches on the backs of their heads. This is because newborn baby hair is not very firmly embedded in the skin and only a small amount of friction is needed to rub it loose. Hair loss may also be due to stress.

By far the most common cause of hair loss in older children is the fungal infection of the scalp known as **ringworm**. This produces circular patches of pink or grey, scaly baldness in the scalp and it is extremely itchy. Another cause of temporary baldness in children is a condition known as *alopecia areata*. Round, bald patches appear suddenly and within a few months fine white hairs break through into the bald area, followed by normal hair. Some children can actually inflict hair loss on themselves with a nervous **tic** or mannerism, compulsively pulling, twisting and breaking their hair. This condition, which is called *trichotillomania*, is often worse when your child is concentrating on something.

Is it serious?

Hair loss is not normally serious, though your child may feel self-conscious until the hair grows back again.

What should I do first?

1 Check any patches of baldness on your child's scalp. If the skin is pink or grey, and scaly, this indicates ringworm. If not, your child could be suffering from alopecia areata.

2 Notice if your child has the nervous tic of pulling and tugging at his hair while concentrating.

Should I consult the doctor?

Consult your doctor as soon as possible if you suspect ringworm. This is infectious but can be easily cleared up with medication. Consult your doctor as soon as possible if you are unsure about the cause of the patches of baldness on your child's head, or if you are worried about the tic.

What might the doctor do?

▶ Your doctor will treat the underlying cause. If your child has ringworm, your doctor will prescribe an anti-fungal ointment for the skin, and tablets for the scalp.

▶ If alopecia areata is the cause, your doctor will advise you that there is no treatment and that the condition is only temporary.

What can I do to help?

▶ If your child has ringworm, keep him away from school until treatment has been started.

▶ Let your child wear a hat if he feels self-conscious about the bald patches.

▶ Check for regrowth regularly and encourage your child not to be disheartened.

▶ Try not to make a fuss about the baldness; treat it as a normal condition. Inform your child's teacher so that your child does not suffer too much teasing.

▶ If your child fiddles with his hair, try not to let him see that it annoys you. Discourage him gently and make sure he doesn't get over-tired or anxious as this can make such tics worse.

SEE ALSO:
Ringworm 210
Tic 242

Hayfever

HAYFEVER IS SIMILAR to **asthma** except that the allergic reaction occurs in the mucous membranes of the nose and eyelids, not in the chest. The condition is also known as allergic rhinitis and causes sneezing, a runny nose and itchy, watery eyes. It occurs in spring and summer and is usually due to a reaction to pollen from flowers, grasses and trees. Most hayfever sufferers are sensitive to more than one pollen and, short of isolation in an air-conditioned room, it is difficult for them to avoid the symptoms. Children who suffer from hayfever can become mouth-breathers because the nose is so blocked. Hayfever tends not to occur before the age of five, but it can start or stop at any time, and it tends to run in families. Some children who are allergic to animals and house dust as well as pollens suffer all year round from hayfever; this condition is called perennial allergic rhinitis.

Is it serious?

Hayfever is periodically troublesome, but it has no serious consequences.

Possible symptoms

▶ Sneezing.
▶ Runny nose with clear discharge.
▶ Itchy, watery, red-rimmed eyes.

What should I do first?

1 If your child is sneezing a lot, check his temperature to make sure he isn't ill with an infection such as **influenza** or a **common cold**.

2 Discourage your child from rubbing his eyes; this will make them worse. Bathe his eyes with cool water to ease the irritation.

Should I consult the doctor?

Consult your doctor as soon as possible if you think your child may be suffering from a more serious infection, or if the hayfever is making your child miserable.

What might the doctor do?

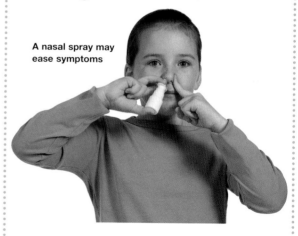

A nasal spray may ease symptoms

▶ Your doctor will probably prescribe an anti-allergy nasal spray or antihistamine spray, elixir or tablets to relieve the symptoms.
▶ If your child's condition is severe, your doctor may arrange for him to have a series of skin tests to track down the allergen that is causing the symptoms of hayfever. Once one or more allergens has been determined, a special vaccine

Continued from previous page

can be made for your child and a course of desensitizing injections given over a period of weeks to protect him. These don't always work, however, and have to be given during the winter.

What can I do to help?

▶ Watch the pollen count each day and, if it is high, discourage your child from playing near freshly mown grassland, for example.

▶ Avoid feathers in your child's bedding and fluff in his clothing.

▶ Keep your house as dust-free as possible. Even if your child isn't allergic to dust, a dusty atmosphere makes hayfever worse.

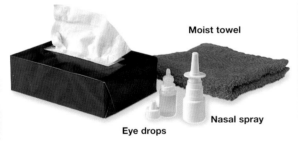

Paper handkerchiefs

Moist towel

Nasal spray

Eye drops

▶ Prepare an emergency pack for outings. It should contain paper handkerchiefs, eye drops to reduce the eye irritation, a moist towel to soothe your child's eyes, and whatever medication has been prescribed.

SEE ALSO:
Asthma 58
Common cold 90
Influenza 167

Head injury

CHILDREN HIT THEIR HEADS FREQUENTLY and in the majority of cases the child has stopped crying and is playing normally within 10–15 minutes of the accident. With some harder knocks to the head, there is **headache** and local swelling; if the skin is broken, the blood flow may be alarming from even a small cut.

When there is no outward sign of injury, a mild headache is probably all your child will complain about. If, however, he lapses into unconsciousness, complains of **dizziness**, or appears stunned and vomits, this may be concussion, when the brain is shaken inside the skull. The symptoms of concussion may not appear for several hours.

Is it serious?

A head injury resulting in unconsciousness, dizziness or **vomiting** should always be treated as serious. If your child has any bleeding or straw-coloured discharge from his nose or ear after a blow to his head, treat this as an emergency because it indicates a skull fracture. If there is a fracture and an open wound, or any bleeding into the brain, the chances of brain damage are higher.

Possible symptoms

- **Headache.**
- **Stunned and dazed state.**
- **Drowsiness.**
- **Period of unconsciousness.**
- **Irritability.**
- **Vomiting.**
- **Discharge of blood or straw-coloured fluid** from the nose and ears.

What should I do first?

1 If your child has fallen on his head or suffered a blow to his head, check for any of the symptoms of concussion or a fracture of the skull, whether or not there is an open wound. Treat any symptoms other than just a mild headache as an emergency and take your child to the nearest casualty department.

2 If your child complains of a headache but seems otherwise alert, let him lie down for an hour in a dark room, but keep a watch on him to check that he doesn't lose consciousness.

3 If the wound is bleeding, press a clean pad or handkerchief on to it for about 10 minutes, or until the bleeding has stopped. If it is a small wound, clean the area with soap and water, place a clean

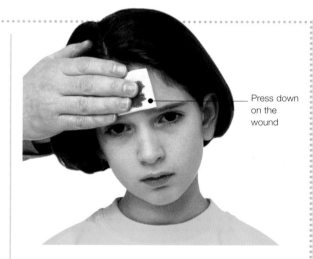

Press down on the wound

pad over it and secure with a bandage to keep pressure on the wound. If the wound is jagged or long, take your child to the nearest casualty department for stitching.

Continued from previous page

4 If there is discharge coming from ears or nose, do not try to stop the flow – put a pad against the ear or nose to absorb it. Take your child to the nearest casualty department.

Should I consult the doctor?

Consult your doctor immediately or take your child to the nearest casualty department if he loses consciousness, even for a short time, if he complains of a severe headache and dizziness, if he vomits or if there is any discharge from his nose or ears. Take your child to the nearest casualty department if there is a cut that needs stitching. Consult your doctor immediately if you are at all worried about your child's behaviour even hours after a head injury, particularly if he is pale, unnaturally quiet and has lost interest in food. Be sure to tell the doctor what sort of fall or incident caused the injury.

What might the doctor do?

▶ If there is any likelihood of a skull fracture, your child will be given a skull X-ray.
▶ If there is a cut, the doctor will stitch it under local anaesthetic.
▶ If there are no signs of a fracture but your child is dizzy and has a headache, the doctor may admit him to hospital for overnight observation.

SEE ALSO:
Cuts and grazes 104
Dizziness 116
Headache 156
Vomiting 257

Headache

ABOUT ONE IN FIVE CHILDREN suffers from recurrent headaches, although a serious physical cause is hardly ever found. Most commonly children complain of pain in their heads after sitting in a hot, stuffy room, if they are worried or anxious about something, if they have a **fever**, or they have **sinusitis** or **toothache**, for example. Some children complain frequently of headache and tummy ache. Such pain is known as abdominal **migraine**.

Is it serious?

Headaches are rarely serious but if a single headache is accompanied by a temperature, neck stiffness, confusion or an intolerance of bright light, this may be a symptom of a more serious illness, such as **encephalitis** or **meningitis**, and you should seek medical advice. Similarly, if your child has had a recent injury to his head, you should get immediate medical attention.

What should I do first?

1 Ask your child if he has pain anywhere else. Run your hands over the area around his cheeks, jaw and ears to see if sinusitis, a **gum boil** (dental abscess), toothache or **earache** are the problem.

2 Check your child's temperature to see if he has a fever. Headache and fever could be among the first symptoms of an infectious illness such as **measles** or **influenza**.

3 Check to see if your child has suffered any injury to his head.

4 If the headaches are frequent, find out if your child is worried about anything, such as his school work.

5 If your child complains of nausea or vomits, this could be a migraine headache.

6 If your child has no other symptoms to concern you, give him a drink and a single dose of paracetamol elixir to relieve the pain, and put him to bed in a darkened room for half an hour.

Should I consult the doctor?

Consult your doctor immediately if the headache is accompanied by a temperature of 38°C (100.4°F) with vomiting, neck stiffness and intolerance of

bright light, or if your child has had a recent head injury. Consult your doctor as soon as possible if the headaches are persistent.

What might the doctor do?

▶ Your doctor will examine your child to try to determine the cause of the headache. The examination may include taking your child's blood pressure and looking at the retina in the eye. Further tests will be carried out only if your doctor finds something wrong apart from the headaches.
▶ If the headache is a symptom of a more serious condition, such as meningitis, your doctor will treat the condition accordingly.

What can I do to help?

If your child complains of a headache at the end of the school day, give him a drink and a nutritious snack and encourage him to go out and play in the fresh air.

SEE ALSO:
Earache 122
Encephalitis 126
Fever 134
Gum boil 149
Head injury 154
Influenza 167
Measles 177
Meningitis 178
Migraine 180
Sinusitis 217
Toothache 245

Heat exhaustion

HEAT EXHAUSTION RESULTS when too much body fluid is lost through sweating, and occurs when the body becomes overheated, either by excessive exposure to sunshine, excessive humidity or through over-exertion. Although a strenuous game can raise the temperature to over 38°C (100.4°F), the rise is usually temporary and the temperature returns to normal quite rapidly. However, if it doesn't, your child will develop the symptoms of heat exhaustion and will become pale and clammy and may complain of **dizziness**, nausea and **headache**.

Possible symptoms

- **Temperature** over 38°C (100.4°F).
- **Pale and clammy skin**.
- **Dizziness**.
- **Nausea**.
- **Headache**.
- **Rapid pulse rate**.
- **Muscle cramps**.

Is it serious?

Heat exhaustion isn't serious as long as you recognize the problem and cool your child down, thus preventing **heatstroke**.

What should I do first?

1 Lay your child down in a cool place with his feet raised a little. Remove most of his clothing.

2 Use tepid sponging (*see page 31*) to cool the skin down quickly. Keep the air in the room as cool as you can.

3 Give your child plenty of fluids – plain water or fruit juice is best.

4 Take his temperature every half hour to make sure that it is coming down.

Should I consult the doctor?

You should not need to consult your doctor if your child is suffering only from heat exhaustion, and is cool and feels better within one hour. Consult your doctor immediately or take your child to the nearest casualty department if, after an hour, he is still extremely hot but his skin is dry. He could be suffering from heatstroke. Consult your doctor immediately if your child's temperature fails to come down after an hour; he may be suffering from some other illness.

What might the doctor do?

- If your child is suffering from heatstroke or an infection, your doctor will deal with this accordingly.
- Your doctor may advise you to keep your child inside during the heat of the day or until he is acclimatized to the hot weather.

What can I do to help?

- Discourage your child from playing active games in strong sunshine.
- Keep a watch on your child if he has a tendency to become exhausted in hot weather.
- Make sure your child wears a sun hat and sunblock cream when playing in the sunshine.

SEE ALSO:
Dizziness 116
Headache 156
Heatstroke 159

Heat rash

HEAT RASH IS A FAINT red **rash** in the areas of the body where the sweat glands are most numerous – on the face, neck, shoulders and in the skin creases, such as the elbows, groin and behind the knees. It is quite common in babies because their sweat glands are still primitive and not efficient at regulating body temperature. Heat rash is not due to exposure to sunlight but arises when the body becomes overheated and the skin responds with excessive production of sweat.

Is it serious?

Heat rash is never serious.

Possible symptoms

Areas affected

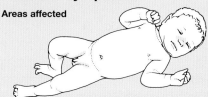

▶ **Faint, red rash** over the face, neck, shoulders and in the creases, such as the elbows, groin and knees.
▶ **Flushed** and hot appearance.

What should I do first?

1 Check your baby's clothing. He may be wearing too many clothes for the air temperature.

2 Undress your baby and bath him in tepid water. Pat him dry to remove most of the moisture. Allow the rest to evaporate – this will help to cool his skin down.

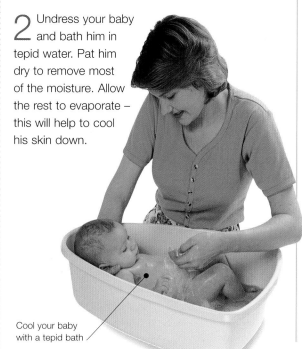

Cool your baby with a tepid bath

Should I consult the doctor?

There is no need to consult the doctor for a heat rash. Consult your doctor as soon as possible if the rash does not disappear 12 hours after the baby has cooled down.

What might the doctor do?

Your doctor will examine your baby to exclude any other reason for the rash, and will probably advise you to dress your baby in natural fibres, which do not trap the sweat.

What can I do to help?

▶ Check that the temperature in your baby's room is not too high. Keep the air flowing by opening a window slightly.
▶ Don't overdress your child in hot weather.
▶ Don't put wool or manmade fibres directly against your baby's skin. Dress him in a cotton vest first.
▶ Consult your doctor or health visitor about keeping your child cool.

SEE ALSO:
Rash 206

Heatstroke

HEATSTROKE, OR SUNSTROKE, is due to exposure to extreme heat, which causes the body's temperature-regulating mechanism to break down. The sweat glands fail to work and the body cannot cool itself in the normal way by producing sweat. Your child's skin will remain dry instead of sweaty, and he may become drowsy with a rapid pulse. He may then become confused and lapse into unconsciousness. If your child is not first acclimatized to the sun and heat, **heat exhaustion** and heatstroke can easily result.

Is it serious?

Heatstroke is very serious and may even be fatal. It should be treated as an emergency, although there are first-aid procedures you should follow while you are waiting for help.

Possible symptoms

▶ **Temperature** as high as 40°C (104°F).
▶ **Hot skin** which remains dry, not sweaty.
▶ **Drowsiness**.
▶ **Rapid pulse**.
▶ **Confusion** followed by **unconsciousness**.

What should I do first?

1 Undress your child completely and lay him down in a cool room.

2 Check his pulse (*see page 26*), and take his temperature to see if he has a fever. If his temperature is as high as 40°C (104°F), consult your doctor immediately, or take your child to the nearest casualty department.

3 If your child's temperature isn't this high, try to bring it down slowly. Play a fan over him to cool him and sponge his whole body with tepid water (*see page 31*).

4 Place an icepack on your child's forehead and give him plenty of cool drinks.

5 Take your child's temperature regularly to make sure it is dropping.

Should I consult the doctor?

Consult your doctor immediately or take your child to the nearest casualty department if his temperature is as high as 40°C (104°F).

What might the doctor do?

The doctor will continue to cool your child's body. There are special drugs that can be given in emergencies to bring the body temperature down.

What can I do to help?

▶ Apply a sunblock cream to your child's skin before he is exposed to the sun. Get him to wear a hat.
▶ Watch your child when he plays in very hot or sunny conditions. An older child will probably rest in the shade, but a young child is often incapable of exercising this much caution, so you must be careful to monitor the time he spends in full sunlight if he has not been acclimatized.

SEE ALSO:
Heat exhaustion 157

Hepatitis

HEPATITIS IS AN INFECTION that causes inflammation of the liver. One form of the illness, hepatitis B, can be transmitted from an infected mother to her child, and also by infected blood. The most common form of the illness in children is the highly contagious acute hepatitis A, caused by the type A virus, found in the stools of a sufferer. If the hands are not washed after going to the toilet, the infection can easily be passed on to others by contaminated food and drink. The virus is also found in the blood and saliva. The first symptom is a loss of appetite. **Influenza**-like symptoms then develop, followed by **jaundice**, with its associated symptoms of yellowing of the skin and whites of the eyes, dark brown urine, and abnormally pale stools.

Is it serious?
Hepatitis itself is rarely a very serious illness in children. However, because it is contagious and can spread quickly through a household or school, it should be treated promptly.

Possible symptoms

▶ **Loss of appetite**.
▶ **Influenza-like symptoms** of headache, fever and aching joints.
▶ **Jaundice** (yellow skin), **dark brown urine and pale stools**.

What should I do first?

1 If your child loses interest in food and has 'flu-like symptoms, keep a check on his skin, urine and stools for any changes in colour.

2 If your child won't eat, give him frequent drinks of diluted fruit juice, or rehydration solution (available in powder form from the chemist) to prevent dehydration and to maintain his energy.

3 If you suspect hepatitis, keep your child home from school.

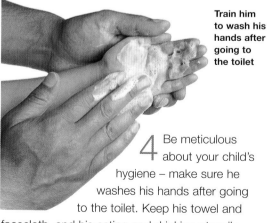

Train him to wash his hands after going to the toilet

4 Be meticulous about your child's hygiene – make sure he washes his hands after going to the toilet. Keep his towel and facecloth, and his eating and drinking utensils, separate from those of the rest of the family.

Continued from previous page

Should I consult the doctor?

Consult your doctor immediately if you suspect your child has hepatitis, especially if jaundice develops.

What might the doctor do?

▶ Your doctor will take a blood sample from your child to test for hepatitis.

▶ Your doctor will recommend bed-rest and isolation measures for at least two weeks, until the 'flu symptoms have passed. After another two weeks your child will probably feel well enough to return to school.

▶ Although there is no specific treatment for hepatitis other than bed-rest, some doctors advise a high-calorie, low-fat diet to reduce the strain on the liver. Others, however, don't consider this worthwhile.

▶ Your doctor may suggest that the rest of the family have a gamma globulin injection to minimize the risk of their contracting the infection.

What can I do to help?

▶ Observe the isolation measures for at least two weeks, or until your doctor says otherwise. Nurse your child in his own room, restrict physical contact with others, and keep his eating utensils, toys and other objects separate from those of the rest of the household.

▶ Maintain high standards of hygiene. Wash out the toilet bowl with disinfectant after your child has used it, wash his eating things separately from those of the family, and continue to keep his facecloth and towel separate, too.

▶ Despite these measures, try not to make your child feel left out. Put a television in his room, allow him books and tapes, and aim to keep him cheerful but quiet. Check with your doctor before you reduce isolation measures and before you send your child back to school.

▶ Post-hepatitis symptoms like lethargy, difficulty in concentrating and moodiness may persist for up to six months, so be patient and understanding with your child.

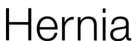
Hernia

A HERNIA RESULTS when a small defect in the muscular wall of the abdomen allows soft tissue to protrude through. This appears as a slight bulge in the skin and can be seen even more clearly if your child coughs or strains. The most common hernia in children is the *umbilical hernia*. This appears near the navel and results from a weakness that occurs in the abdominal wall at birth. An *inguinal hernia* appears lower down in the groin and is most common in boys, the defect occurring after the testicles have descended into the scrotum. Umbilical hernias rarely need any treatment; they heal spontaneously. Inguinal hernias need to be corrected by minor surgery.

Is it serious?
A hernia is not usually a serious problem unless the bowel is trapped.

Possible symptoms

Areas affected

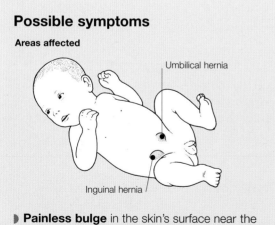

Umbilical hernia

Inguinal hernia

▶ **Painless bulge** in the skin's surface near the navel or in the groin; the bulge increases in size when the child coughs, sneezes or cries.
▶ **Vomiting** with sharp abdominal pain if the bowel has become trapped.

What should I do first?
Try to push the hernia gently inwards. Most hernias respond to gentle pressure by sliding back inside the muscular wall.

Should I consult the doctor?
Consult your doctor immediately if you notice a bulge in your baby's abdomen before he is six months old. Consult your doctor immediately if a hernia becomes hard, the bulge won't go back with the application of gentle pressure and there is accompanying abdominal pain and vomiting.

What might the doctor do?
If the hernia is hard or won't go back, your doctor will refer you to a paediatric specialist as the hernia will probably have to be repaired surgically. The operation for a hernia repair is simple. If your child has an inguinal hernia, your doctor may recommend surgical repair to avoid any trapping of the bowel.

What can I do to help?
▶ Check an umbilical hernia regularly, at bathtimes, for example, to make sure that the hernia is not enlarging, that it is not hard and that it goes back when gently pushed.
▶ Discuss future action with your doctor and decide together whether to let the hernia heal spontaneously or whether surgery is necessary.
▶ Take your child for regular check-ups, as decided with your doctor.

Hives

HIVES, URTICARIA OR NETTLE RASH is a skin condition. The **rash** that results is easy to recognize: the skin erupts into white lumps on a red base. These are known as weals. The weals can be as small as pimples or centimetres across. Hives can be caused by skin contact with an allergen, such as primulas, or it can result from eating certain foods, most commonly strawberries and shellfish, or from taking certain drugs, particularly penicillin and aspirin. Hives is most common after a nettle sting. Each crop of weals is extremely itchy and lasts up to an hour. It then disappears, to be replaced by more weals elsewhere on your child's face or body.

Is it serious?

Hives is not serious but, if it appears on the face, especially in or around the mouth, and is accompanied by swelling, get medical assistance immediately. This allergic reaction is known as *angio-neurotic oedema* and, if the swelling spreads to the tongue or the throat, it can cause severe breathing problems.

Possible symptoms

Classic appearance of rash

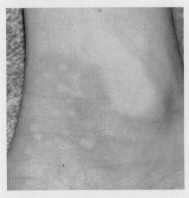

▶ **White lumps** on a red base.
▶ **Extremely itchy rash**.
▶ **Weals** that disappear within an hour or so to be replaced elsewhere by other weals.
▶ **Swelling** on the face.

What should I do first?

1 Apply calamine lotion to the weals in order to soothe the skin.

2 Give your child a tepid bath, which will help to relieve itching.

Should I consult the doctor?

Consult your doctor immediately if hives on your child's face causes swelling, particularly in and around the mouth. Consult your doctor as soon as possible if the weals have not gone after several days, or if your child is miserable with the itchiness.

What might the doctor do?

▶ Your doctor may prescribe antihistamine tablets or medicine to relieve the itchiness of your child's skin.
▶ Your doctor may give your child an injection of adrenalin if the swelling is causing him to have breathing problems.

What can I do to help?

If your child has frequent attacks, make a note of any new foods he might have eaten. Provided it is not an essential food for a growing child, you can exclude the suspected allergen for a week or two, then reintroduce it and watch for a reaction.

SEE ALSO:
Itching 170
Rash 206

Hydrocephalus

THE TERM "HYDROCEPHALUS" means water on the brain, and this condition results when there is an excessive build-up of the fluid that surrounds the brain. This fluid, known as cerebrospinal fluid or CSF, carries nutrients to the brain and acts as a protective, fluid buffer. If the circulation of CSF is blocked for some reason, or if the fluid is produced in too great a quantity, the build-up of fluid increases pressure inside the brain. The brain tissue becomes thinner and the bones of the skull stretch to accommodate the excess fluid. The pressure on the brain can cause brain damage and, if untreated, more than 50 per cent of hydrocephalic infants die.

The symptoms of hydrocephalus depend on the age at which it develops in the child. If it is present at birth, the head is abnormally large because the skull bones have been pushed apart by the fluid; the baby in such cases will probably also suffer from **spina bifida**. In milder forms of hydrocephalus, the head may be normal at birth but grow at an excessive rate in the following months.

Hydrocephalus can also develop later in childhood as the result of a tumour, or an infection such as **meningitis**, when there may be no appreciable enlargement of the head, although the pressure of the fluid on the brain may cause the symptoms of **headache** and **vomiting**.

Possible symptoms

- **Abnormal head size** at birth, or rapid growth of it in following months.
- **Veins standing out** on scalp.
- **Swollen fontanelle**.
- **Headache**.
- **Vomiting**.

What can be done?

If the condition is present at birth, this will normally be noticed by the doctor at delivery, or at regular check-ups when your baby's head is measured to check the size. A careful initial evaluation by a paediatrician is necessary to determine the exact cause of the build-up of fluid. In mild cases, drugs may be used to prevent excess production of CSF. Otherwise, provided the hydrocephalus is not too advanced, the condition will be relieved surgically. Under anaesthetic, a fine tube with a one-way valve is inserted into a hole in the skull. The other end is usually inserted into the peritoneal (abdominal cavity), thus draining the fluid from the brain directly into the bloodstream. After these treatments the baby's head gradually returns to normal; about 40 per cent of hydrocephalic infants then go on to develop near-normal intelligence. (If at some stage after the operation your child becomes irritable and is vomiting, a blockage of the tube will be suspected. The tube will be replaced or the blockage removed.)

For help and advice contact the Association for Spina Bifida and Hydrocephalus (see page 324).

Hyperactivity

THE WORD "HYPERACTIVE" is the broad term formerly used to describe children who have Attention Deficit Disorder (ADD) and Attention Deficit Hyperactivity Disorder (ADHD) – behavioural conditions that include disruptive behaviour, poor attention span, sleeplessness and excitability.

Although certain food colourings and flavourings have been found to contribute to hyperactivity, proper handling by parents can solve most of the problems of individual behaviour in a child.

Possible symptoms

▶ **Disruptive behaviour**.
▶ **Restlessness**.
▶ **Short attention span**.
▶ **Sleeplessness**.
▶ **Foolhardiness and unpredictability**.

Is it serious?

There are few degrees of hyperactivity in children that are abnormal or serious.

What should I do first?

1 Try to determine whether your child is bored or restless for some reason. Intelligent children need a lot of stimulation.

2 Don't exaggerate the problem. Most parents would agree that their pre-school child is hyperactive some of the time.

Should I consult the doctor?

Consult your doctor for advice if you find your child difficult to live with, or if his behaviour is interfering with his schooling. Your health visitor may also be able to offer advice.

What might the doctor do?

It is difficult to find two doctors who agree on the origin, features or even the fact of hyperactivity. If minor behavioural problems are combined with any form of learning disability, such as **dyslexia**, the confusion is compounded. Your doctor may refer your child to a child psychiatrist to establish whether or not he has ADD/ADHD. If learning difficulties are also present, these are more likely to be detected when your child begins school. Your doctor will not prescribe any drugs unless a definite diagnosis is made.

What can I do to help?

▶ The essential approach for parents with hyperactive children is proper handling. You should both adopt the same approach so that your child cannot manipulate either of you.
▶ Learn to live with your child by treating him as an exciting, unpredictable, but nevertheless normal child. While your child is young, this will be exceedingly difficult at times, but by the time he goes to school he should have learned, with your help, to concentrate.
▶ You will need to be more vigilant if your child is foolhardy, and more inventive at providing games, so that he doesn't become bored.

SEE ALSO:
Dyslexia 120
Sleeplessness 219

Impetigo

IMPETIGO IS A BACTERIAL SKIN INFECTION that is most often seen around the lips, nose and ears. It is caused by common skin organisms (*staphylococcus* and *streptococcus*), which are carried in the nose and on the skin. The rash starts as small **blisters**, which break and crust over to become yellow-brown scabs. The condition is most often seen in school-age children and is contagious.

Is it serious?
Impetigo rarely has serious effects but, because it is highly contagious, it should be treated immediately.

Possible symptoms

Common sites

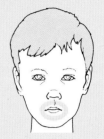

▶ **Tiny blisters** around the nose and mouth or ears, which ooze and harden to form crusty, yellow-brown scabs.

What should I do first?

1 If the rash on your child's face starts to weep, stop him from touching it. Gently wash away any crusts with warm water and pat dry with a paper towel before applying an antibiotic cream prescribed by your doctor. Keep your child's facecloth and towel separate from those of the rest of the family to avoid spreading the infection.

2 Keep your child away from school until you have visited the doctor.

Should I consult the doctor?

Consult your doctor as soon as possible if you suspect impetigo.

What might the doctor do?

▶ Your doctor will prescribe an antibiotic cream which should clear up the impetigo within five days.
▶ Your doctor might also prescribe a course of antibiotics to be taken by mouth to eradicate the infection from your child's body, or a nasal cream to prevent the infection being spread from there.

What can I do to help?

▶ Before applying the ointment, wash away any yellow crusts with warm water and pat dry with a paper towel.
▶ Be meticulous about hygiene. Wash your hands before and after administering the treatment, and encourage your child to keep his hands away from his face. Keep his fingernails short to reduce the risk of spreading the infection to other parts of the body.
▶ Be very strict with your child if he sucks his thumb, bites his nails or picks his nose. Any of these can spread the infection.
▶ When the infection has cleared, keep the area moist with emollient cream.

SEE ALSO:
Blister 67
Nephritis 189

Influenza

INFLUENZA ('FLU), like the **common cold**, is caused by a virus and has no known cure. It lasts around three to four days. Unless there is a secondary infection, treatment of the symptoms is all that is necessary in most cases.

Is it serious?

It is rare for serious complications to occur with influenza. However, natural resistance is reduced and a secondary infection, such as **pneumonia**, **otitis media**, **bronchitis** or **sinusitis**, may result. Influenza is always serious in a child who has **asthma**, or a condition such as **diabetes mellitus**.

Possible symptoms

- **Runny nose**.
- **Sore throat**.
- **Cough**.
- **Temperature** above 38°C (100.4°F).
- **Shivering**.
- **Aches and pains**.
- **Diarrhoea, vomiting or nausea**.
- **Weakness and lethargy**.

What should I do first?

1 Check your child's temperature every three to four hours. If it has not come down after 36 hours, call your doctor.

2 Give your child paracetamol elixir and put him to bed.

3 Don't force your child to eat, but make sure he gets plenty of water or diluted fruit juice to drink.

4 If a rash appears just after the onset of 'flu symptoms, your child may have **measles** and not influenza.

Should I consult the doctor?

Consult your doctor immediately if your child's temperature fails to come down within 36 hours, if you notice a deterioration in your child's condition after 48 hours, or if you suspect measles. Watch out for a worsening cough, which may suggest a chest infection; earache, which may suggest otitis media; or yellow pus discharge from the nose, which may indicate sinusitis.

What might the doctor do?

If there is a secondary infection, your doctor will prescribe an antibiotic accordingly.

What can I do to help?

- Your child should rest in bed in a warm room. As soon as he feels better, let him get up, but make him rest if his temperature rises again.
- Dispose of used paper handkerchiefs and wash used linen handkerchiefs in boiling water.
- You might consider protecting your child with an annual influenza vaccine.
- If, after your child should have recovered, his temperature rises and he vomits, consult your doctor immediately. A rare but serious illness, Reye's syndrome, could be the cause.

SEE ALSO:
Asthma 58
Bronchitis 73
Common cold 90
Cough 98
Diabetes mellitus 111
Fever 134
Measles 177
Otitis media 198
Pneumonia 202
Reye's syndrome 208
Sinusitis 217
Sore throat 222

Ingrowing toenail

WHEN A TOENAIL FAILS TO GROW STRAIGHT out from the nailbed, but instead curves over into the sides of the toe, it is referred to as an ingrowing toenail. This occurs most often to the nail of the big toe, and causes pain and discomfort. An ingrowing toenail is more likely to occur if the toe is broad and plump, if the toenail is cut down at the sides instead of straight across, if the toenail is small, or if tight shoes and socks push the nail into the skin. If untreated, the nail will penetrate the skin, possibly becoming infected, causing painful inflammation and a pussy discharge around the edges of the nail.

Is it serious?
An ingrowing toenail is painful but it is not serious.

What should I do first?

1 Examine the skin around the nail to see if the nail has penetrated the skin.

2 Cut a tiny V shape in the top edge of the nail to relieve pressure on the sides of the nail.

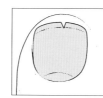

3 Apply an antiseptic cream to the sides of the nail to prevent infection.

4 If there is any sign of redness or pus, stop your child walking and get him to lie down with his foot propped up. Apply a sterile dressing to the toe.

Should I consult the doctor?
Consult your doctor as soon as possible if the nail has penetrated the skin, if you notice any redness or pus around your child's toenail, or if ingrowing toenails are a recurrent problem.

What might the doctor do?
▶ Your doctor may prescribe antibiotic tablets to clear up the infection, and an antiseptic cream to apply to the affected toe. Your doctor may also prescribe an astringent lotion to toughen up the skin around the toenail.

▶ If the problem is recurrent, your doctor may refer your child to an orthopaedic surgeon to see whether the ingrowing edge of the toenail should be removed. This is a minor operation.

What can I do to help?

Incorrect   Correct

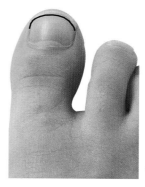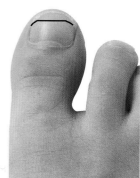

▶ Cut your child's toenails straight across at the top and not too short. Cut them regularly; don't let them get too long.
▶ Make sure your child's shoes and socks are not too tight and allow him enough space to wriggle his toes.
▶ If your child's toenail becomes infected, don't put socks on him; cut the toe out of an old shoe or let him wear sandals while the infection is clearing up.

Intussusception

INTUSSUSCEPTION IS A CONDITION that occurs when part of the small intestine telescopes inside the intestine ahead of it, rather like a finger in a glove being turned inside out. The twisted intestine swells and this causes a blockage. In an effort to overcome this blockage, the affected intestine goes into spasm. There is no known cause for intussusception and it can happen at any age; however, it most often affects baby boys under 12 months of age who have previously been in excellent health. The baby may suddenly cry out as the muscular spasms begin and may vomit and be pale and feverish. In between spasms, he may appear quite normal and pass normal bowel motions for the first few hours. However, as the attacks continue, the bowel motions characteristically look like redcurrant jelly because they contain mostly blood and mucus.

Is it serious?
Though rare, intussusception is a serious condition. If left untreated, it can be fatal.

Possible symptoms
▶ **Severe abdominal pain**, possibly accompanied by screaming.
▶ **Vomiting**.
▶ **Paleness**.
▶ **Slight fever**.
▶ **Bowel motions, containing blood and mucus**, which resemble redcurrant jelly.

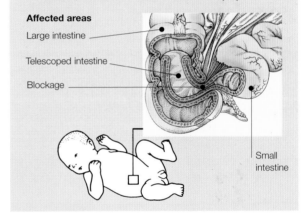

Affected areas
Large intestine
Telescoped intestine
Blockage
Small intestine

What should I do first?

1 If your baby has a number of spasmodic attacks when he screams and pulls his legs up to his stomach in pain, yet he appears quite well in between attacks, consult your doctor immediately.

2 Check your baby's bowel motions for any blood and mucus.

3 In between the attacks, take your baby's temperature to see if he has a fever.

Should I consult the doctor?
Consult your doctor immediately if your baby has a number of attacks of abdominal cramps, or if you notice the presence of any blood or mucus in your baby's bowel motions.

What might the doctor do?
Your doctor will refer your baby to hospital for a barium enema to confirm the diagnosis of intussusception. This is a painless investigation in which fluid is pumped into the intestines through your baby's rectum; the condition of the intestines can then be seen on X-ray. The barium enema sometimes causes the condition to right itself; if it does not, your baby will have an operation to push the intestine back into its normal position.

SEE ALSO:
Colic 88
Vomiting 257

Itching

ITCHING IS NEARLY ALWAYS A SYMPTOM of some underlying skin problem (**eczema**, **ringworm**), the result of an infestation (**scabies**, fleas or **worms**), sensitivity to some foodstuff or drug, skin contact with an irritant (**hives**), or the result of an infectious disease (**chickenpox**). Sometimes nervous tension and worry can cause itching, and scratching can make the itchiness even worse.

Is it serious?
Itching is rarely serious but it should not be ignored.

What should I do first?

1 Try to determine the cause of the itching. The site may give you a clue. For example, itching around the anus and genitals could indicate worms or **thrush**, itchiness in the hair, ringworm, on the feet, **athlete's foot**, or between the fingers, scabies.

2 Check any pets your child comes into contact with for fleas.

3 Check to see if your child has eaten any new foods recently.

4 Note whether your child is taking any new medicines.

5 Try soothing the itching with calamine lotion or give your child a cool bath with a handful of bicarbonate of soda dissolved in the water.

Should I consult the doctor?

Consult your doctor as soon as possible if you can find no apparent reason for the itching or if your child is having difficulty sleeping because of constant itchiness.

What might the doctor do?

◗ Your doctor will examine your child and determine the cause of the itching. If itching is a symptom of another condition, he will treat this accordingly. He may prescribe antihistamine tablets, paracetamol elixir or cream to curb the itching.

◗ If your child is having difficulty sleeping, your doctor may prescribe a mild sedative.

What can I do to help?

◗ Dress your child in cotton underwear so that fabrics such as wool and nylon, which irritate, do not touch his skin.
◗ If you have recently changed your washing powder or fabric conditioner, change back to the old brand and see if the irritation subsides. Rinse clothes well.
◗ Use a mild soap and shampoo for your child.

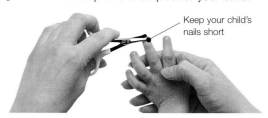

Keep your child's nails short

◗ To stop your child scratching, put mittens on him whenever possible, and keep his nails short to prevent infection should he break the skin by scratching too hard.

SEE ALSO:
Athlete's foot 60
Chickenpox 82
Chilblains 83
Eczema 124
Hives 163
Ringworm 210
Scabies 212
Thrush 240
Worms 263

Jaundice

JAUNDICE IS A SYMPTOM of an underlying disease, and it causes a yellow coloration of the skin and of the whites of the eyes.

The condition is due to the presence of yellow bile pigment, *bilirubin*, in the blood. Bile pigment is made during the normal breakdown of old red blood cells but, when certain illnesses are present, the bile pigment accumulates in the blood, tingeing the skin yellow. Possible causes of this condition include **hepatitis** (liver infection), a blockage or malformation of the bile duct, and certain types of **anaemia**.

The yellowish skin coloration is often accompanied by dark brown urine. This is because bile pigment overflows from the blood into the urine. There may also be pale stools because the pigment is no longer present in the intestinal contents to darken their colour.

Jaundice also occurs in one-third of babies during the week after birth, when it is called "physiological jaundice". In nearly all such cases there is no under-lying disease. The condition is merely due to the baby's liver and digestive system adapting to life outside the womb. Physiological jaundice is more common in breastfed babies and, once followed up by your doctor, is usually nothing to worry about.

Is it serious?

Jaundice should be treated seriously because it is usually a symptom of an underlying complaint.

Possible symptoms

▶ **Yellowish coloration** of the skin and of the whites of the eyes.
▶ **Dark brown urine**.
▶ **Pale-coloured stools**.
▶ **Nausea and loss of appetite**.

What should I do first?

1 Look to see if your child's urine is a darker colour and check if his stools are abnormally pale.

2 If your child feels sick and will not eat, give him frequent drinks to prevent dehydration.

3 Be meticulous about hygiene until you have consulted your doctor; your child may have hepatitis, which is contagious.

Should I consult the doctor?

Consult your doctor immediately if you suspect your child is jaundiced. Consult your doctor immediately if your baby seems yellow or unusually suntanned. A baby who is jaundiced must be checked by a doctor since excess bilirubin can damage internal organs; he must also be checked for any underlying disease.

What might the doctor do?

▶ The underlying disease will be identified and treated as necessary. If it is hepatitis, your child may need to be isolated.
▶ Your child will need regular check-ups at the hospital clinic for some weeks or months after the problem has cleared up, to ensure that there are no after-effects.

What can I do to help?

▶ Ensure that your child keeps to any special diets and treatments.
▶ Be sympathetic. Your child may have difficulty understanding why he has to eat special food, and he may feel tired and depressed for some weeks.

SEE ALSO:
Anaemia 53
Appetite, loss of 55
Hepatitis 160

Kawasaki syndrome

FIRST REPORTED IN THE 1960s by Doctor Tomisaku Kawasaki of Japan, Kawasaki syndrome is an acute illness that affects almost every system in the body and one that is becoming increasingly common in Western countries. The syndrome usually affects children under the age of five, although cases have been reported in older children.

Also known as mucocutaneous lymph node syndrome, Kawasaki syndrome is an inflammatory process with no known cause, although it is believed to be due to an infection. Its seriousness cannot be underestimated: in around 20–40 per cent of cases, serious heart complications can arise and, in 1–2 per cent of these, the illness has proved fatal.

There is no cure as yet for Kawasaki syndrome but medication, if given by a paediatrician within the first 10 days of fever, may help prevent possible heart complications. Most children make a complete recovery from Kawasaki syndrome after about three weeks but, for those who sustain heart damage, the condition is long-standing and can occasionally lead to sudden death.

Possible symptoms

- **High temperature** present for five days or more.
- **Red eyes**.
- **Cracked, red lips** and strawberry-like tongue.
- **Skin rash** all over body.
- **Swelling of the lymph glands** in the neck, usually on one side.
- **Swelling and/or redness of the hands and feet**, finally with peeling of skin on hands and feet.
- Other possible symptoms include **swollen and painful joints**, **mood changes**, **extreme irritability**, **loss of appetite**, **vomiting**, **diarrhoea**, **abdominal pain** and **jaundice**.

What can be done?

Consult your doctor if your child has a fever that lasts more than 24 hours, or if you suspect that any of the accompanying symptoms indicate Kawasaki syndrome. Do not give your child aspirin. Your doctor may admit your child to hospital for monitoring and prompt treatment should any of the more serious complications arise. Your child may be given aspirin and gamma globulin intravenously under strict medical supervision to reduce the risk of heart complications.

For help and advice contact the Kawasaki Syndrome Support Group (see page 324).

Laryngitis

LARYNGITIS IS AN INFLAMMATION of the larynx, or voice box. Many minor viruses, and occasionally bacteria, can enter the body through the throat and quickly infect the larynx. The most obvious symptoms of laryngitis are hoarseness and a dry **cough**, and sometimes **fever.**

Is it serious?

Laryngitis is rarely serious and lasts less than seven days, even if it is part of a more serious infection, such as **tonsillitis** or **bronchitis**. However, in young children a swollen larynx can obstruct the passage of air causing breathing difficulties and **croup**, which is a serious complication. If laryngitis develops into croup, you should seek urgent medical treatment.

Possible symptoms

▶ **Hoarseness** or loss of voice.
▶ **Dry cough**.
▶ **Slight fever**.
▶ **Sore throat**.
▶ **Croup**, a barking type of cough.

Cross-section of the throat

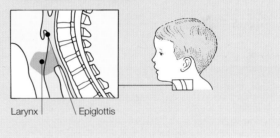

Larynx | Epiglottis

What should I do first?

1 If the hoarseness is not accompanied by any other symptoms of a respiratory tract infection, such as bronchitis, keep a check on your child's temperature. If it rises above 38°C (100.4°F), there may be another infection present.

2 Listen closely to identify the barking cough of croup.

3 Keep the air in your child's room moist if possible. Open a window to allow air to circulate. This is usually an effective atmosphere for suppressing a dry cough.

Should I consult the doctor?

Consult your doctor immediately if you think your child has croup. Consult your doctor as soon as possible if your child has a fever or you think he has contracted another infection.

What might the doctor do?

If there is a bacterial infection such as bronchitis or tonsillitis, your doctor will prescribe antibiotics.

What can I do to help?

▶ Discourage your child from talking out loud. You could make a game of it and have the whole family talking in whispers.
▶ Give your child plenty of warm drinks to soothe his throat. Try hot lemon and honey or heat any fruit-juice drink by diluting it with hot water.

SEE ALSO:
Bronchiolitis 72
Cough 98
Croup 101
Fever 134
Tonsillitis 243

Leukaemia

LEUKAEMIA IS A RARE FORM OF CANCER caused by the rapid overgrowth of millions of primitive white blood cells. The cancerous white blood cells prevent the normal growth of red blood cells, leading to **anaemia**; they cause a lack of mature white blood cells, which reduces immunity to infection; and they prevent the growth of platelets, which help in the blood-clotting mechanism of the body. Quite often the first indication of leukaemia is the anaemic condition of the child and his failure to recover quickly from an infectious illness.

Possible symptoms

▶ **Anaemia** – paleness, fatigue and shortness of breath.
▶ **Susceptibility to infection**.
▶ **Pain in the limbs**; if in the legs, perhaps seen as a limp.
▶ **Purpura** – a purplish-red rash which doesn't disappear with pressure.
▶ **Tendency to bruise easily**.
▶ **Recurrent nosebleeds**.

What can be done?

At one time the outlook for children with leukaemia was not good, but over the last decade therapy has improved the chances of a complete cure for 60–80 per cent of those children suffering from the most common type of childhood leukaemia.

All children with the disease will be treated by a paediatrician who is experienced in childhood leukaemic diseases. Several drugs are given at the same time, some by mouth and some by injection. In the most common type of childhood leukaemia, radiotherapy and special drugs may be used to kill the cancer cells in the brain. A blood transfusion may be given at the beginning of the treatment. If the number of white blood cells falls to a very low level, your child will be isolated against infection, and all visitors will need to wear masks and gowns. After several weeks, your child should be allowed to return home to lead as normal a life as possible. Regular check-ups will be necessary to keep track of the condition.

The important role for you as parents is to support your child through the long and arduous treatment by keeping up his morale with the prospect of an eventual cure. Children with leukaemia must not be exposed to the common childhood infectious diseases, such as **chickenpox**, unless they are already immune, so you will need to screen your child's playmates carefully. Chickenpox vaccine is offered to children with leukaemia.

For help and advice contact the Leukaemia Society (see page 324).

SEE ALSO:
Anaemia 53
Chickenpox 82

Lice

THE HEAD LOUSE IS A TINY INSECT which infests the hair on the human head. The adult louse lays its eggs (nits) at the root of the hair, to which they become firmly attached. This distinguishes them from dandruff, which can be flaked off easily with a fingernail. The eggs hatch after 7–10 days and the lice bite the scalp to get blood. Your child's head will be itchy where the lice bite, particularly after strenuous exercise when he is hot. Your child can become infested by contact with another infested child or adult.

Are they serious?

Lice and nits are irritating, but they can be eradicated and are therefore not serious.

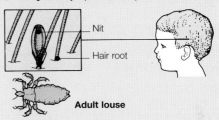

Possible symptoms

▶ **Itchy scalp**, particularly when the head is hot.

Nit

Hair root

Adult louse

▶ **Tiny, pearly-white eggs** covering the roots of the hair.

What should I do first?

1 If your child scratches, inspect the roots of the hair for nits. If you find them, you must keep your child away from school or nursery until you have administered the treatment. You should inform the headteacher of the outbreak so that he can inform the health authorities.

2 Ask your chemist or health visitor to explain the wet-combing ("bug-busting") method to you. This involves combing wet hair first to remove adult lice and nits and then applying a medicated lotion or shampoo. This method prevents lice from becoming resistant to treatment. Some anti-lice products cannot be used by asthmatics, so you should consult your pharmacist if necessary. There are lotions available that contain an ingredient called malathion, and these are left on the hair overnight.

3 Examine the heads of the rest of your family for nits, and treat with the wet-combing method and an appropriate shampoo or lotion. If anyone in your family has been in contact with someone who

has lice, it is quite likely that the insects have transferred from one head to another.

4 After treatment, remove any dead eggs with a fine-toothed comb.

Should I consult the doctor?

Consult your doctor as soon as possible if the treatment doesn't work – you may not have administered the treatment properly – or if you are not sure your child has head lice.

What might the doctor do?

Your doctor or health visitor will question you about any self-help treatment you have used. He may prescribe another shampoo.

What can I do to help?

▶ Repeat the treatment seven days later in case any eggs remain.
▶ Clean the child's headgear, brushes or combs with the anti-louse shampoo.

SEE ALSO:
Itching 170

Limp

YOUR CHILD IS LIMPING if he is not taking the full weight of his body on one leg as he walks. The cause, on investigation, may be obvious, such as a **cut**, a **blister** or a **splinter** on the sole of the foot or the heel, a protruding toenail, an **ingrowing toenail**, tight shoes, wrinkling of the inner soles in his shoes or a pebble in a shoe. A persistent limp which has no such obvious cause may be a symptom of some other, more serious, problem.

Is it serious?

Limping for no apparent reason should always be treated seriously in a child. An unexplained limp can be a symptom of the rare form of blood cancer, **leukaemia**. If the limp is accompanied by swelling or tenderness of the joints, it may be caused by **rheumatic fever**, **arthritis** or **osteomyelitis**. These could have long-term complications and should therefore be treated seriously.

What should I do first?

1 Look for obvious injuries and examine any areas that your child claims are painful.

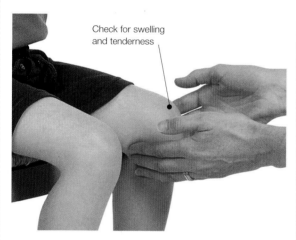

Check for swelling and tenderness

2 Check to see whether the joints are swollen and inflamed.

3 If you suspect your child may have a **broken bone**, don't hesitate to get medical attention. The injury may not always be obvious.

Should I consult the doctor?

Consult your doctor immediately for a thorough investigation of the limp if you can't find a reason for it, or if you suspect a broken bone. Consult your doctor immediately if any of your child's joints is swollen or tender.

What might the doctor do?

❯ Your doctor will examine your child's leg thoroughly and may refer your child to a paediatric orthopaedic surgeon to try to discover the cause of the problem.

❯ If a bone in your child's leg is broken, your doctor will refer your child to the nearest hospital for an X-ray and to have the leg put into plaster.

What can I do to help?

Never give up if your child has a limp. Continue taking your child to your doctor for investigation and be persistent until the cause is found.

Measles

MEASLES IS AN INFECTIOUS CHILDHOOD disease, caused by a virus, which has become less common since routine immunization was introduced. It is very contagious and has an incubation period of between eight and 14 days. The first indication of measles is usually symptoms similar to those of the **common cold**, with a **fever** that becomes increasingly higher, and small, white spots inside the mouth, on the lining of the cheeks (Koplik's spots). Your child's eyes may also be red and sore. The initial symptoms are followed about three days later by small, brownish-red spots behind the ears; these spots merge together to form a rash over the face and torso.

Is it serious?

Measles is an unpleasant childhood illness but it is not usually serious. However, in rare cases your child may develop complications, such as **otitis media**, **pneumonia** or **encephalitis**.

Possible symptoms

▶ **Runny nose and dry cough**.
▶ **Headache**.
▶ **Fever**, rising as high as 40°C (104°F).
▶ **Small, white spots** inside the mouth.
▶ **Red, sore eyes** and intolerance of bright light.
▶ **Brownish-red rash of small spots**, starting behind the ears and spreading to the torso.

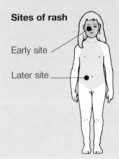

Sites of rash

Early site

Later site

What should I do first?

1 Check your child's temperature. If he has a fever, try to bring it down with tepid sponging (*see page 31*). If his eyes are sore, bathe them with cool water.

2 Make sure he drinks plenty of fluids by offering small amounts regularly.

Should I consult the doctor?

Consult your doctor immediately to confirm the diagnosis, or if your child gets worse after seemingly recovering from measles, or if he complains of **earache**.

What might the doctor do?

▶ Your doctor will advise you to keep your child in bed for as long as his temperature remains high.

He will examine your child's ears to check that there is no ear infection. If there is, he will prescribe a course of antibiotics.

▶ Your doctor may prescribe eye drops for your child's eyes if they are sore.

What can I do to help?

▶ Don't send your child back to school until the rash has faded.

▶ Have any other children inoculated against measles. The MMR (measles, mumps and rubella) vaccination is given at 12–15 months and a pre-school booster three years later.

SEE ALSO:
Common cold 90
Earache 122
Encephalitis 126
Fever 134
Otitis media 198
Pneumonia 202

Meningitis

MENINGITIS IS AN INFLAMMATION of the membranes (meninges) that cover the brain and spinal cord, and most frequently results from an infection, either viral or bacterial. Viral meningitis occurs most commonly after **mumps**, but it is not a very serious illness. Bacterial meningitis, however, is serious, but can be treated successfully with antibiotics if it is diagnosed early enough. The symptoms of meningitis are **fever**, a stiff neck, lethargy, **headache**, **drowsiness** and intolerance of bright light; in rare cases, there may also be a purple-red rash. Meningitis can be difficult to diagnose in babies and children, whose inability to communicate what they are feeling may lead to a delay in diagnosis. Under the age of 18 months, the fontanelle will bulge slightly. After that age it will have closed.

Babies and children are now routinely immunized against the strain of bacterial meningitis known as Group C meningococcal meningitis. However, this does not protect against other forms of bacterial, or viral, meningitis. It is still very important to be aware of the signs of meningitis.

Is it serious?

Bacterial meningitis is a very serious disease and, if it is left untreated, it can prove fatal.

Possible symptoms

▶ **Fever**, as high as 39°C (102.2°F).

▶ **Stiff neck**.

▶ **Lethargy**.

▶ **Headache**.

▶ **Inability to tolerate bright light**.

▶ **Bulging fontanelle**.

▶ **Drowsiness and confusion**.

▶ **Vomiting**.

▶ **Purple-red rash** anywhere on the body, which does not fade when pressed with a glass.

Cross-section of the meninges

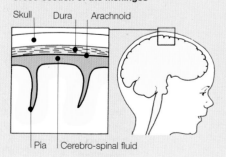

Skull | Dura | Arachnoid

Pia | Cerebro-spinal fluid

What should I do first?

1 If you suspect meningitis, or your child has just had mumps, bend your child's head forward so that his chin touches his chest to see if there is any stiffness or pain in his neck.

2 If your child is under two years old, see if he screws his eyes up in bright light. Feel the fontanelle to see if it bulges outwards.

Purpura rash on light skin

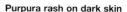

Purpura rash on dark skin

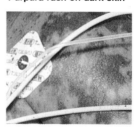

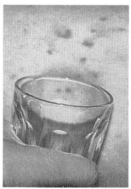

3 Check for a rash, known as a purpura rash, which doesn't fade when pressed with a glass. If present, take your child to the nearest casualty department and insist on being seen at once.

Continued on next page

Continued from previous page

Should I consult the doctor?

Consult your doctor immediately if you suspect meningitis, or take your child to the nearest accident and emergency department and insist on being seen at once.

What might the doctor do?

▶ Your doctor will refer your child to hospital for a lumbar puncture. This involves testing a sample of spinal fluid, taken under local anaesthetic.

▶ If your child is suffering from bacterial meningitis, he will be given high doses of antibiotics intravenously. Viral meningitis clears up on its own, but your child will be given painkilling drugs to relieve the symptoms and steroids to help speed recovery.

What can I do to help?

▶ It is the health authority's responsibility to check that the school is informed of your child's meningitis. You can check that the school has been informed.

SEE ALSO:
Drowsiness 118
Encephalitis 126
Fever 134
Headache 156
Mumps 184
Vomiting 257

Migraine

MIGRAINE IS A SEVERE, recurrent **headache** (felt on one or both sides of the head) that is accompanied by **vomiting** and, in children, by abdominal pain. For this reason, it is often referred to as abdominal migraine. Migraine tends to run in families and starts in late childhood or in early adolescence. Headaches in younger children are not usually migraine headaches. It is not known what sets off a migraine headache but tension and certain foods, such as cheese and chocolate, are possible causes.

Quite often a migraine headache is preceded by an "aura", a series of strange sensations, such as flashing lights, peculiar smells and numbness on the affected side of the head. Most children can pinpoint these sensations clearly.

Possible symptoms

- **Severe headache** on one or both sides.
- **Vomiting**.
- **Nausea**.
- **Abdominal pain**.
- **Paleness**.
- **Withdrawn, quiet behaviour**.
- **Aura**, involving strange visual and physical sensations, preceding the attack.

Is it serious?

Migraine is not serious, but it is debilitating.

What should I do first?

1 Put your child to bed in a cool, darkened room if he complains of headache and nausea. If the headache persists, it is best to give him paracetamol elixir.

2 Put a bucket next to your child's bed in case he needs to vomit.

3 If your child complains of abdominal pain check for **appendicitis** (*see page 54*).

Should I consult the doctor?

Consult your doctor immediately if your child is suffering severe abdominal pain, to exclude the possibility of appendicitis. Consult your doctor as soon as possible if your child suffers from recurrent migraine headaches.

What might the doctor do?

Your doctor will ask your child to describe the headache. Your doctor may prescribe painkilling drugs for an acute attack. If your child's headaches are frequent, your child may be given drugs to take immediately an attack begins, or, in severe cases, to be taken regularly to prevent attacks.

What can I do to help?

If the headaches are frequent, keep a diary of your child's diet to try to pinpoint a possible trigger food. Avoid any suspect foods for a couple of weeks to see if there is any reduction in headaches.

SEE ALSO:
Appendicitis 54
Headache 156
Vomiting 257

Milia

MILIA IS A RASH of tiny creamy white spots that appear on the nose and cheeks of a newborn baby within the first three weeks of life. The spots occur because the baby's sebaceous glands are not well-enough developed to function properly. They remain until the sebaceous glands mature, usually within the first three months. The spots are not itchy and give rise to no unpleasant symptoms in the baby.

Is it serious?

Milia is never serious and resolves itself naturally without treatment.

Possible symptoms

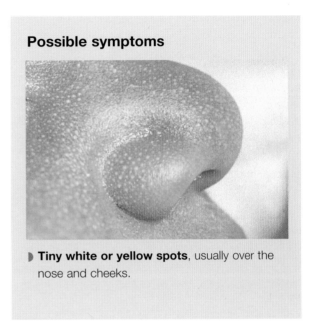

▶ **Tiny white or yellow spots**, usually over the nose and cheeks.

What should I do first?

1 Don't squeeze the spots. Though they may appear to have very tiny yellow heads, they are not infected and the skin of a baby is too fragile to take any pressure or squeezing.

2 Don't put any creams or lotions on the spots.

Should I consult the doctor?

There should be no need to consult your doctor unless you are concerned about the cause of the rash. Talking to your health visitor may provide the reassurance you need.

What might the doctor do?

Your doctor will reassure you and almost certainly not interfere with the milia.

What can I do to help?

▶ You can ignore the milia as the spots will disappear in time.

▶ Try not to be vain about your baby, even if you feel the spots make him appear ugly. Milia is very common in newborn babies, so try to relax and wait until they disappear.

Mouth ulcers

CHILDREN SUFFER FROM A VARIETY of mouth ulcers, all of them painful, though most are relatively harmless. *Aphthous ulcers* are usually small and creamy-white and appear on the tongue, the gums or the lining of the mouth. They may be so painful that your child will be reluctant to eat. These ulcers are sometimes associated with stress and may come in crops during a particularly anxious time such as starting school. A *traumatic ulcer* usually starts as a sore patch on the inside of the cheeks, possibly after an injury by biting or by the rubbing of a rough tooth. It enlarges to form a painful yellow crater and may take 10–14 days to heal completely. White, painful blisters on the roof of the mouth, on the gums and inside the cheeks can be the result of a primary infection with the **cold sore** virus. White, curd-like blisters could indicate a **thrush** infection.

Are they serious?
Mouth ulcers are rarely serious but, because they are painful, they can interfere with your child's eating.

Possible symptoms
▶ **Small, creamy-white, painful, raised areas** found anywhere on the tongue, gums or lining of the mouth.
▶ **Large red area** with a yellow centre, particularly inside the cheeks.
▶ **White blister-like spots** inside the mouth, sometimes accompanied by a fever.
▶ **Loss of appetite** because eating is painful.

Classic site of aphthous ulcer

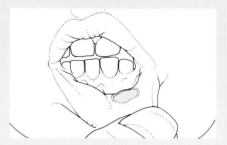

What should I do first?

1 If your child complains of a sore mouth or tongue, check to see whether there are any areas of soreness.

2 If the ulcer is large and is inside the cheek, check for a jagged tooth that might be rubbing the cheek lining and causing the injury.

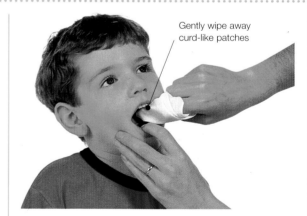

Gently wipe away curd-like patches

3 If the ulcers resemble white curds, try to wipe them off with a handkerchief. If this leaves red, raw patches, the ulcers could be caused by thrush.

Continued from previous page

4 Smear an antiseptic jelly or glycerine over the ulcers with your fingertip, or give your child some paracetamol elixir.

5 If your bottlefed baby has a traumatic ulcer on the roof of his mouth, check the teat. It may be too hard for your baby's tender mouth.

Should I consult the doctor?

Consult your doctor as soon as possible if the ulcers are very painful, or if your home treatment (*above*) doesn't help. Consult your doctor as soon as possible if the mouth ulcers are recurrent. If the ulceration is caused by a jagged tooth, take your child to the dentist to have the tooth smoothed off.

What might the doctor do?

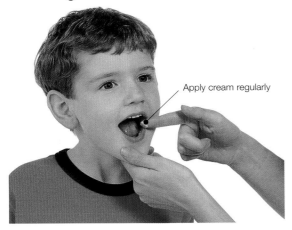

Apply cream regularly

▶ Your doctor will probably prescribe an anti-inflammatory cream for aphthous ulcers. The cream is not dissolved by saliva and therefore clings to the ulcers and speeds healing.
▶ If your child suffers from recurrent mouth ulcers, your doctor will refer him to hospital for blood tests to see if there is an underlying cause for the condition, other than stress.

What can I do to help?

▶ Liquidize foods to minimize chewing when the ulcers are most painful. Let your child feed through a straw if he wants.
▶ Don't give your child any salty or acidic foods. These will cause pain. Ice lollies and smooth, bland foods are best.
▶ Discourage your child from biting his lips or cheeks. This can lead to injury of the mouth and lip lining and eventually to ulceration.

SEE ALSO:
Cold sore 87
Thrush 240

Mumps

MUMPS IS AN INFECTIOUS CHILDHOOD DISEASE, now less common since routine immunization was introduced, and mostly affecting children over the age of two. It is caused by a virus and has an incubation period of 14 to 21 days. Your child will seem generally unwell for a day or two before the major symptoms appear. The salivary glands in front of and beneath the ears and chin swell up and there may be **fever**. The swelling can appear first on one side of the face, then the other, or on both sides at once, and cause pain when swallowing. Your child will complain of a dry mouth because the salivary glands have stopped producing saliva. A less common symptom is the swelling of the testes or ovaries, causing local pain in boys and abdominal pain in girls.

Is it serious?

Mumps is a mild disease. However, if before, during or after swelling, your child has a severe headache and a stiff neck, this could be **encephalitis** or **meningitis**, which are serious complications.

Possible symptoms
Affected areas

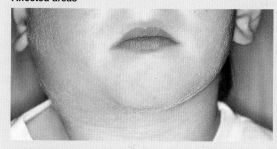

▶ **Swelling of the glands** on either or both sides of the face just below the ears and beneath the chin.
▶ **Pain** when swallowing.
▶ **Dry mouth**.
▶ **Fever**.
▶ **Headache**.
▶ **Swollen, painful testes** in boys, **lower-abdominal pain** in girls.

What should I do first?

1 Check your child's temperature to see if she has a fever. If she has, try to bring it down with tepid sponging (*see page 31*).

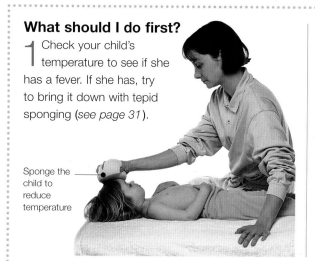

Sponge the child to reduce temperature

2 Liquidize your child's food and feed her through a straw if she is having difficulty eating.

3 Give her plenty to drink and encourage her to rinse out her mouth to alleviate the dryness.

4 Put your child to bed with a hot-water bottle wrapped in a towel to hold against the affected side.

Should I consult the doctor?

Consult your doctor as soon as possible to confirm the diagnosis of mumps, or if your son's testes are very painful or your daughter is suffering abdominal pain. Consult your doctor immediately if, after 10

Continued from previous page

days, your child's condition has worsened and he has a headache and a stiff neck.

What might the doctor do?

▶ There is no specific treatment for mumps. Your doctor will advise you to keep your child away from school until five days after the swelling has gone down.

▶ If the testes are swollen, your doctor will advise complete bed-rest until the swelling has subsided and he will probably prescribe paracetamol elixir for the pain of your son's swollen testes or if your daughter has abdominal pain from swollen ovaries.

What can I do to help?

Be inventive with liquid foods, such as egg-enriched milkshakes, soups and yogurt, which slip down easily.

SEE ALSO:
Encephalitis 126
Fever 134
Meningitis 178

Muscular dystrophy

MUSCULAR DYSTROPHY IS THE TERM GIVEN to a group of disorders which are usually inherited and result in a gradual wasting and weakening of the muscle fibres. The most common form of the disease in children is Duchenne muscular dystrophy, which affects only boys. The boy will be slow at developing muscular power. He will be late for his age to sit, walk and run, and about 25 per cent of boys suffering from this form of muscular dystrophy will have some form of mental handicap.

The disorder is usually diagnosed by the time the child is three years old. As mobility deteriorates your child will walk with a waddling gait and an arched back because of the weakness of the pelvic muscles; he will have difficulty climbing stairs; his calf muscles, though weakened, will appear overdeveloped and the muscles in the upper arm will also be abnormally large. Walking becomes impossible by the age of about 12. Because there is no known treatment, 75 per cent of sufferers die by the age of 20.

Because the cardiac muscles of muscular dystrophy sufferers also weaken, this increases the risk of serious or persistent chest infections, which can result in sudden death.

Possible symptoms

- **Late development** in ability to sit, walk and run.
- **Waddling gait**.
- **Difficulty standing upright**.
- **Difficulty climbing stairs**.
- **Overdeveloped muscles**, particularly noticeable in the calves.
- **Deformation** of the spine.

What can be done?

There is no effective treatment for muscular dystrophy. Sufferers may need to attend a school for the physically disabled as they will usually be confined to a wheelchair by the age of 12. Until this time, the child should be kept active and walking as long as possible, without strenuous exercise, though, as this hastens the muscle deterioration. The use of lightweight splints and calipers can prolong walking. Too much bed-rest is not advisable as this speeds up muscular disintegration. Physiotherapy treatment is available to limit the physical disability.

As Duchenne muscular dystrophy is carried by women, you should seek genetic counselling before deciding to have a baby if there is any family history of muscular dystrophy. If a pattern of inheritance can be found, there is a 50 per cent chance of a male child being affected and the same chance of a female child being a carrier. Early in pregnancy, chorionic villus sampling can be carried out. This involves extracting a sample of the developing placenta to be examined for defective cells and to determine the child's sex. The pregnant woman can then decide whether to terminate her pregnancy. In the near future, more precise tests for muscular dystrophy will be available early in pregnancy.

For help and advice contact the Muscular Dystrophy Group (see page 324).

Nappy rash

NAPPY RASH IS A SKIN CONDITION that affects the area normally covered by a baby's nappy, and can occur whether the nappies used are fabric or disposable. The skin may be slightly red, or broken and inflamed with pus-filled spots.

There are several causes of nappy rash, but it is most commonly caused by urine and stools being left in contact with the skin for too long. The bacteria in the baby's stools break down the urine and release ammonia, a strong irritant. These bacteria grow best in an alkaline environment, and because the stools of bottlefed babies are alkaline – unlike those of breastfed babies, which are acidic – bottlefed babies are much more likely to suffer from ammoniacal nappy rash. In such cases the rash starts around the genitals, and, if left untreated, the skin becomes tight and shiny and pustules may develop. There is always a strong smell of ammonia from the nappy.

Nappy rash can also be caused by inadequate drying after bathing your baby. In such cases the nappy rash is usually confined to the skin creases at the tops of the thighs. If the rash covers most of the nappy area, and you use fabric nappies, nappy rash

may be due to an allergic reaction to chemicals in the washing powder used to wash them, or to fabric conditioner. Nappy rash may also be a sign of seborrhoeic **eczema**.

A rash that starts around the anus and moves over the buttocks and on to the thighs may not be nappy rash at all but a **thrush** infection.

Is it serious?

Nappy rash is not serious and can be easily prevented and treated at home.

Possible symptoms

▸ **Redness** over nappy area.
▸ **Redness**, which starts around the genitals and is accompanied by a strong smell of ammonia.
▸ **Tight, papery skin** with inflamed spots that have pus-filled centres.
▸ **Redness**, which starts around the anus and moves over the buttocks and on to the thighs.

What should I do first?

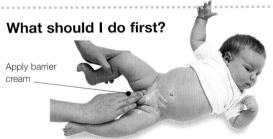

Apply barrier cream

1 As soon as you notice any redness on your baby's bottom, wash his bottom with warm water and dry thoroughly. Apply barrier cream, such as zinc oxide ointment, to prevent the urine from irritating his skin. If your baby wears disposable nappies only a small amount of cream is needed.

2 Change nappies and wash your baby's bottom frequently (at least every two to three hours and as soon as he's had a bowel motion). Leave off the nappy whenever possible.

3 Use one-way disposable nappy liners next to your baby's skin as these are designed to let urine pass through to the nappy while remaining dry next to the baby's bottom.

4 Don't use talcum powder around your baby's genitals because it cakes when wet and may irritate the skin.

Continued on next page

Continued from previous page

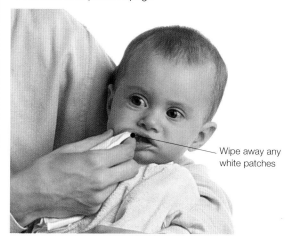

Wipe away any white patches

5 Check inside your baby's mouth. If you notice white patches, try to wipe them off with a clean handkerchief. If they leave raw, red patches, your baby has oral thrush and this may have caused the nappy rash.

Should I consult the doctor?

Consult your doctor as soon as possible if the measures above fail to clear the nappy rash within two or three days, or if you think your baby has thrush.

What might the doctor do?

❯ Your doctor or health visitor will determine the cause of the nappy rash and will make sure you've been using the most suitable home treatment. He or she may suggest alternatives.

❯ If the nappy rash has become infected, your doctor may prescribe an antibiotic ointment.

❯ If your baby has the first signs of eczema, your doctor will question you about any washing powders or fabric conditioners you use to wash your baby's nappies and may advise you to change to another brand if your present brand contains a biological component. He may prescribe a cortisone ointment to be used sparingly.

❯ If the nappy rash is caused by thrush, your doctor will prescribe an anti-fungal cream.

What can I do to help?

❯ Continue to change your baby's nappies frequently, and always after a bowel motion.

❯ Try to use plastic pants as rarely as possible. They stop air from circulating around your baby's bottom.

❯ Wash your baby's fabric nappies thoroughly. Sterilize in nappy sterilizing solution, wash in very hot water and rinse them thoroughly to get rid of all traces of detergent and ammonia.

❯ If the condition is recurrent, change the type of nappies you use from one brand of disposables to another brand, or from disposable nappy to cloth nappy (or vice versa).

SEE ALSO:
Eczema 124
Thrush 240

Nephritis

NEPHRITIS IS A DISEASE THAT AFFECTS the kidneys, and it develops after a streptococcal infection such as **tonsillitis**. To combat this infection the body produces antibodies but, due to a defect in the body's immune system, these antibodies may go on working after the infection has passed and begin to harm the kidneys, which become inflamed and cease to function normally. The condition comes on suddenly in children and produces symptoms of reddish-brown urine and mild swelling of the face, ankles and abdomen.

Is it serious?

If nephritis goes untreated it can develop into a more serious disorder known as nephrotic syndrome.

Possible symptoms

▶ **Reddish-brown urine**.
▶ **Slight swelling** of the face, ankles and abdomen (oedema).
▶ **Headache**.
▶ **High blood pressure**.

What should I do first?

1 If your child has recently had a **sore throat** and you notice that he has reddish-brown urine, check to see if he has eaten any beetroot. This can cause red colouring of the urine.

2 If you notice that your child's face is puffy and swollen, check his ankles and abdomen for swelling.

Should I consult the doctor?

Consult your doctor immediately if you notice reddish-brown urine (and it is not related to something your child may have eaten) or if your child has any unusual swelling of the face, ankles or abdomen.

What might the doctor do?

▶ Your doctor will test your child's urine, take his blood pressure and take a sample of his blood for analysis.

▶ Your child will probably be admitted to hospital for bed-rest, and a special diet will be suggested to reduce salt, fluid and protein levels.

▶ If a streptococcal infection is still present, your child will be prescribed antibiotics. His blood pressure will be closely monitored, too.

▶ Once your child's urine has returned to normal, he will be allowed home. There is usually a complete recovery in one to two weeks.

▶ If there is a chronic condition, your child will have regular check-ups.

What can I do to help?

Take your child to see your doctor whenever he has a severe sore throat or has any other streptococcal infection such as **impetigo**.

SEE ALSO:
Impetigo 166
Rheumatic fever 209
Sore throat 222
Tonsillitis 243

Nightmares

EVERYONE DREAMS, AND MOST children have occasional unpleasant dreams or nightmares. Your child may wake screaming in a panic or sobbing uncontrollably. He will seem to be in a state half-way between consciousness and sleep, with his eyes open, though he will not be in touch with reality and he may not even recognize you or understand what you are saying to him.

Nightmares can occur for a number of reasons. If your child has a high temperature, or is uncomfortable because of illness, he may wake up hot and frightened in the night. If he has gone to bed over-tired, he may wake crying within an hour or two of going to sleep. He may have seen a frightening television programme just before going to bed; he may be scared of the dark, or dislike being alone in his bedroom. In normal children, if nightmares occur with any frequency, the underlying cause is usually anxiety about home life, such as the arrival of a new baby, or about incidents at school.

Are they serious?

Nightmares are not serious and do not require medical attention unless they occur very frequently.

What should I do first?

Go to your child immediately; don't let him get too hysterical. Turn on the light, hold him close to you and speak quietly to soothe him. Don't raise your voice and scold him; this may make him hysterical. Don't ask him why he woke up frightened, or what his dream was about. Stay with your child until he drifts back to sleep.

Should I consult the doctor?

Consult your doctor for advice if the nightmares are frequent (every night, for example) and your child is losing sleep because of them.

What might the doctor do?

▶ Your doctor or health visitor will reassure you that your child will sooner or later grow out of the habit of having nightmares.
▶ If your child is having severe difficulty in sleeping, your doctor may decide to prescribe a sedative in very rare instances.

What can I do to help?

▶ If your child is old enough to explain, ask him what he thinks might have caused the nightmare but wait until the following day to do so.
▶ Try to reduce your child's anxiety by reassuring him. If you can guess the cause of his tension, such as the arrival of a new baby, do your best to allay his fears.

Nose, foreign body in

IF THERE IS A FOREIGN BODY in your child's nose, it is most likely to have been pushed in by your child or a playmate. The problem may not be noticed by you or your child at first, but after two or three days there will be a **nosebleed**, or a blood-stained, foul-smelling discharge from the affected nostril.

Is it serious?

If the foreign body cannot be easily removed from your child's nose, on no account attempt to remove it yourself. Instead, you should consult your doctor immediately or take your child to the nearest hospital.

If the foreign body can be easily removed from the nose, it is not serious and should have no after-effects. The situation becomes serious, however, if your child actually inhales the object into his lungs, as this may partially block his air passages and cause her breathing difficulties, **croup** or **choking**.

Possible symptoms

▶ **Nosebleeds**.

▶ **Smelly, blood-stained discharge** from the nostril.

▶ **Red, swollen, tender area** over the nose.

▶ **Peculiar odour** on your child's breath, sometimes said to smell like ripe cheese.

What should I do first?

1 If your child is old enough to understand, ask her to hold a finger against the good nostril (or do this for her) and to blow the affected one to dislodge the foreign body. Don't ask a young child to do this – she might sniff the object back into her air passages.

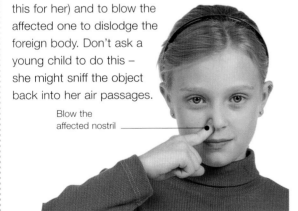

Blow the affected nostril

2 Alternatively, lay your child on her back on a flat surface and shine a light on her face. If the object can be seen near the entrance to the nose, and if it is soft, remove it with tweezers. If it moves further up the nostril, leave it alone. If your child has breathing problems, treat this as an emergency (*see page 284*).

Should I consult the doctor?

Consult your doctor immediately or take your child to the nearest hospital if you cannot easily remove a foreign body from your child's nose.

What might the doctor do?

If possible, your doctor will remove the foreign body with a pair of forceps. If your child is very young, or refuses to stay still, he may have to be taken to hospital and have the foreign body removed under general anaesthetic.

What can I do to help?

Try not to allow a child under the age of three to play with toys or objects small enough to swallow or put up his nose.

SEE ALSO:
Croup 101
Nosebleed 192

Nosebleed

A NOSEBLEED OCCURS when a small area of blood vessels on the inner surface of the nose ruptures. This can be caused by hard nose-blowing or sneezing when your child has a **common cold** or **hayfever**, by a knock on the nose, by picking the nose, or by a foreign body in the nose; in this last case the blood will be accompanied by a foul-smelling discharge. The blood loss can look dramatic, but is usually very little.

Is it serious?

A nosebleed is hardly ever serious. However, if your child has frequent nosebleeds which don't stop easily, or if his nose bleeds after a blow to the head, medical advice should be sought.

What should I do first?

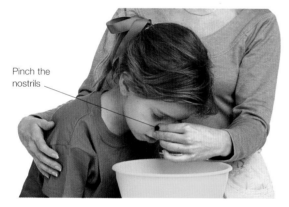

Pinch the nostrils

Don't try to staunch the blood by pushing anything into the nostrils. Sit your child down with her head forward over a basin or sink. Apply firm pressure to both nostrils, gripping her nose between your thumb and forefinger just where the bone ends. Squeeze for 10 minutes or until the bleeding stops. Don't let your child put her head back during a nosebleed. This allows blood to drip down the back of the nose into the stomach and can cause irritation and vomiting.

Should I consult the doctor?

Consult your doctor immediately if the nosebleed fails to stop after 30 minutes and your child is dizzy and pale. Consult your doctor as soon as possible if you think there may be a foreign body in your child's nose, or if the nosebleeds are frequent.

What might the doctor do?

▶ If your child has suffered a blow to the head, your doctor will probably arrange for an X-ray to discount the possibility of a fractured skull.
▶ If the nosebleed has failed to stop, your doctor will pack your child's nose with gauze to stem the blood flow. This will be done under a local anaesthetic. The gauze can be removed after a couple of hours.
▶ If your child has a foreign object stuck in her nose, your doctor will remove it, under local anaesthetic if necessary.
▶ If the nosebleeds are frequent, your doctor may refer you to an ear, nose and throat specialist for assessment. If the recurrent nosebleeds are caused by a fragile blood vessel the specialist may cauterize it. This involves burning off the end of the vessel, and is done under a general anaesthetic.

What can I do to help?

Don't let your child blow his nose for at least three hours after a nosebleed as the bleeding might start again.

SEE ALSO:
Common cold 90
Hayfever 152
Nose, foreign body in 191

Obesity

A CHILD IS TERMED OBESE, or seriously overweight, if he is 20 per cent heavier than the average for his height and age (*see page 304*). A child is not obese if he merely has a protruding tummy or a round, chubby-cheeked face, both of which are quite common in children under the age of five. If you are concerned that your child might be overweight, you should consult your health visitor or doctor.

Obesity in babies and children is rarely due to any kind of family trait or hormonal disease. It is nearly always due to bad feeding habits, chiefly overfeeding by parents. It's for this reason that parents of a fat child rarely see that there's a weight problem.

Is it serious?

Obesity in children is serious. There will be an emotional strain on the child when he is teased by his playmates. More importantly, fat children tend to grow into fat adults who run higher-than-normal risks of heart disease, high blood pressure and joint disorders.

Possible symptoms

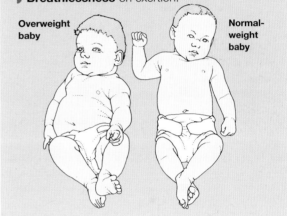

▶ **Twenty per cent or more average weight** for height and age.
▶ **Rolls of fat** around the thighs, upper arms, breasts and chin.
▶ **Breathlessness** on exertion.

Overweight baby

Normal-weight baby

What should I do first?

1 Weigh your child and check the charts on page 304 to see if he is much heavier than normal for his age.

2 Examine your child for rolls of fat around his upper arms and thighs, and see whether there are overdeveloped breasts.

3 Look at his diet. Do you give him high-calorie foods such as syrup drinks, lots of refined foods and sugar products? Compare your child with his playmates – is he as physically active?

Should I consult the doctor?

Consult your doctor as soon as possible if you think your child has a weight problem. If you are overweight yourself, you may be confusing your child's natural plumpness with the more serious problem of obesity. Your doctor can advise you.

What might the doctor do?

▶ Your doctor will examine your child. In the rare cases in which obesity is due to a glandular disorder your doctor will refer your child to an endocrinologist (a specialist in hormonal disorders) for investigation.
▶ If no disease is suspected, your doctor will give you advice on diet and advise you to encourage your child to use up more energy.

Continued on next page

Continued from previous page

What can I do to help?

❭ Consider whether obesity is a family problem. If you plan changes in your child's diet, you should adopt these yourself to set an example. Find out about how to eat healthily.

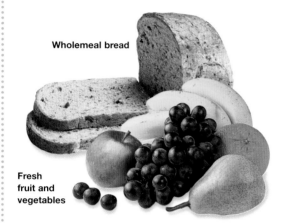

Wholemeal bread

Fresh fruit and vegetables

❭ Don't put your child on a special diet to lose weight. Instead, change his diet to include more unrefined, fibre-rich foods such as wholemeal flour, brown rice, fresh fruit and vegetables. Cut out refined flours and sugar in cooking, and avoid cakes, biscuits, sweets and sugary drinks.

❭ Try not to fry food; grill or steam instead. Cut the fat off the meat before cooking.

❭ Always make up feeds using the correct amount of formula.

❭ Don't give your baby snacks of rusks or biscuits, both of which are full of sugar; give him dried wholemeal toast or pieces of celery or apple instead.

❭ Dilute fresh fruit juice with water, and avoid carbonated and squash drinks.

❭ Encourage your child to be active. Don't confine a toddler to a playpen or pushchair; let him use up his energy by crawling or walking. Play lively games with him.

Osteomyelitis

OSTEOMYELITIS IS AN EXTREMELY rare bacterial infection of the bone. Although it can affect any bone in the body, those of the arms and legs are the most commonly affected. The infection may arise because of an injury to the bone itself, or it may be carried in the blood from an infected cut elsewhere in the body. Pus forms in the bone and the area becomes tender and painful. Within a day or two the skin over the bone swells, and, if left untreated, a pus-filled abscess will form on the skin's surface.

Is it serious?

Osteomyelitis is always serious and can result in bone deformity or stiffness.

Possible symptoms

▶ **Extreme pain and tenderness** over an affected bone, usually in the arms or legs.
▶ **Red, swollen area** after a day or two, which may develop into a pus-filled abscess.
▶ **Reluctance to use or move** the affected part.
▶ **Limping** if the infection is in a leg.
▶ **High temperature**.
▶ **Loss of appetite**.

What should I do first?

1 If your child suddenly complains of pain in a limb, try to find out whether he has knocked himself or suffered an injury to the affected part.

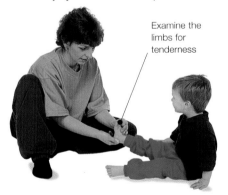

Examine the limbs for tenderness

2 Try to determine how painful the area is by pressing it gently and noting your child's reaction.

3 Take your child's temperature to find out whether he has a fever.

4 Put your child to bed to rest the affected part.

Should I consult the doctor?

Consult your doctor immediately if your child has a fever and is in great pain for no apparent reason.

What might the doctor do?

▶ Your doctor will probably admit your child to hospital for blood tests and X-rays to make a definite diagnosis. If osteomyelitis is confirmed, your child will be given antibiotics.
▶ If an abscess has formed, the pus-infected bone and skin will be cleaned out surgically under an anaesthetic. The cavity left behind may take some time to heal completely but new bone usually forms within six months.

What can I do to help?

If possible, try to stay with your child in hospital. When he is discharged, help him to exercise the affected limb according to instructions given by the hospital physiotherapist.

SEE ALSO:
Limp 176

Otitis externa

OTITIS EXTERNA IS AN INFECTION of the external ear canal – the passage that leads from the ear flap (pinna) to the eardrum. The infection may be caused by a foreign body in the ear, by a **boil** in the canal, or as the result of damage to the skin from over-vigorous cleaning or scratching. The infection is more common in children who swim a great deal. The symptoms of the infection are **earache**, inflammation, swelling, itchiness, dry, scaly skin or a discharge.

Is it serious?

As the external ear canal does not contain the ear's delicate hearing mechanisms, the infection is relatively minor. However, otitis externa should always be treated because the infection could spread to the bones of the skull. Any discharge from the ear should be treated seriously as this could be a symptom of the serious middle-ear infection, **otitis media**.

Possible symptoms

▶ **Earache**.
▶ **Redness and tenderness** of the ear flap and external ear canal.
▶ **Pus-filled boil** in the canal.

Area affected

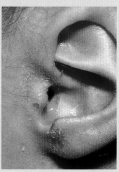

▶ **Discharge** from the ear.
▶ **Itchy, dry, scaly** ear.

What should I do first?

1 Look at the ear and into the external ear canal to check for any signs of infection or foreign objects. Remove the foreign object if you can do so easily.

2 Do not push or poke anything into your child's ear, and discourage him from touching or scratching it if it's sore.

3 Ask your child to open his mouth as wide as possible to see if this causes pain.

4 Pull back gently on the ear flap to see if this causes pain.

5 Clean away any discharge with warm water and soap.

6 Give your child a dose of paracetamol elixir to relieve pain, and place a cotton-wool pad over the ear to absorb any discharge.

Should I consult the doctor?

Consult your doctor as soon as possible if you notice any discharge from your child's ear or if you suspect infection of the external ear canal.

What might the doctor do?

▶ Your doctor will examine your child's ear with an otoscope and may then clean out the ear with a probe. He will probably prescribe antibiotic ear drops or tablets to clear up the infection.

Continued from previous page

▶ If there is still a foreign body in your child's ear, your doctor will remove it or refer your child to hospital for its removal.

▶ If the pain is the result of a boil, your doctor may lance it and drain the pus away; this will relieve the pain almost immediately.

What can I do to help?

▶ Give your child junior paracetamol tablets or paracetamol elixir on the advice of your doctor if the condition is still painful.

▶ Prevent water from entering the ear during bathing until the infection has cleared. Don't let your child go swimming.

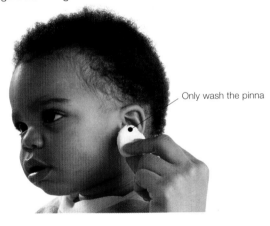

Only wash the pinna

▶ Don't interfere with your child's external ear canal. Wash around the pinna but never poke cotton-wool swabs into the area to clear wax, for example. Wax is not abnormal. It is a natural lubricant, keeping infection at bay. Any cotton wool or twisted piece of facecloth will only push the wax further into the canal or damage the lining, increasing the chances of infection.

▶ Never use patent eardrops unless your doctor advises them.

Otitis media

OTITIS MEDIA IS INFECTION of the middle ear. The infection causes fluid to build up in the middle ear, producing **earache** and sometimes **deafness**. It is common in young children because the tube connecting the throat with the ear, the Eustachian tube, is relatively short, and because children spend a lot of time lying down. This means that any bacteria or viruses that invade the nose or throat have only to make a short journey to reach the middle ear. The infection may also result when enlarged adenoids block the entrance to the Eustachian tube. If the tube is blocked, mucus will not be able to drain away and may become sticky and glue-like, producing a condition known as **glue ear**.

Is it serious?
Otitis media is both painful and serious. If left untreated it can result in permanent loss of hearing.

Possible symptoms
▶ **Severe pain in the ear**; in a baby, the pulling or rubbing of an ear accompanied by crying.
▶ **Temperature** of over 39°C (102.2°F).
▶ **Vomiting.**
▶ **Partial deafness.**
▶ **Pussy discharge** from the ear.

Cross-section of the ear

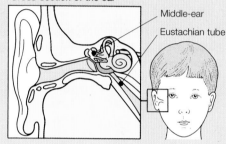

Middle-ear

Eustachian tube

What should I do first?

1 Take your child's temperature to establish whether he has a fever.

2 Keep your child comfortable and cool. If the pain in the ear is severe, a well-wrapped hot-water bottle placed against it may relieve the pain.

3 Give your child junior paracetamol tablets or elixir to relieve the earache.

4 Check for any discharge from the ear.

Should I consult the doctor?
Consult your doctor immediately if you suspect a middle-ear infection. Consult your doctor as soon as possible if you suspect any hearing loss.

What might the doctor do?
▶ Your doctor will examine your child's ear with an otoscope and will probably prescribe antibiotics to clear up the infection. If there is any build-up of fluid in the Eustachian tube, your doctor may also prescribe a drug to reduce swelling so that the fluid can drain away naturally down the throat.
▶ If the attacks are recurrent, your doctor will refer your child to an ear, nose and throat (ENT) specialist for assessment.

What can I do to help?
Check your child's hearing regularly (*see page 108*).

SEE ALSO:
Deafness 108
Earache 122
Glue ear 145

Paronychia

A PARONYCHIA IS AN INFECTION of the fold of the skin at the side of a fingernail or toenail. The bacteria that cause the infection are able to enter the skin if it is soggy because of prolonged immersion in water, or if the nail or adjacent skin is constantly picked at or bitten. While pus is building up in the nail fold the area will be painful.

Is it serious?

A paronychia is not serious and can be easily treated. Sometimes a fungus such as *Candida albicans*, which causes thrush, can complicate a paronychia and give rise to a chronic condition that has a greater risk of deformity and requires prolonged treatment.

Possible symptoms

▶ **Redness and swelling** around the nail fold.
▶ **Pus** under or next to the nail.
▶ **Throbbing pain**.

Area affected

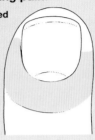

What should I do first?

1 If your child complains of a throbbing pain around a nail and you can see that pus has collected under the skin, don't try to let the pus out yourself – you may damage the nail bed.

2 Apply a warm compress or a pad of cotton wool soaked in warm water to bring the pus to a head. It should then burst or drain away naturally.

3 Protect the finger or toe from knocks with a thick pad of cotton wool and a plaster.

Should I consult the doctor?

Consult your doctor as soon as possible if the pus does not drain within a few hours of coming to a head, or if the pain is severe.

What might the doctor do?

▶ If pus has collected, your doctor will probably lance it and let the pus drain away. This is usually done under a local anaesthetic. Sometimes if the condition is severe, a small piece of nail has to be removed under anaesthetic to allow the pus to drain. This relieves the pain immediately.
▶ If there is an acute infection, your doctor will prescribe antibiotics to be taken by mouth, or in cream form to be spread on the nail, to eradicate the bacterial infection.
▶ If the paronychia fails to improve, your doctor may refer your child to a dermatologist to see whether or not there is a fungal infection. If so, your child may be prescribed anti-fungal cream or tablets.

What can I do to help?

▶ Keep your child's nails short and file any rough pieces that your child may bite to make smooth.
▶ Discourage your child from biting or picking at his nails or at the skin around the edge of the nails.

SEE ALSO:
Thrush 240

Penis caught in zip

THIS SITUATION MAY ARISE if your son is hurrying after going to the toilet, or is not paying attention to what he's doing when he gets dressed, and catches both skin and fabric in the teeth of the zip.

Is it serious?

There should be no serious complications, but the pain your child will be suffering means that you should treat this as an emergency.

What should I do first?

Don't touch the penis or the zip unless you are sure that you can separate the two quickly and easily. If your child will let you, place a cold compress, or ice cubes tied in a clean cloth, over the zip and penis. This should numb the area and relieve the pain while you get help.

Should I consult the doctor?

Consult your doctor immediately, or take your child to the nearest hospital.

What might the doctor do?

Your doctor will apply a local anaesthetic cream to your child's penis. Because this can be painful, try to distract your son's attention while it is being done. When the penis is thoroughly numb, your doctor will cut the bar of the zip allowing the rows of teeth to come apart.

What can I do to help?

▶ Apply a thin smear of antiseptic cream to the damaged penis three or four times a day to soothe the area and prevent infection. Let your child apply it himself, if he wants to.

▶ Leave the skin open to the air as much as possible to promote healing and prevent rubbing.

▶ Give your child a bowl of warm water to pour over his penis as he urinates to stop the stinging. He will probably complain that it is painful to pass urine for about 48 hours.

▶ Keep your child quiet and calm so that he doesn't accidentally knock himself. There will be bruising and swelling for about four or five days.

▶ Give your child paracetamol elixir if he is in pain.

Phimosis

PHIMOSIS IS THE NAME given to an abnormal tightness of the foreskin which prevents it from being drawn back over the tip of the penis. Phimosis can result in infections such as **balanitis** because the penis cannot be properly cleansed; it may also cause problems with urination and pain with erections. If the foreskin fails to loosen naturally, circumcision is usually recommended.

Is it serious?

Abnormal tightness of the foreskin after the age of five should be treated seriously because of the pain and discomfort it may cause, and because of the increased risk of infection.

Possible symptoms

- **Foreskin cannot be drawn back** over the tip of the penis.
- **Urine does not come out in a steady stream**; it either dribbles out slowly or the foreskin balloons with the pressure of the urine, which sprays out in all directions.

What should I do first?

Never attempt to force the foreskin back, especially if your child is under five years old.

Should I consult the doctor?

Consult your doctor as soon as possible if you are concerned about the condition or if the foreskin has not loosened naturally by the time your child is five or six years old. Consult your doctor as soon as possible if either you or your child have forced the foreskin back and it will not slide forwards again.

What might the doctor do?

- Your doctor may refer you to a surgeon for permanent correction of the condition by circumcision. Your child will be admitted to hospital, and the foreskin will be removed under a general anaesthetic. Your child will be discharged from hospital within 24 hours.
- Your doctor will return the foreskin to its normal position if it has been pulled back and won't return naturally.

What can I do to help?

- Try not to worry about the condition if your son is under five years old; it may correct itself in time.
- Make sure your child bathes frequently. A warm bath is the best way to keep an uncircumcised penis clean and to prevent infection. Retraction of the foreskin to clean the penis should not be necessary.
- If your child has just been circumcised, give him baths with a handful of salt in them twice a day for a couple of days to promote healing.
- Let him go about with no pants on – anything rubbing on a recently circumcised penis will make it sore.
- Give your newly circumcised child a bowl of warm water to pour over his penis when he urinates. There will be some pain urinating for about 48 hours after the circumcision operation.

SEE ALSO:
Balanitis 62

Pneumonia

PNEUMONIA IS THE TERM used to describe inflammation of the lungs. It may be caused by viral or bacterial infection, or by a foreign body which has been inhaled into the lungs. In young children, the occurrence of pneumonia is nearly always due to an upper respiratory infection such as a **common cold** or **influenza** spreading to the lungs. It can also be caused by **bronchitis** (when it is known as bronchopneumonia). Certain underlying conditions predispose to bronchopneumonia: these include **asthma**, **cystic fibrosis**, **whooping cough** and **measles**.

Older children may contract a type of pneumonia known as lobar pneumonia, where one or more of the lobes of the lungs may be infected by the *pneumococcus* bacterium. This form of pneumonia can start without warning, even when there is no other infection present.

The common symptom of all types of pneumonia is difficulty in breathing; with bronchopneumonia there will also be a noticeable deterioration of an existing illness and a high temperature.

Is it serious?

Pneumonia is always serious.

Possible symptoms

▶ **Difficulty in breathing**: the nostrils flare, the chest wall sinks with every breath, and efforts to breathe produce grunting sounds.
▶ **Dry cough**.
▶ **Fever**, up to 39°C (102.2°F).
▶ **Vomiting and diarrhoea**.
▶ **Pain in the chest**, made worse by deep breathing.

What should I do first?

1 If your child has an upper respiratory infection or an infectious illness and his condition worsens instead of getting better, look out for a dry cough and breathing difficulty.

2 Take your child's temperature to see if he has a **fever**. If he has, try to bring his temperature down with tepid sponging (*see page 31*).

3 Give your child plenty of fluids to prevent him becoming dehydrated.

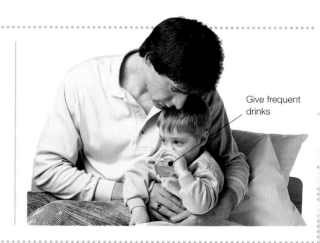

Give frequent drinks

Continued from previous page

Should I consult the doctor?

Consult your doctor immediately if your child's condition worsens and breathing becomes difficult. Any breathing problems in a child warrant immediate medical attention.

What might the doctor do?

▶ Your doctor will examine your child and he may prescribe antibiotics. If your doctor is in any doubt about the presence of pneumonia, your child may be sent to hospital so that he can be supervised and given a chest X-ray and oxygen if necessary.
▶ Your doctor will advise you about nursing procedures if your child is to be treated at home.

What can I do to help?

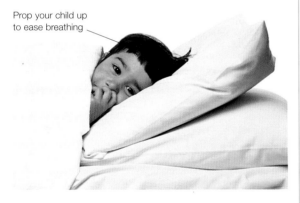

Prop your child up to ease breathing

▶ Prop your child up in bed; this may help his breathing.
▶ Keep the room moderately warm and well-ventilated, but not hot and stuffy.
▶ Give your child plenty of fluids. When he feels like eating, give him foods that are easy to digest such as yogurt, fruits and soups.
▶ If he is feverish and too lethargic to go to the bathroom for a wash, give him a sponge-down to refresh him.

SEE ALSO:
Asthma 58
Bronchitis 73
Common cold 90
Cystic fibrosis 106
Fever 134
Influenza 167
Measles 177
Whooping cough 261

Poliomyelitis

POLIOMYELITIS (POLIO) IS A VIRAL INFECTION of the spinal cord and nerves. Polio has the same symptoms as many other viral infections, with a **fever**, **sore throat**, **headache** and stiff neck. In many cases, the disease does not progress to paralysis and there is a complete recovery without polio even being suspected. If it does progress, however, there is, most commonly, paralysis of the lower limbs, making walking difficult or even impossible. The disease is carried in the stools of an infected person and can quickly reach epidemic proportions. It is now entirely preventable with an immunization course of three doses of a vaccine taken by mouth.

Possible symptoms

▶ **High temperature**, rising to 39°C (102.2°F).
▶ **Sore throat**.
▶ **Headache**.
▶ **Pain and stiffness** in the neck.
▶ **Vomiting**.
▶ **Weakness**.
▶ **Paralysis of muscles**, usually in the lower limbs, or in the chest, causing breathlessness.

Is it serious?

Polio is always serious. If it is not diagnosed and progresses, permanent paralysis will occur.

What should I do first?

If you know of any cases of polio in your community, be on the alert if you notice that your child has the symptoms of influenza with a stiff and painful neck and a fever.

Should I consult the doctor?

Consult your doctor immediately if your child has 'flu-like symptoms and then has difficulty in moving his limbs or becomes breathless – even if he has been immunized against polio.

What might the doctor do?

▶ Your doctor will admit your child to hospital for assessment if polio is suspected. Absolute quiet and bed-rest are the only treatments for polio, since antibiotics have no effect on viral illness. Your child may be returned home if you can manage the special nursing he will require.

▶ If your child is nursed at home, your doctor and physiotherapist will advise you about the diet and exercise regime your child should follow.

What can I do to help?

Immunize your baby against polio within the first year of life. (The polio vaccine is given with the "triple vaccine", DTP, on the standard immunization schedule.) Even though polio is no longer the menace it once was, there is no reason for complacency. Risks from the vaccine are virtually unknown.

SEE ALSO:
Fever 134
Headache 156
Influenza 167
Sore throat 222

Pyloric stenosis

PYLORIC STENOSIS IS A CONGENITAL CONDITION – that is, it is present at birth. The ring of muscle (*pylorus*) which links the stomach to the duodenum thickens and narrows, preventing the contents of the stomach from passing through it to the intestine. The cause of this is not known, but when the baby is about one month old the symptoms begin. Food builds up in the stomach, which contracts powerfully in an attempt to force the food through the thickened pylorus. Because this is impossible, milk is vomited up violently after a feed. This is known as projectile vomiting, and the unpleasant-smelling milk curds and mucus can be thrown a metre or two (up to two yards) away. Projectile vomiting should not be confused with possetting, in which a baby naturally regurgitates milk after a feed.

Is it serious?

Pyloric stenosis is serious. The vomiting eventually leads to **dehydration** and a failure to thrive.

Possible symptoms

▶ **Projectile vomiting** after a feed, beginning at around four weeks of age.
▶ **Failure to thrive**.
▶ **Weakness and listlessness**.
▶ **Lack of bowel movements**.

Cross-section of the pylorus

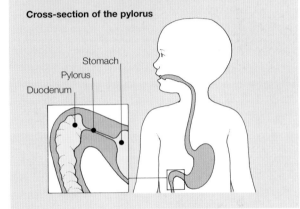

Stomach
Pylorus
Duodenum

What should I do first?

1 If your baby vomits violently after three consecutive feeds, consult your doctor immediately.

2 While you are waiting for medical attention, feed your baby frequent but small amounts of milk to keep up his fluid levels.

Should I consult the doctor?

Consult your doctor immediately if your baby vomits violently after every feed.

What might the doctor do?

▶ If pyloric stenosis is suspected, your doctor will refer your baby to hospital. A paediatrician will examine your baby's abdomen during a feed to see if the enlarged pylorus can be felt.
▶ A simple surgical operation to widen the thickened pylorus will be performed, giving a complete cure.

What can I do to help?

Stay with your baby in hospital. After the operation you will be advised to feed your baby gradually increasing amounts of milk. Forty-eight hours after the operation, his feeding routine should be back to normal.

SEE ALSO:
Dehydration 109
Vomiting 257

Rash

A SKIN RASH CAN BE A SYMPTOM of infection, either in the skin or elsewhere. It can also be an allergic reaction to something on the skin, or a reaction to an irritating chemical or to physical damage.

Many childhood infectious diseases, including **chickenpox**, **German measles** and **measles**, have a rash as one of their main symptoms. Localized rashes may be the result of a skin infestation by **scabies** mites or **ringworm** fungus. A child who is allergic to a drug may break out in a rash when he takes the drug. Nettles and certain other plants cause a rash on contact with the skin. Babies may suffer from heat rash, milk rash, **nappy rash** and sweat rash.

The skin condition known as purpura looks like a rash and is usually the result of a serious disorder, such as **leukaemia** or **hepatitis**. It can also indicate a disorder of the capillaries and meningococcal **meningitis**. If there is a problem with the blood's clotting mechanism, tiny areas of bleeding tend to occur in the skin. These look like small, spidery "spots", but they do not itch. There are no other skin changes.

Purpuric marks can be distinguished from other rashes by pressing the side of a drinking glass gently on them; if the marks are still visible, this indicates purpura. A purpuric rash may be brought on by infection or sensitivity to certain drugs.

Is it serious?

Skin rashes themselves are hardly ever serious, although they may be irritating. However, you should never ignore a rash, particularly a purpuric rash, since it may indicate a serious underlying illness or a sensitivity to a drug.

What should I do first?

1 Note where the rash occurs on your child's body, and whether it has spread from one area to another. He could have one of the common infections, such as chickenpox, measles or German measles.

2 Take his temperature to see if he has a fever.

3 Check whether your child has eaten something for the first time, such as shellfish or strawberries, or whether he has started a course of medicine, such as penicillin, for example.

4 Check whether your child has any symptoms of infestation, especially if his skin is very itchy between the fingers. This could indicate scabies.

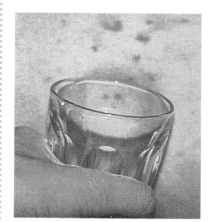

Test for purpura

5 Press a drinking glass against your child's skin to see if the rash remains visible; the rash could be purpuric.

6 If the rash is itchy, use calamine lotion to relieve the irritation.

Continued from previous page

Should I consult the doctor?

Consult your doctor as soon as possible for an accurate diagnosis of your child's rash. Consult your doctor immediately if the rash is purpuric and your child has a fever: these two symptoms together could indicate meningitis.

What might the doctor do?

❱ Your doctor will examine your child carefully to determine the cause of the rash, which will then be treated accordingly.

❱ If the rash is purpuric, your doctor will arrange for a blood test to determine the cause.

What can I do to help?

❱ If the rash is itchy, baths with a handful of bicarbonate of soda added to the water will ease the irritation.

❱ Keep your child's skin cool to reduce irritation.

❱ Discourage your child from scratching the rash. Keep his hands clean and his nails short to prevent damage to the skin if he does scratch it.

Reye's syndrome

REYE'S SYNDROME IS A CHILDHOOD ILLNESS in which the child suddenly becomes ill with **vomiting** and **fever**. The body's reaction to the illness causes the brain to become inflamed, so your affected child may also become delirious and even lapse into unconsciousness and then a coma. Reye's syndrome usually occurs a few days after a child has had **chickenpox** or **influenza**, and it is particularly associated with these illnesses when aspirin was used to relieve symptoms, or to reduce temperature.

The cause of Reye's syndrome is only now becoming clear: a virus or some other poisonous agent damages cells in various parts of the body. However, only certain children seem susceptible. It is thought that susceptibility may be related to the body's inability to deal with certain chemical substances, especially fats.

Is it serious?

Reye's syndrome is very serious and can result in death if it is not identified quickly. It is, however, rare.

Possible symptoms

▶ **Uncontrollable vomiting**.
▶ **Fever**.
▶ **Delirium**.
▶ **Drowsiness or unconsciousness**.

What should I do first?

1 If your child is recovering from chickenpox or influenza and he starts to vomit, take his temperature to see if he has a fever.

2 If he does have a fever, consult your doctor immediately. While waiting for medical help, *do not* give him any form of aspirin. Try tepid sponging (*see page 31*) to lower his temperature.

3 Consult your doctor immediately if your child has been vomiting and subsequently becomes drowsy or difficult to rouse.

Should I consult the doctor?

Consult your doctor immediately, or call an ambulance if there is any delay, if your child has a fever or has become drowsy and difficult to rouse.

What might the doctor do?

▶ If your doctor suspects Reye's syndrome, he will admit your child to hospital immediately. Usually many tests are necessary to confirm the diagnosis but, if there is any doubt, the doctor will remove a tiny piece of liver under local anaesthetic, using a hollow needle (a procedure called a liver biopsy). This sample will then be analysed for abnormal fat distribution, which is characteristic of the illness.
▶ Your child will be treated in an intensive care unit and given intravenous glucose. Various measures will be taken to control swelling of the brain.

What can I do to help?

▶ Stay with your child in hospital if possible.
▶ Be prepared for a long convalescence. Ask about any special precautions that should be taken to avoid a recurrence of the syndrome.

Rheumatic fever

RHEUMATIC FEVER IS A RARE DISEASE characterized by inflammation of the joints and the heart. It is caused by an allergic response to streptococcal bacteria, which exist in the throat, where they cause such infections as **tonsillitis**.

Rheumatic fever usually begins within a week or two of a throat or ear infection (for example, **otitis media**) and produces symptoms of general ill health, with fever and aching joints. In some cases there may be a circular, blotchy red rash on the trunk and limbs. Rheumatic fever is now less common because streptococcal infections are usually treated with antibiotics at an early stage.

Is it serious?

Rheumatic fever can have serious consequences. The earlier the treatment, the less likelihood there is of any heart disease in later life.

Possible symptoms

▸ **Fever**.
▸ **Swollen, painful joints**.
▸ **Blotchy, circular rash** on the trunk and limbs.
▸ **Chest pain**.
▸ **Listlessness**.
▸ **Loss of appetite**.

Areas affected

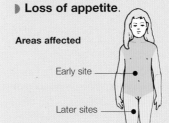

Early site

Later sites

What should I do first?

1 If your child has recently had tonsillitis or an ear infection, and complains of pain in his joints when he should be getting better, check to see if he has a fever.

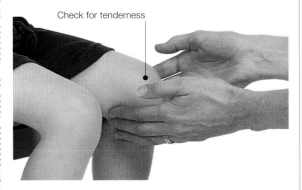

Check for tenderness

2 Feel for swelling and tenderness by pressing on and around the major joints.

3 Look for a circular rash on your child's trunk and limbs.

Should I consult the doctor?

Consult your doctor immediately if you suspect rheumatic fever.

What might the doctor do?

▸ Your doctor will admit your child to hospital for bed-rest and medication.
▸ After he has recovered, your child will be given penicillin for many years to prevent a recurrence of rheumatic fever.

SEE ALSO:
Otitis media 198
Sore throat 222
Tonsillitis 243

Ringworm

RINGWORM IS A FUNGAL INFECTION of the skin and hair that shows itself as bald patches in the hair, and as round, reddish or grey scaly patches on the skin. As the infection spreads, the edges of the ring remain scaly, and the centre begins to look more like normal skin. Ringworm is a condition that is usually contracted from animals, such as a household pet, or from other infected humans.

Is it serious?
Though not a serious disorder, ringworm is unattractive and irritating. Ringworm is also contagious and must therefore be treated promptly.

Possible symptoms
▶ **Red or grey scaly rings** on any part of the body, particularly in warm, moist areas, and on the scalp, where they produce bald patches.
▶ **Itchiness** in the ringed areas.

What should I do first?

1 If your child is scratching, check all over his body for the distinctive rings of ringworm.

2 Do not try to treat it yourself and wash your hands after examining your child. Discourage him from touching the infected areas.

3 Keep your child away from school until you have visited the doctor.

Should I consult the doctor?
Consult your doctor as soon as possible as ringworm is contagious as well as irritating for your child.

What might the doctor do?
Your doctor will prescribe an anti-fungal cream for the skin and oral anti-fungal medicine (tablets or liquid) for the scalp and hair. The tablets will have to be taken for at least four weeks.

What can I do to help?
▶ Throw out any brushes, combs or headgear your child may have used while infected. Disinfectant will not destroy the fungi.
▶ Keep your child's facecloth and towel separate from those of the rest of the family to avoid spreading the infection.
▶ If your pet is a possible source of ringworm, take it to the vet for treatment as soon as possible.
▶ Ringworm on the skin clears up quickly, but treatment of the scalp may take a couple of weeks. Get your child some form of headgear to hide the bald patches if he is bothered by them.
▶ Always make sure that you and your child wash your hands carefully before and after touching the affected areas.

SEE ALSO:
Hair loss 151
Itching 170

Roseola infantum

ROSEOLA INFANTUM IS A RELATIVELY common viral infection which causes **fever** and a **rash** in young children; it is contagious, and has symptoms that may be mistaken for **scarlet fever**. It starts with the sudden onset of a high fever which lasts for three days. As the fever subsides, a rash of flat red or pink spots appears, first on the torso, then spreading to the limbs and neck. The rash fades after about 48 hours with no other side effects.

Is it serious?

Roseola infantum is not a serious condition, though the temperature can rise high enough to cause a febrile **convulsion**.

Possible symptoms

▶ **Fever** with temperature of 39–40°C (102.2–104°F) for three days, with no apparent symptoms.

Sites of rash

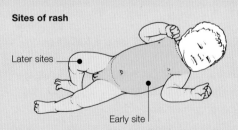

Later sites

Early site

▶ **Rash** of separate, flat red or pink spots, which appears first on the trunk, then spreads to the limbs and neck, after the fever has subsided.

What should I do first?

1 Check your child's temperature. If it is high, try to reduce it with tepid sponging (*see page 31*).

2 Note where the rash starts and to which parts of the body it spreads.

Should I consult the doctor?

Consult your doctor as soon as possible for a definite diagnosis of the condition. Consult your doctor immediately if your child's temperature fails to come down after 48 hours, or if your child has a febrile convulsion.

What might the doctor do?

▶ There is no specific treatment for viral illnesses, only treatments for the symptoms. Your doctor will advise you on how to reduce your child's fever and will recommend that you keep your child in bed until the rash appears.
▶ If your child has had a febrile convulsion before, your doctor may prescribe drugs to prevent possible convulsions.

What can I do to help?

Take your child's temperature at regular intervals. If it rises, try to bring it down, first by tepid sponging or, if this fails, by paracetamol elixir.

SEE ALSO:
Convulsion 94
Fever 134
Rash 206
Scarlet fever 213

Scabies

SCABIES IS AN IRRITATING, ITCHY RASH caused by a tiny mite. The burrowing and egg-laying of these mites produce a rash which nearly always affects the hands and fingers, particularly the clefts between the fingers. It may also affect the ankles, feet, toes, elbows and the area around the genitals. When the eggs hatch, they are easily passed to another person by direct contact. They can also be picked up from bedding or linen that is infested with the mites.

Is it serious?

Scabies is not serious but it is a contagious condition and could run through a family or a school class if not treated promptly.

Possible symptoms

▶ **Intense itchiness**.

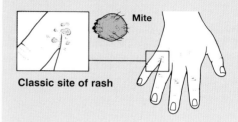

Classic site of rash

▶ **Fine, short lines** that end in a black spot the size of a pinhead, most often found between the fingers.
▶ **Scabs** on the itchy areas.

What should I do first?

1 If your child is scratching a lot, look for the fine lines of the mites' burrows.

2 If you suspect scabies, keep your child away from school until you have administered the treatment prescribed by your doctor.

3 Try to discourage your child from scratching. This may hinder the doctor's diagnosis and cause sores to form that could become infected.

Should I consult the doctor?

Consult your doctor as soon as possible if you suspect scabies or if your child is scratching a lot.

What might the doctor do?

Your doctor will prescribe a lotion in sufficient quantity for the whole family to be treated.

What can I do to help?

▶ After thorough washing, you should paint the whole body below the neck with the lotion and leave to dry. Do not wash it off for 24 hours. To ensure disinfestation, repeat the procedure for a further 24 hours in a day or two.
▶ Carry out the treatment for other members of the family simultaneously.
▶ Launder or air all bedding and clothing to eradicate the mite. The mite does not live for longer than five or six days after it is removed from human skin.

SEE ALSO:
Itching 170
Rash 206

Scarlet fever

SCARLET FEVER IS ONE OF THE LESS common infectious diseases of childhood, even though it is caused by the widespread streptococcus bacterium (the same bacterium that causes **tonsillitis**). Scarlet fever is similar to tonsillitis, except that it produces a rash as well as a **sore throat**. The incubation period is one to five days, after which the symptoms manifest themselves. After three days of a sore throat, inflamed tonsils, **fever**, **vomiting** and possibly abdominal pains because of swollen glands near the bowel, a rash of small spots that merge with one another appears on the chest and neck, and then the whole body. The rash may be itchy but is distinctive because it does not affect the area surrounding the mouth. The tongue may also be red and furry. The rash fades after five days, but the skin flakes off for up to two weeks.

Is it serious?

Scarlet fever is rarely serious. However if your child is sensitive to the bacterium the infection can cause inflammation of the kidneys (**nephritis**) or of the joints and heart (**rheumatic fever**). However, these complications are rare.

Possible symptoms

▶ **Sore throat**.
▶ **Inflamed tonsils**.
▶ **Fever**, as high as 40°C (104°F).
▶ **Vomiting**.
▶ **Abdominal pains**.

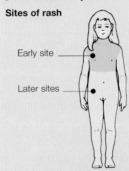

Sites of rash

Early site

Later sites

▶ **Rash of small spots** starting on the chest and neck, then merging together over the whole body, except the area around the mouth.
▶ **Strawberry-red patches** on a furry tongue.

What should I do first?

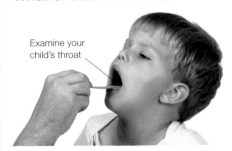

Examine your child's throat

1 Check your child's throat to see if the tonsils are red and swollen (*see page 243*). Check his tongue to see if it is furry with bright red patches.

2 Check your child's temperature to see if he has a fever. If he has, put him to bed and try to bring his temperature down with tepid sponging (*see page 31*).

3 Give your child plenty of cool drinks as well as giving paracetamol elixir to soothe his throat if he is in pain.

Should I consult the doctor?

Consult your doctor as soon as possible if you suspect scarlet fever.

Continued on next page

Continued from previous page

What might the doctor do?

Your doctor will prescribe antibiotics to minimize the severity of the illness and prevent complications. Your doctor will advise you about the complications that can follow a streptococcal infection, so that if certain symptoms occur after your child should have recovered you can consult your doctor immediately.

What can I do to help?

▶ Bed-rest is not usually necessary but keep your child warm and quiet.

▶ Scarlet fever is not generally a severe illness and your child should be well enough to return to school seven days after the onset of the symptoms.

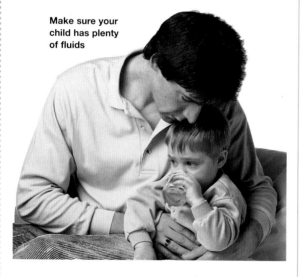

Make sure your child has plenty of fluids

▶ Give your child plenty of fluids if he has lost his appetite, or if he has a sore throat that makes swallowing painful.

▶ Liquidize his foods if this makes swallowing easier for him.

SEE ALSO:
Fever 134
Nephritis 189
Rheumatic fever 209
Sore throat 222
Tonsillitis 243
Vomiting 257

Scoliosis

SCOLIOSIS IS A SIDEWAYS CURVATURE of the spine, very often so slight that it is not observed until a child is approaching adolescence. The spinal deformity may be present from birth; it may be the result of injury to, or a weakness of, muscles in the back such as that caused by **muscular dystrophy**; or it may be the result of infection such as **tuberculosis** (now extremely rare) affecting the spine. Scoliosis can also develop at any time in otherwise perfectly healthy children and may be triggered off by a fast growth spurt, by one leg being longer than the other, or by poor posture. The condition is much more common in girls than in boys.

Is it serious?
Scoliosis should always be treated seriously. Early diagnosis is necessary to prevent deformity. Untreated, the condition can also affect the lungs, resulting in breathing difficulties.

Possible symptoms

▶ Looked at from behind, **one shoulder is slightly lower than the other**.
▶ **Lopsidedness** when your child bends forward.

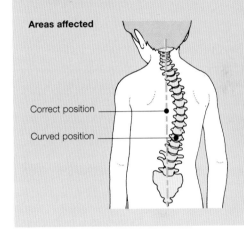

Areas affected

Correct position

Curved position

What should I do first?
Ask your child to stand up straight with his heels together, then to bend forward from the waist. If there is a curvature, your child's back will remain curved sideways.

Should I consult the doctor?
Consult your doctor as soon as possible if you suspect scoliosis.

What might the doctor do?
▶ Your doctor may refer your child to an orthopaedic specialist who will monitor the curvature. Depending on the severity of the condition, the specialist may decide that it is necessary for your child to wear a back brace, perhaps for 23 hours a day, until he has stopped growing.

▶ Physiotherapy may be used to correct posture.

What can I do to help?
▶ Seek help from a scoliosis self-help group in your area; your doctor may be able to give you an address. If your child has to wear a brace, this can be a frightening experience. Communication with other parents experienced in coping with the problem may help.
▶ Treat the condition as casually as possible. Don't draw attention to it.

SEE ALSO:
Muscular dystrophy
186
Tuberculosis 249

Sickle cell anaemia

SICKLE CELL ANAEMIA IS AN inherited condition caused by an abnormal form of haemoglobin in the blood. The inheritance is recessive; that is, both parents carry an abnormal gene but are themselves healthy. The risk of a child having sickle cell anaemia in such a family is one in four. The anaemia that results from the blood condition is not present at birth, but develops in the first six months.

Haemoglobin is the protein contained in red cells in the blood. Its function is to pick up oxygen from the blood and carry it to various parts of the body. Sickle cell anaemia occurs when the inherited haemoglobin causes the red blood cells to become sickle-shaped as a result of abnormally low oxygen levels. In a child with this condition the blood flows through the blood vessels less smoothly than in a normal child. If the blood clogs the vessels, your child will experience pain in the area of the blockage, a worsening of anaemia, **jaundice** and an increased susceptibility to infections such as coughs and colds. People of African descent are most prone to this disease.

Possible symptoms

▶ **Anaemia**.
▶ **Fatigue**.
▶ **Mild jaundice** – yellowing of the whites of the eyes.
▶ **Pain in the limbs and abdomen**, wherever blockages occur in the blood vessels.
▶ **Susceptibility to infection**.

What can I do to help?

Sickle cell anaemia does not affect a child's intelligence, and most children with this condition can attend ordinary schools. However, as your child may suffer an acute attack (known as a crisis) at school, when he will have severe joint and abdominal pain, his teachers should be alerted to the need to get immediate medical attention for him, if necessary.

A sickle crisis can be precipitated by strenuous activity, particularly in the cold and damp. It will be treated with painkilling drugs. It is essential for your child to be fully immunized against all infectious diseases and to take any prescribed vitamin supplements. Affected children should take penicillin regularly to prevent certain bacterial infections. As the condition is inherited, it is important for potential carriers to seek genetic counselling before deciding to have a baby. A blood test will show if the prospective parents are carriers of the disease.

For help and advice contact the Sickle Cell Society (see page 324).

Sinusitis

SINUSITIS IS AN INFECTION OF the cheek and forehead sinuses. These are air-filled spaces grouped around the eyes and nose which make the skull bones light, and give the voice resonance. Infections of the sinuses are rare in babies because their sinuses are not fully developed, but in older children some degree of sinusitis often accompanies a **common cold**, **cough** or **sore throat**.

Because the sinuses are lined by the same mucous membrane as the nose, and are connected to the upper throat, infection in these areas can be easily spread to them. The sinuses also drain through small holes into the nose and, when your child has a cold, the possibility of these holes becoming blocked and infected increases. A yellow-green discharge from the nose is often the sign that your child has sinusitis.

Is it serious?

Sinusitis is not serious although it can become chronic if not treated efficiently and quickly.

Possible symptoms

▶ **Yellow-green discharge of pus** from the nose where previously there was a clear, runny discharge.
▶ **Pain** over the cheeks.
▶ **Pain** on moving the head.
▶ **Slight fever**.
▶ **Blocked nose**.

Affected areas

Frontal sinuses

Maxillary sinuses

What should I do first?

1 If your child has a cold, cough or a sore throat, watch out for a change in the colour of his nasal discharge.

2 Check to see if there is a **foreign body** lodged in your child's nose. The discharge will then be foul-smelling and stained with blood. Seek medical help immediately if you cannot easily remove the object.

3 If the cause is not a foreign object, relieve your child's blocked nose by giving him an inhalation of menthol crystals dissolved in boiling water. Take care that your child doesn't knock over the bowl and scald himself.

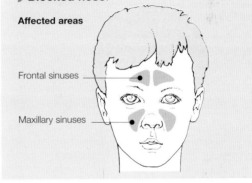

Give menthol inhalations

Continued on next page

Continued from previous page

Should I consult the doctor?

Consult your doctor as soon as possible if the yellow-green nasal discharge continues for more than two days.

What might the doctor do?

▶ Your doctor will prescribe antibiotics to eradicate the infection. He may also prescribe special nose drops for your child to take whenever he has a cold, so that the sinuses keep draining, thus preventing a recurrence of sinusitis.

▶ If the infection persists, your child will be prescribed a prolonged course of antibiotics to prevent the sinusitis from becoming chronic.

▶ If sinusitis is recurrent, your doctor will refer your child to an ear, nose and throat specialist to see whether surgical draining of the sinuses is indicated.

What can I do to help?

▶ If your child complains of a headache or fever, give him paracetamol elixir.

▶ Continue giving your child menthol inhalations to relieve the symptoms of sinusitis.

▶ Don't overheat your child's bedroom. Try to keep the air cool and humid because a dry atmosphere makes the symptoms of sinusitis worse.

Sleeplessness

SLEEPLESSNESS MAY BE A PROBLEM for parents when their child is very young. Your baby may sleep a less than normal amount from the first weeks of life: 12 hours instead of the accepted norm of 16–20 out of 24. These 12 hours may be taken in short, unpredictable bursts so that you never have more than a few hours' consecutive sleep yourself. Sleepless babies are usually full of life, interested in everything that's going on, affectionate and sociable. As long as your baby is happy and cheerful when he's awake, he is normal and does not need medical attention.

The sleep patterns of toddlers can be very different. Some need to sleep for an hour or two during the day until they are four or five years old, while others need no daytime nap, and sleep only eight hours at night and wake early in the morning. Usually, however, a child that needed little sleep as a baby needs little sleep as a toddler. Providing a child can cope with school work and normal daily routine and is cheerful and bright, the sleep he takes is the amount of sleep he needs.

Is it serious?

Sleeplessness – that is, less than eight hours in a 24-hour day – is hardly ever serious, though it may seem serious and disruptive to parents.

What should I do first?

1 Face up to the fact of your baby's relative sleeplessness and sort out a shift system for the first months so that you and your partner don't become overtired.

2 If your baby wakes and cries in the night, go to him, comfort him and be cheerful. Try not to pick him up and take him into bed with you straight away, unless you think he is ill or frightened. If he continues to cry or call out, stay with him for a while so that he doesn't feel you are deserting him.

3 Have plenty of toys and books and a drink by your toddler's bed so that he can entertain himself if he wakes early.

Should I consult the doctor?

Consult your doctor as soon as possible if you are exhausted and the sleepless nights are affecting you or your baby's health. Your health visitor can also be an excellent source of support and advice.

What might the doctor do?

If your baby is fit and well, but you are not, your doctor may prescribe a sedative for your baby to give you a break and to try to get him into a more established sleep routine.

What can I do to help?

▶ Make sure your baby's room is warm and snug.
▶ Try not to become resentful about your baby's wakefulness. Accept it as a fact of life and take practical steps to make sure you get enough sleep yourself. Sleep whenever your baby sleeps, get friends round to help look after the baby and look for support groups in your area.
▶ Take your baby to bed with you if you really want to; there is no danger of spoiling your baby by doing this.
▶ Never use bed as a punishment with an older child. Sleeping will then be associated with punishment, and this will make your child even less willing to go to bed.
▶ Never give your baby or child a sedative without your doctor's advice.

Sleepwalking

Sleepwalking, when a child wanders about the house while asleep, is a sort of "mobile dreaming". A sleepwalking child does not walk about with his eyes closed and his arms held straight out in front of him as is popularly supposed. His eyes will be open but he will be asleep; he won't see you and won't understand anything you say to him. Many children go through a short phase of sleepwalking but this soon passes. Sleepwalking may be associated with **nightmares** if your child is unduly troubled about something. If he has had frequent nightmares and you have tried to ignore them, he may be walking in his sleep to find you and seek reassurance.

Is it serious?

Sleepwalking is not serious unless your child is in physical danger, for example, from falling down a stairway or walking into a glass door.

What should I do first?

If you find your child sleepwalking, don't try to waken him. Instead, lead him slowly and gently back to bed.

Should I consult the doctor?

There is no need to consult your doctor unless sleepwalking becomes very frequent and you need reassurance that nothing is seriously wrong.

What might the doctor do?

▶ Your doctor will question you about the frequency and nature of your child's sleepwalking and will ask you if he has had any nightmares.
▶ Your doctor may recommend that you and your child speak to a child psychiatrist to help to find the cause of the problem if your child is sleepwalking frequently.

What can I do to help?

▶ Protect your child – for instance, by putting a barrier at the top of the stairway at night, and by making sure that no windows are left open.
▶ Try to reassure your child if you think you know the underlying cause of the sleepwalking.

SEE ALSO:
Nightmares 190

Snake bite

ANY BITE FROM A SNAKE, whether poisonous or not, will be extremely frightening for your child. In Britain, the only poisonous snake is the adder, recognizable by the zig-zag markings along its back. It is important to note the snake's markings wherever possible so that the correct anti-venom can be administered.

Is it serious?

A snake bite should always be treated as serious. Prompt treatment is necessary in case the bite was from a poisonous snake. However, deaths from snake bites are rare, even in countries where there are many poisonous snakes.

Possible symptoms

▶ **Swelling and pain** at the site of the bite.
▶ One or two **puncture marks**.
▶ **Pain or numbness** spreading through the rest of the limb.

What should I do first?

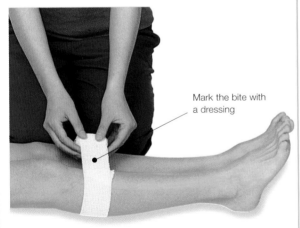

Mark the bite with a dressing

1 Clean the skin around the puncture mark and place a dressing over it. This will help to identify the wound when you get to hospital.

2 Get your child to the nearest hospital. If possible, lay your child down flat as you do so. Don't move or raise the affected part above the level of the heart; this will only spread the venom into the bloodstream more quickly.

3 Keep your child calm and still, and warm if she seems clammy and pale.

4 Don't apply a tourniquet or suck out the poison in cases of snake bite. This is now thought to be inadvisable.

Should I consult the doctor?

Take your child to the nearest hospital or call an ambulance if your child has been bitten by a snake.

What might the doctor do?

▶ Your child will be given an anti-venom injection if the snake was recognized as, or is thought to be, poisonous.
▶ Your child will be given a tetanus booster, if this is necessary.

What can I do to help?

▶ Give your child paracetamol elixir to ease the pain.
▶ If you are in an area where poisonous snakes are prevalent, seek advice as to whether you should keep an emergency anti-venom kit at home.

Sore throat

A SORE THROAT IS USUALLY A SYMPTOM of an infection of the respiratory tract. While a baby or young child may not be able to tell you about the raw feeling in his throat, you will notice that he has difficulty swallowing. Sore throats can occur because of inflammation of the tonsils (**tonsillitis**), caused by the *streptococcus* bacterium, or more usually by a virus, such as the **common cold** or **influenza**. If there is inflammation elsewhere, as there is in the larynx when your child has **laryngitis**, this can also give a raw feeling in the throat. If the glands in the neck are swollen, with **mumps**, for example, this may be felt by your child as pain in the throat.

Is it serious?

Most sore throats are not serious. However, if your child is allergic to the streptococcus bacterium and he has a streptococcal infection in the throat, this could have effects elsewhere in his body. Possible serious complications include **nephritis** and **rheumatic fever**.

What should I do first?

1 If your child complains of a sore throat, or if he has difficulty swallowing and is off his food, examine his throat in a good light, with his head held back and the tongue depressed gently with the handle of a clean spoon. Ask him to say a long "aaah". This will open up the throat so that you can see if there is any inflammation or if the tonsils are enlarged.

2 Run your fingers down either side of your child's neck and under his chin to check for any swelling in the glands – the glands will feel like large peas under the skin.

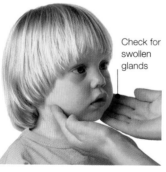

Check for swollen glands

3 Take your child's temperature to establish whether he has a **fever**.

4 If your child has a sore throat and is otherwise unwell, keep him away from school until you have seen your doctor.

Should I consult the doctor?

Consult your doctor if your child has a sore throat and other symptoms of illness or if the sore throat persists for more than a few days. Streptococcal infections of the throat should be treated promptly to avoid complications.

What might the doctor do?

Your doctor will examine your child to determine the cause of the sore throat. If it is a streptococcus bacterium, your doctor will prescribe antibiotics.

What can I do to help?

▶ Give your child paracetamol elixir to ease the pain.
▶ Soothe your child's sore throat with cold drinks or hot lemon drinks.
▶ Give your child plenty of liquids. If he isn't eating because it hurts to swallow, liquidize foods where possible.

Spina bifida

IN A CHILD BORN WITH SPINA BIFIDA, the bones of the spine (the vertebrae), which normally protect the spinal column, fail to join up properly, leaving a gap, so that in extreme cases the nerves of the spinal column are exposed. The condition most commonly affects the lower region of the spine and can be relatively minor – with just a dimple, or a brown, hairy mole growing from the bottom of the spine – or very serious, when the spinal cord is underdeveloped and the gap in the spine is covered by a large red membrane instead of skin. The symptoms reflect the severity of the condition. These may range from no symptoms at all, except for the skin markings, to complete paralysis of the lower limbs and incontinence. With a moderate to severe form of spina bifida, the development and function of your child's lower body will never be quite normal and he may be physically stunted, and walk with a limp. Nine out of 10 spina bifida babies also have **hydrocephalus** – a condition in which excessive fluid accumulates in the brain. Spina bifida is one of the most common congenital disorders.

Possible symptoms

▶ **Part of the spinal cord exposed**.
▶ **Dimple or brown, hairy mole** at the base of the spine.
▶ **Swelling** over part of the spine – covered by skin or large red membrane.
▶ **Paralysis** of the lower body.
▶ **Excessively large head**.
▶ **Incontinence**.

What can be done?

Severe cases of spina bifida are recognized at birth. The degree and extent of paralysis will be assessed as soon as possible by a paediatrician, and a brain scan will be performed to see if excessive fluid is present on the brain. In very severe cases, the paediatrician may have to tell the parents that their child will be paralysed below the waist, and that there could be mental retardation as well. Surgery can be carried out to correct the skin defect and prevent infection, but this will not restore function to the spinal cord. A drainage-valve operation can also be performed to control the hydrocephalus. If no action is taken in such severe cases, the babies usually die peacefully within weeks of birth.

Less severe cases are referred for surgery and then a programme of rehabilitation and physiotherapy. Checks will be made at frequent intervals on bladder control, kidney function and hip-joint development.

If there is a family history of spina bifida, it is important to make a special search for this during pregnancy. This can be done by ultrasound scanning and by measuring the alphafetoprotein levels in the mother's blood and, if necessary, in the amniotic fluid. If the tests are positive, you will be given the option of terminating the pregnancy.

Folic acid in the diet has been shown to reduce the risk of spina bifida and is recommended to women who are pregnant or planning a pregnancy.

For help and advice contact the Association for Spina Bifida and Hydrocephalus (ASBAH) (see page 324).

Splinter

A SPLINTER IS A TINY SLITHER of material that becomes embedded in or under the skin. It may be wood, metal, glass, a thorn or a prickle. Generally, it is hardly ever necessary to get medical help; most splinters can be removed at home.

Is it serious?

A splinter is rarely serious. However, splinters that cause deep wounds, particularly if they do not bleed much, can be serious because they carry the risk of **tetanus** infection.

What should I do first?

1 Find out, if possible, what material is embedded in the skin. If it is glass, the entire surface of the splinter will be capable of cutting into your child's flesh, so don't try to remove it yourself; seek medical aid.

2 If the splinter is not of glass and the end is sticking out of the skin, remove it with tweezers. Sterilize them first by passing the ends through a flame. Allow them to cool, then distract your child so that he doesn't flinch too much when you gently pull out the splinter.

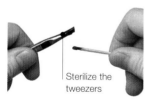

3 If the splinter is under the skin, sterilize a sewing needle with a flame or by standing it in surgical spirit or antiseptic lotion for a few minutes.

Sterilize the tweezers

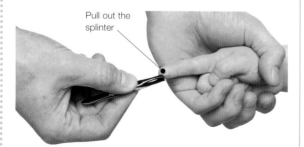

Pull out the splinter

4 Place a piece of ice over the splinter area so that the skin is lightly numbed, then use the sterile needle to gently break the skin's surface and expose the splinter. Once the end of the splinter is free, pull it out with a sterilized pair of tweezers.

5 Clean the area with soap and water and apply an antiseptic cream. Don't put a plaster on unless your child asks for one.

6 If you experience any difficulty while trying to remove a splinter, abandon the attempt and obtain medical help.

Should I consult the doctor?

Consult your doctor immediately if the splinter is glass, if it is deep in the skin, if it's contaminated with garden material (which increases the risk of tetanus), or if you cannot remove it easily yourself.

What might the doctor do?

▶ If the splinter is a piece of glass, or if it is deep in the skin, your doctor will remove it under a local anaesthetic.
▶ If there is any garden material embedded in or around the wound, your doctor may give your child a tetanus booster injection.

SEE ALSO:
Tetanus 238

Sprain

A SPRAIN IS THE TEARING of the tough, strap-like structures (ligaments) that support a joint and limit its movement. The sprain usually occurs because of overstretching or a sudden twisting action which wrenches the joint beyond its normal movement. The tearing causes bleeding into the joint, which results in swelling, pain and a bad bruise. (If no ligaments are torn and only muscle fibres are over-stretched, it is known as a strain.) The most common sites of a sprain are the ankle, knee and wrist. Because the ligaments are near to the skin's surface in these joints, and there is little but hard bone beneath them, swelling shows rapidly and your child will not be able to take any weight on the sprained joint.

It is rare for young children to suffer a sprain because their joints are so supple. Sprains are, however, quite common in the six to 12 age group.

Is it serious?

A sprain is painful but not serious, though it can be difficult to determine without an X-ray whether the injury is a sprain, a **broken bone** or a dislocated joint.

Possible symptoms

▶ **Swelling and tenderness**.
▶ **Pain** when the affected joint has to bear any weight.
▶ **Bruising**.

Common site of pain

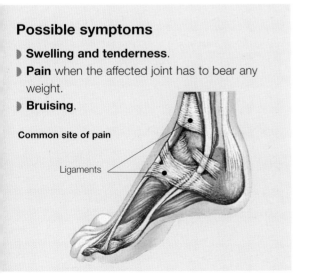

Ligaments

What should I do first?

1 If the affected joint or limb is not misshapen (which could indicate a dislocation or fracture), lay your child down and raise the injured part.

2 Apply a cold compress to the joint to reduce the swelling.

3 Support the joint with a firm crepe bandage applied over a thick wad of cotton wool. Check the bandage regularly to make sure that subsequent swelling has not made it too tight.

4 Encourage your child to rest the joint for at least 24 hours.

Should I consult the doctor?

Consult your doctor immediately if there is intense pain and the affected joint or limb is misshapen, suggesting a dislocation or fracture. Consult your doctor as soon as possible if, after 48 hours, the swelling has not subsided or if your child still complains of severe pain and cannot bear any weight on the injured part.

What might the doctor do?

▶ If your doctor suspects a dislocation or fracture, your child will be referred to a hospital casualty department.
▶ If the injury is a sprain, your doctor will strap the damaged joint with a firm bandage.

SEE ALSO:
Broken bone 70

Squint

IT IS QUITE COMMON FOR THE EYES of newborn babies to move independently of each other until the age of six weeks. At about this time, the baby's eyes should become permanently aligned. If this doesn't happen, and one or both eyes wander, this is known as a squint or crossed-eyes. This condition is most commonly caused by an imbalance of the eye muscles. It may also be associated with other vision defects such as long or short sight. The brain compensates for the wandering eye by blocking out what is seen by it.

Is it serious?

A squint that persists is serious because the child could lose sight from that eye.

Possible symptoms

Common form of squint

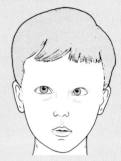

▶ **Eyes appear to be looking in different directions**.

What should I do first?

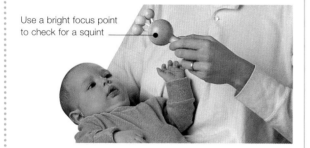

Use a bright focus point to check for a squint

If you think that your baby's eyes wander out of focus, check this by getting him to follow your finger or a colourful toy. See if both eyes track the object together or if one eye wanders to one side. Your health visitor will check your child's vision at routine health assessments. You should contact her if you have any concerns.

Should I consult the doctor?

Consult your doctor as soon as possible if the squint persists after your baby is three months old.

What might the doctor do?

▶ Your doctor will treat the condition by blacking out the strong eye with a pad or patch. This forces the muscles of the wandering eye to work and become stronger. The treatment usually corrects the laziness in the eye within four or five months.
▶ If your child is older, an eye specialist will teach him simple eye exercises to strengthen the eye muscles.
▶ If your child's squint is associated with some vision defect, and spectacles are required, you will be referred to an optician.
▶ If the squint persists, surgery may be performed to correct muscular imbalance. This will not be contemplated until your child is at least two years old.

What can I do to help?

▶ Have your child's eyes checked annually.
▶ If you are concerned about your child's eyes, ask to be referred to an ophthalmologist for another opinion.

SEE ALSO:
Vision problems 255

Stammering

STAMMERING IS A SPEECH DISORDER in which the flow of words is interrupted while the child struggles to start a word. It is perfectly normal in a child who is learning to speak, when excitement, a profusion of ideas and the inability to form sentences properly may result in jerky speech. Nearly all children grow out of this phase by the time they reach school age. If stammering continues beyond this time, there is nearly always an underlying emotional problem such as fear, anxiety or tension – usually caused by parental concern. Stammering does tend to run in families.

Is it serious?

Stammering is not serious and can be controlled, if not cured. However, drawing unnecessary attention to the stammer may make your child feel self-conscious and worsen the problem.

What should I do first?

1 Resist the temptation to give your child the word you think he needs. Give him plenty of time to express himself.

2 Check to see if there is any cause for anxiety or stress in your child's life and do your best to deal with it.

Should I consult the doctor?

Consult your doctor as soon as possible if your child is obviously embarrassed and upset by the stammering, and it is causing him to contort his lips, tongue and face when he tries to express himself.

What might the doctor do?

▶ Your doctor may reassure you that the stammer will soon disappear.
▶ Your doctor may decide to refer your child to a speech therapist for assessment and therapy. If therapy is started early on, there is a very good chance of eliminating the stammer completely from your child's speech.

What can I do to help?

▶ Your child needs your help to prevent him losing confidence in himself. Never ridicule or draw attention to your child's stammering. Try to be open and frank about discussing it and never show embarrassment.
▶ If your child is old enough to understand, discuss with him the possibility of therapy. Ask him if he would like professional help and see how he responds to the suggestion. He may be quite happy to live with his stammer.
▶ Don't push your child or interrupt him when he's talking. If he asks for help with a word, then give it.
▶ Suggest that your child imposes a rhythm when speaking and that he speaks slowly to accentuate the rhythm of his sentences. Stammerers don't stammer while they are singing or reciting poetry.

Sticky eye

STICKY EYE IS A MILD EYE INFECTION that is quite common in the first week of a baby's life. It is nearly always due to a foreign substance getting into the eye during delivery, possibly a drop of amniotic fluid or blood. Your baby's eye will ooze pus and when he wakes from sleep, the eye will be gummed up with it. In some instances, sticky eye can be caused by very narrow tear ducts in newborn babies and infants.

Is it serious?
Sticky eye is not serious. There is no danger to your baby's eyes, but sticky eye should be treated promptly to prevent the more serious infection of **conjunctivitis** from developing.

Possible symptoms
▶ **Pus** coming from the inner corner of one or both of the eyes.
▶ **Eyelashes** stuck together after sleep.

What should I do first?

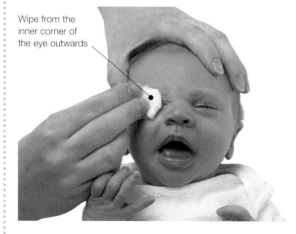

Wipe from the inner corner of the eye outwards

1 Wash both eyes with warm, boiled water, using a clean piece of cotton wool for each eye. Start at the inner corner of the eye and move outwards.

2 Put your baby down to sleep with the infected eye uppermost. The other eye may otherwise become infected from the sheet.

Should I consult the doctor?
Consult your doctor immediately if your baby's eyeball is red. This could be conjunctivitis. Consult your doctor as soon as possible if the sticky eye does not improve within 24 hours.

What might the doctor do?
If there is an infection, your doctor will prescribe eye drops or an eye ointment to apply to the eye three or four times a day.

What can I do to help?
▶ Bathe your baby's eyes frequently whenever you notice a discharge.
▶ Change his bedlinen regularly to avoid contaminating his eyes.

SEE ALSO:
Conjunctivitis 91

Stings

Most stings, whether from insects or jellyfish, cause only local irritation and pain. In the rare cases where there is a severe allergic reaction to a sting, shock may develop (*see page 306*). This is known as *anaphylactic shock*. Bee and wasp stings make a small puncture hole in the skin; bees leave their stings behind but wasps rarely do. Jellyfish stings cause a localized burning sensation.

Are they serious?

A sting is rarely serious. However, if it causes an allergic reaction with severe swelling leading to loss of consciousness; if it is in the mouth or throat, where swelling could lead to breathing problems; if it is caused by a Portuguese man-of-war jellyfish sting; or if your child is stung by a number of insects (in which case the amount of poison in his body could be more than he can cope with), then it should be treated as an emergency.

Possible symptoms

▶ **Small puncture mark**, with or without the sting left behind.

▶ **Localized swelling** and irritation.

▶ **Red swelling** with pieces of jellyfish still adhering to the skin.

▶ **Breathing difficulties**.

▶ **Signs of shock** – rapid pulse, clammy and pale skin, shortness of breath, sweating and faintness.

Appearance of
bee sting

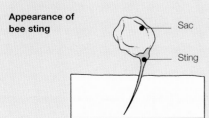

Sac

Sting

What should I do first?

Calm your child and keep him as still as possible to slow down the poison's rate of spreading.

If your child is stung by a bee or wasp

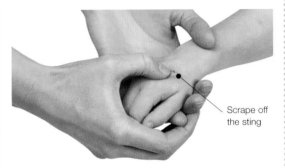

Scrape off
the sting

1 If the sting is still in the skin, scrape it off with the blade of a knife or a fingernail. Avoid squeezing the sac at the top of the sting because this will force more poison into your child's body.

2 To reduce the pain and swelling, apply a cold compress of diluted vinegar for wasp stings and bicarbonate of soda and water paste for bee stings. Don't rub the area; just lay the compress on top. You can also apply calamine lotion.

If the sting is in the mouth or throat

1 If the sting is visible, remove it with a pair of tweezers. Avoid squeezing the sac at the top of the sting because this will force more poison into your child's body. Give your child cold water to drink or a cube of ice to suck. If not visible, seek medical aid.

2 If the area swells quickly, place your child in the recovery position (*see page 287*) and get medical help immediately.

Continued on next page

Continued from previous page

If your child is stung by a jellyfish

1 Use dry sand to wipe away any bits of the jellyfish stuck to your child's skin.

2 Wash the area with water or soap and water if available.

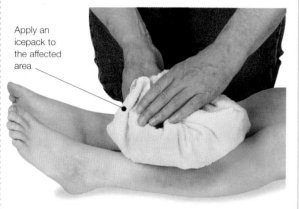

Apply an icepack to the affected area

3 Relieve the pain and irritation with calamine lotion or ice.

Should I consult the doctor?

Take your child to the nearest casualty department if he has an allergic reaction, if he has been stung more than once by an insect, or if he has been stung by a Portuguese man-of-war jellyfish. Consult your doctor immediately or go to the nearest casualty department if your child develops any symptoms of shock (*see page 306*), has breathing difficulties, or if he has been stung in the throat or mouth and you can't remove the sting, or if the area is swelling.

What might the doctor do?

▶ The hospital doctor will treat your child for shock.
▶ If your child has suffered an allergic reaction to a sting, your doctor may prescribe antihistamine tablets, depending on the severity of the reaction.

If your child's reaction was severe, your doctor may prescribe antihistamine in a syringe (an "epi-pen") for you to adminster if your child is stung again. He may also give your child a series of desensitizing injections to prevent the same reaction in future.
▶ Your doctor will remove the sting from your child's mouth if you've been unable to do so, and will control any swelling in the area.

What can I do to help?

▶ Make up an emergency pack of antihistamine medication if your child suffers from an allergic reaction to insect stings. Carry it with you on holidays and outings.
▶ Keep a proprietary brand of aerosol sting reliever with you on picnics and outings. The quick relief of pain and itching will reduce any fear your child may build up about insects like wasps or bees.
▶ Have a bracelet or medallion engraved for your child to wear stating that he is allergic to stings and should be given immediate medical treatment.

Stye

A STYE IS A PUS-FILLED SWELLING on the margin of the eyelid. It is caused by the inflammation of one of the hair follicles from which the eyelashes grow, and it nearly always appears on the lower eyelid. It usually comes to a head and bursts within four or five days. Styes are encouraged by rubbing and pulling at the eyelashes and may be associated with a general irritation of the eyelids known as **blepharitis**. Styes are not highly infectious, but they can be conveyed from one eye to the other.

Is it serious?

A stye is usually harmless and can be treated at home.

Possible symptoms

Common site

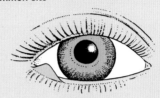

▶ **Swollen, sore, red area on the lower eyelid**, which enlarges to become pus-filled.

What should I do first?

1 If the spot on the eyelid is merely red and sore, leave it alone and discourage your child from touching or rubbing it. If the stye is painful and unsightly, keep the eyelid still with a pad of gauze or a clean, ironed handkerchief held loosely in place with a bandage.

2 If the stye is pus-filled and painful, apply a warm compress, or a ball of cotton wool squeezed out in hot water, for a few minutes every two or three hours. This will soothe the pain and bring the stye to a head.

3 Once the stye has come to a head, your aim is to release the pus and ease the pain. If you can see the eyelash at the centre of the stye, try to pull it out gently with a pair of tweezers. If it won't come out, leave it, and continue with the warm compresses. As soon as the eyelash comes out, the pus will drain away and the stye will get better quickly. Bathe the pus away with warm water and cotton wool.

4 Note whether the eyelids are red-rimmed, with dandruff-like flakes clinging to the eyelashes. This may be blepharitis.

Should I consult the doctor?

Consult your doctor as soon as possible if the home treatment does not improve the stye within four or five days, if the eyelid becomes generally swollen, or if the stye is accompanied by blepharitis.

What might the doctor do?

If there is an infection of the eyelid or the eye itself, your doctor will prescribe an antibiotic ointment or eye drops. If the stye is accompanied by blepharitis, your doctor may prescribe an ointment to clear it up.

What can I do to help?

▶ Keep your child's facecloth and towel separate from those of the rest of the family to avoid spreading any infection.
▶ Wash your hands before and after treating the stye and discourage your child from touching the area.

SEE ALSO:
Blepharitis 66

Sunburn

SUNBURN IS INFLAMMATION of the skin caused by excessive exposure to the ultra-violet rays in sunlight. It is always due to misjudgement or carelessness on the part of the parent. The best cure is prevention. Even adults should give all but deep olive or black skins a chance to gradually acclimatize to the sun. It is necessary to be strict with children who may not appreciate the dangers. Your child's sunburn can result in tender and damaged skin that may blister or peel off. Even in mild sunshine, the effects of the sun can be increased if you are near water, snow or sand, where the rays are reflected off the bright surface.

Is it serious?

Sunburn can be serious if a large area of the skin is burned. The skin may lose its ability to regulate body temperature so that your child's temperature soars and **heatstroke** results. There is also a major long-term risk of skin cancer.

Possible symptoms

▶ **Red, hot, tender skin**.
▶ **Blisters**.
▶ **Itchiness** prior to peeling skin.

What should I do first?

1 Apply a soothing lotion such as calamine, or a cold compress, to any tight, red skin to cool it down and help to reduce irritation.

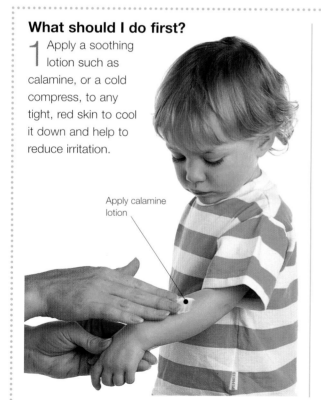

Apply calamine lotion

2 When you're inside, don't put any clothing on the sunburned areas; leave them exposed to the air. Cover sunburned areas when you are outside.

3 If blisters appear and your child complains of pain, give him paracetamol elixir.

4 Take your child's temperature to see if he has a fever. If his temperature is over 39°C (102.2°F), consult your doctor immediately and try to reduce the fever with tepid sponging (see page 31).

5 Keep your child out of direct sunlight for at least 48 hours.

Should I consult the doctor?

Consult your doctor if blisters form on your child's sunburned skin and he is feverish and unwell. Consult your doctor immediately if your child has a fever but his skin is dry and he seems confused and drowsy. This could be heatstroke, which should be treated as an emergency (see page 159).

Continued from previous page

What might the doctor do?

▶ In a mild case of sunburn, your doctor may prescribe a soothing cream.

▶ If blisters have formed and your child is feverish, your doctor may prescribe an anti-inflammatory cream to help the skin to heal more quickly.

▶ If your child is suffering from heatstroke your doctor will treat this accordingly.

What can I do to help?

▶ Draw the sheets on your child's bed tightly so that nothing scratches his tender skin.

▶ To prevent sunburn, keep all but the toughest parts of your child's skin covered up for the first few days of bright sunlight. From then on, apply a total-sunblock lotion to all the exposed parts of his body. Try to ensure that your child wears UV-resistant clothing whenever he is in the sun. You should keep all parts of your child's skin protected at all times in sunlight, either with clothes or with sunscreen, due to the increased risk of skin cancer.

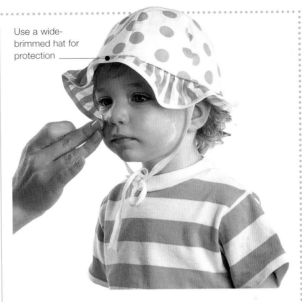

Use a wide-brimmed hat for protection

▶ Cover your child's lips and nose with a sunblock and protect the nape of his neck with a wide-brimmed hat.

▶ Remember to apply the sunblock again after your child has been swimming.

SEE ALSO:
Heatstroke 159

Teething

TEETHING IS THE TERM USED to describe the eruption of a baby's first teeth. Teething usually begins at about the age of six or seven months, with most of the first teeth breaking through before your baby is 18 months old. Your baby will produce more saliva than usual and will dribble; he will try to cram his fingers into his mouth and chew on his fingers or any other object that he can get hold of. He may be clingy and irritable, have difficulty sleeping and he may cry and fret more than usual. Most of these symptoms occur just before the teeth erupt. It is important to realize that the symptoms of teething do not include bronchitis, nappy rash, vomiting, diarrhoea or loss of appetite. These are symptoms of an underlying illness, *not* of teething.

Is it serious?

Teething and the symptoms associated with teething are never serious.

Possible symptoms

▶ **Increased saliva and dribbling**.
▶ **Desire to bite** on any hard object.
▶ **Irritability and increased clinginess**.
▶ **Sleeplessness**.
▶ **Swollen red area** where the tooth is being cut.

Order of appearance
1 1st incisors
2 1st incisors
3 2nd incisors
4 2nd incisors
5 1st molars
6 1st molars
7 Eye
8 Eye
9 2nd molars
10 2nd molars

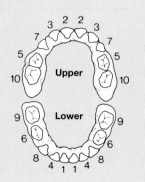

What should I do first?

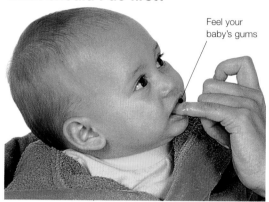

Feel your baby's gums

If you can't work out why your child is so irritable, and he has no other symptoms of illness, feel his gums. If a tooth is coming through, you will feel a hard or sharp lump and the gum area will be swollen and red.

Should I consult the doctor?

You should not need to consult your doctor unless your baby has other symptoms which cannot be attributed to teething, or you are unduly worried.

What might the doctor do?

Your doctor will give you advice on how to cope with the symptoms of teething and will perhaps prescribe a mild analgesic to be used for a short time to relieve the irritation.

What can I do to help?

▶ Nurse your baby often. A teething baby needs your comfort and closeness. Don't think that the arrival of teeth means a necessary speeding-up of the weaning process. Babies with teeth can still be breastfed with no discomfort to the mother.

Continued from previous page

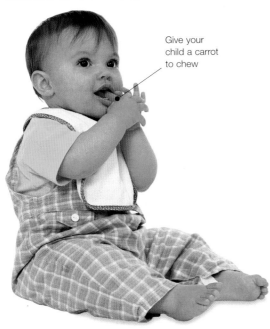

Give your child a carrot to chew

▶ Distract your child with a chilled teething ring (never freeze the ring or your baby may get **frostbite**) or a piece of carrot or apple – something with a firm texture. Stay with your baby so that he doesn't choke on the food.

▶ Try not to resort to analgesics such as paracetamol elixir. Over the course of the teething process, doses of such painkillers could become too large. Only use analgesics on your doctor's advice.

▶ Rub the swollen gum with your finger. Try to avoid teething jellies that contain local anaesthetics as these have only a temporary effect and they can cause an allergy.

▶ If your child refuses food, encourage him to eat by giving him cold, smooth foods such as yogurt, ice cream or jelly.

SEE ALSO:
Crying 102
Frostbite 139
Sleeplessness 219

Temper tantrums

TEMPER TANTRUMS ARE NORMAL in children between the ages of two and four years. They arise because the child hasn't acquired the judgement to match his will, nor has he the linguistic skills to argue or to explain what he wants. Clashes with parents tend to become frequent towards the end of the second year, leading to the time known as the "terrible twos". Tantrums take many forms, but usually the child throws himself on the floor, kicking and screaming, banging his feet against the walls or perhaps holding his breath with frustration. The child's actions show no regard for his own safety and he can easily hurt himself on hard objects.

Are they serious?

Temper tantrums are not in themselves serious, though they may happen at inconvenient times and in embarrassing situations. Even if your child holds his breath until he becomes blue in the face, he will not be able to harm himself. There is an automatic reflex that forces the body to take a breath when it is running short of oxygen, and this cannot be overriden by willpower.

What should I do first?

1 Stay calm. Even if your child's anger affects you, don't let him see that you are upset. Your child can easily catch your mood.

2 Ignore your child as much as possible. Walk away, but don't go out of sight. A tantrum loses much of its effect if there is no audience. However, move sharp pieces of furniture and breakable objects so that no harm can come to your child.

3 If this doesn't work, try holding your child on your lap while he calms down. He may fight to get away, or he may realize that comfort and sympathy are really what he wants.

Should I consult the doctor?

There is usually no need to consult your doctor about temper tantrums. If your child continues to throw tantrums after the age of five, however, or if you are finding them difficult to cope with, ask your doctor or health visitor for advice.

What might the doctor do?

Your doctor or health visitor will ask you about the frequency and nature of the tantrums and whether they are accompanied by other behavioural problems. Your doctor or health visitor may refer you to a child psychiatrist for further assessment.

What can I do to help?

▶ Remember that the tantrums are directed against you. Your child is trying to gain your attention. Tantrums can be difficult to deal with in a public place when your child may sense that he will have impact. But if you show that the tantrums never succeed, they should stop.

▶ Try to anticipate problems and forestall clashes with the use of distraction tactics. As your child grows up, he will be better able to tolerate delays and accept compromises.

▶ Don't ask your child why he is angry during a tantrum. He won't be able to reason with you.

▶ Don't slap your child to bring him out of a breath-holding attack. Just leave him and it will come to an end naturally.

Testicles, undescended

THE TESTICLES GROW AND DEVELOP inside the abdomen, near the kidneys. Shortly before a boy is born, they move down or "descend" into their normal position in the bag of skin called the scrotum. For testicles to develop normally at adolescence and produce sperm, it is necessary for them to hang outside the body. This is because sperm production can proceed only at a temperature that is slightly below the body's internal temperature. If the testicles – or, more usually, one testicle – fail to descend, sperm will not be produced normally, but the hormone testosterone (which produces male characteristics, such as a deeper voice and body hair) will be. Theoretically, one descended testicle could be sufficient to produce sperm and male hormones but, if your son's testicles have failed to descend by the age of two, the problem should probably be corrected surgically.

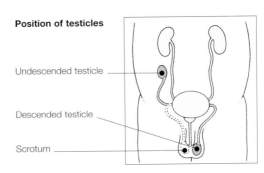

Position of testicles

Undescended testicle

Descended testicle

Scrotum

Are they serious?

Undescended testicles are generally not considered a serious matter, but there is an increased risk of cancer of the testes, and of infertility

What should I do first?

When a baby boy is born, a paediatrician will examine his testicles to see if they have descended. If not, you will be advised of the fact and reassured that they may descend naturally. If your baby's testicles did not descend at birth, feel for them occasionally in the scrotum. If they have descended, they will feel small – each about the size of a pea. Warm your hands before you do this, otherwise the testicles may temporarily retract into the abdomen.

Should I consult the doctor?

Your doctor will be aware of your baby's problem and will check the scrotum regularly.

What might the doctor do?

Your doctor will probably take action before your son is three years old. If a boy's testicles fail to descend, many surgeons recommend operating before the age of two-and-a-half to three years.

What can I do to help?

▶ Stay with your child in hospital when he has the operation to lower his testicles.
▶ Keep your son as quiet and calm as possible when he returns after the operation. If he engages too soon in any boisterous play, he could easily damage the scrotum.

Tetanus

TETANUS IS A SERIOUS BACTERIAL INFECTION caused by the bacterium *Clostridium tetani*. The bacterium is commonly found in farm and garden dirt, gravel and rusty metal, and it usually enters the body through a cut caused by anything from a rose thorn to a sharp piece of metal. The bacterium, which thrives in the low-oxygen environment created by a deep cut, makes a poison or toxin that causes the muscles of the body to go into spasm (uncontrollable contraction). The jaw muscles are often affected first, hence the common name for the illness, lockjaw. This is followed by spasm of muscles throughout the rest of the body. These symptoms of tetanus can occur any time from a week to several months after the wound was sustained.

Tetanus is entirely preventable if your child has a course of injections within the first five years of life, updated every five years. Because of this programme, tetanus is very rare.

Is it serious?

Tetanus is very serious. Sometimes the breathing muscles go into spasm, and even with intensive care this can result in death.

Possible symptoms

▶ **Muscle stiffness and cramp**, at first around the jaw and mouth.
▶ **Sore throat**.
▶ **Difficulty in swallowing or breathing**.

What should I do first?

1 Always examine any wound your child receives to see if it is deep and dirty. Clean the wound thoroughly with an antiseptic solution or soap and water, removing the dirt where you can.

2 Take your child to your doctor or the nearest hospital for a tetanus injection if your child has not already been immunized.

3 If your child complains of muscle stiffness, especially of the jaw and neck, seek medical attention at once.

Should I consult the doctor?

Consult your doctor immediately, or take your child to the nearest hospital, if your child has a deep cut from a possibly contaminated source or if he develops symptoms of tetanus.

What might the doctor do?

▶ The doctor will clean a deep or dirty wound and give your child a booster injection if he is already immunized. If your child is not immune, an injection of anti-tetanus globulin will be given to provide immediate protection against the poison.
▶ If tetanus develops, the treatment includes a course of antibiotics and nursing in an intensive care unit. The child's breathing is supported by a respirator while the disease runs its course, which may be several weeks.

What can I do to help?

All babies should receive a course of three tetanus injections (usually as part of the "triple vaccine", DTP) in the first year. This provides a good immunization against the toxin. Tetanus is also given as a pre-school booster and is repeated after 10 years to maintain protection.

Thalassaemia

THALASSAEMIA IS A FORM OF genetically inherited anaemia. It occurs mostly in people from the mediterranean area but it can also affect people from India and south-east Asia. Thalassaemia can be passed on to a child if both parents carry the faulty gene (or trait). The parents themselves may not be anaemic but there is a one in four chance that their child will suffer from the disease. If he does, his body cannot make normal haemoglobin, the substance in the blood that makes the red cells red and carries oxygen through the body. The problem reveals itself when the child is about three months old with symptoms of severe anaemia: fatigue, breathlessness and pallor; he will then become increasingly inactive. A child with thalassaemia will also have difficulty feeding, and his abdomen will become swollen as the spleen and liver enlarge. A less severe form of the condition, known as thalassaemia minor, does not cause these symptoms and requires no treatment.

Possible symptoms

▶ **Fatigue**.

▶ **Breathlessness**.

▶ **Pallor** of the lips, tongue, hands, feet and other parts of the body.

▶ **Loss of appetite** accompanied by a swollen abdomen.

What can be done?

Your doctor will take a blood sample for testing. If a disease such as thalassaemia is suspected, your child will be referred to hospital for more blood tests. If thalassaemia is confirmed, blood transfusions will usually be necessary – usually every four to six weeks – to prevent your child from being incapacitated by severe anaemia.

Later in childhood, your child may need an operation to remove his spleen. This will reduce the need for such frequent transfusions. There is a problem if your child has to have too many transfusions: iron can build up in the body and damage the liver, pancreas and heart. This "iron overload" is the major threat of the disease and many sufferers have died in their teens; with new treatment, however, prospects are better. Many children with thalassaemia now receive injections of a drug which helps the body to get rid of the iron. In some cases this treatment is carried out overnight by means of a continuous injection into the skin.

A child with thalassaemia should lead as normal a life as possible. There should be no need to restrict physical activity, but he will need support and encouragement with the repeated transfusions. Ask your doctor or the hospital to put you in touch with other families with a similar problem so that you can learn how others cope.

If you are from a race particularly susceptible to this disease, ask your doctor to carry out a blood test on both you and your partner before you conceive, in order to find out if one or both of you might be a carrier of the thalassaemia trait. It is now possible to test the fetus at an early stage in pregnancy to detect thalassaemia so that a termination of the pregnancy can be offered.

For help and advice contact the United Kingdom Thalassaemia Society (see page 324).

Thrush

THRUSH IS AN INFECTION caused by the fungus *candida albicans*. Under normal circumstances, this fungus is kept under control by other bacteria that also live in the intestines. If the balance is disturbed – for example, when your child is on antibiotics or his natural resistance is low because of illness – the fungus can overgrow, causing infection in any part of the gastro-intestinal tract. Thrush most often affects the mouth, causing white patches to appear on the tongue, roof of the mouth and inside the cheeks. It can also affect the anus. In babies, anal thrush is sometimes confused with **nappy rash** because it forms red patches with little red spots within them. It does not, however, respond to the usual self-help treatments.

Is it serious?

It is rare for thrush to give rise to serious symptoms but, as it does not respond to self-help treatment, you should get medical advice.

Possible symptoms

▸ **Creamy yellow or white frothy patches** inside the cheeks, on the tongue and on the roof of the mouth, which become raw or bleed when wiped off.
▸ **A pimply red rash** around the anus.

What should I do first?

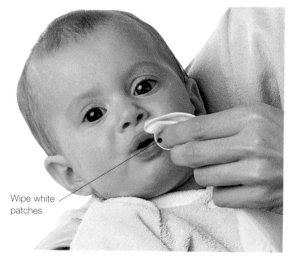

Wipe white patches

1 If your child refuses to eat, check his mouth for any white patches. Try to wipe them off with a clean handkerchief. If they don't come away easily or if they leave raw patches underneath, or bleed, your child probably has oral thrush.

2 Avoid giving your child spicy foods and cool all cooked food to lukewarm. Natural yogurt is the best food to give until you have consulted your doctor.

3 Change your baby's nappies frequently. The fungus may be in his stools and this could give rise to thrush around the anus.

Should I consult the doctor?

Consult your doctor as soon as possible if you suspect your child has thrush.

What might the doctor do?

▸ Your doctor will prescribe a liquid anti-fungal medication to be dropped on to the affected area in your child's mouth if he has oral thrush.
▸ Your doctor will prescribe an anti-fungal cream if there is a rash around the anus.

Continued from previous page

What can I do to help?

▶ If you are breastfeeding, you may need treatment to avoid cross-infection or reinfection.

▶ Feed your child with mild, liquidized foods if he has oral thrush.

▶ Keep your child's hands clean so that the infection does not spread from the anus to the mouth, or vice versa.

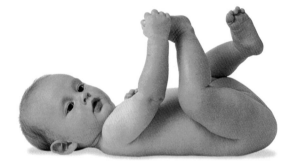

▶ Leave your baby's bottom exposed to the air as much as possible if he is still in nappies.

SEE ALSO:
Nappy rash 187

Tic

A TIC IN A CHILD IS AN HABITUAL, jerky movement of the body or face that can become a mannerism. It is not the result of neuralgia as are the facial tics seen in elderly people. The most common tics in children are a slight twitching of the eye or of the corner of the mouth, wiggling the nose or blinking. Other habits include tossing the hair back off the forehead, fiddling with the hair, clearing the throat and sniffing; even head-banging can be seen as a tic. Tics of all kinds are usually transient and they often appear when a child is particularly stressed or fatigued and will disappear when the child settles back to normal. In young children, some sort of tic is fairly common and is not usually indicative of any problem.

Is it serious?

A tic is not serious, although it can be irritating.

Possible symptoms

▶ **Habitual, jerky movements** of parts of the face or body.

What should I do first?

Don't over-react to a tic; you may increase your child's anxiety and make it worse. Play it down and pretend not to notice, even though it may be irritating to you.

Should I consult the doctor?

Unless the tic is interfering with everyday life, or it is causing a problem at school, you really should not need to consult a doctor.

What might the doctor do?

If you do seek advice, your doctor will reassure you that there is no long-term problem.

What can I do to help?

▶ A tic is nearly always worse when a child gets tired, so make sure he has plenty of rest.
▶ Learn to control your irritation so that you don't increase your child's tension.
▶ If your baby is a head-banger, make sure he isn't left alone to get bored. Put bumper pads around his cot so that he can't hurt himself.

Tonsillitis

TONSILLITIS IS AN ACUTE INFECTION of the tonsils, usually caused by a viral infection. Positioned on either side of the back of the throat, the tonsils form the body's first line of defence by trapping and killing bacteria, thus preventing them from entering the respiratory tract. In the process, the tonsils themselves can become infected and inflamed, causing the symptoms of a **sore throat**, **fever** and swollen glands. The adenoids, positioned at the back of the nose, are nearly always affected as well.

Babies under the age of one rarely suffer from tonsillitis; the infection occurs mainly among children of school age, when the relatively large tonsils and adenoids are exposed for the first time to infectious microbes. As resistance to the infection increases and the adenoids become smaller, so attacks of tonsillitis should lessen. Most children cease to suffer from tonsillitis from around the age of ten.

Is it serious?

Tonsillitis is not serious unless repeatedly accompanied by **otitis media**, which could lead to permanent deafness. There are also the rare complications of **nephritis** and **rheumatic fever**.

Possible symptoms

▶ **Sore throat**, possibly bad enough to cause difficulty in swallowing.

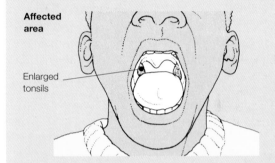

Affected area

Enlarged tonsils

▶ **Red and enlarged tonsils**, possibly covered in yellow spots.
▶ **A temperature** of over 38°C (100.4°F).
▶ **Swollen glands** in the neck.
▶ **Mouth-breathing, snoring and a nasal voice** when the adenoids are affected.
▶ **Unpleasant breath**.

What should I do first?

1 If your child complains of a sore throat or you notice that he has difficulty eating, examine his throat in a good light, with his head held back and the tongue depressed gently with the handle of a clean spoon. Ask him to say a long "aaah". This will open up the throat, and after a second or two you should be able to see whether his tonsils are red, enlarged or covered with yellow spots.

2 Take your child's temperature to establish whether he has a fever.

3 Check to see if your child's glands are swollen by running your fingers down the sides of his neck and under his chin – swollen glands will feel like large peas under the skin.

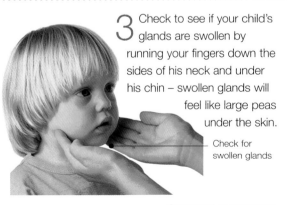

Check for swollen glands

Continued on next page

Continued from previous page

4 If your child is old enough, ask him if he has earache. In a young child, note whether he pulls or rubs one of his ears. Check the ear to see if there is any discharge.

5 Give your child plenty of cool drinks to soothe his throat.

Should I consult the doctor?

Consult your doctor as soon as possible if you suspect tonsillitis.

What might the doctor do?

▌ Your doctor may take a throat swab (which is quite painless), to be sent to a laboratory for identification of the organism that is causing the infection. Your doctor may prescribe antibiotics if a bacterial infection seems likely. There is no specific medication for viral tonsillitis.

▌ Your doctor will examine your child's ear and eardrum to check for any ear infection. If there is any sign of infection, antibiotics may be prescribed.

▌ If your child suffers from frequent attacks of tonsillitis, or if enlarged adenoids are causing recurrent middle-ear infections, you may be referred to a specialist to see whether the tonsils and adenoids should be removed. The circumstances under which the operation might be performed would take the following account:

a *Age* The operation is seldom performed before a child is four years old.

b *The onset of tonsillitis* The length of time that your child has been suffering from recurrent attacks of tonsillitis or earache is important. Most doctors would wait two years before deciding to operate.

c *Effect on the child* Tonsillectomy is advisable if the attacks are so frequent that they affect your child's education because he is absent from school so often, or if his health is deteriorating because he cannot eat well.

What can I do to help?

▌ Treat your child as you would for a fever. Bed-rest is not necessary but keep him in a warm room.

▌ Keep your child's fluid intake up by offering him regular drinks.

▌ Liquidize your child's foods if he finds swallowing difficult, but don't force him to eat. Give him his favourite foods, especially those that slip down easily like ice cream or yogurt.

▌ Never give your child a gargle for a sore throat. This has been shown to spread infection from the throat to the middle ear.

Toothache

TOOTHACHE IS THE PAIN WHICH RESULTS when a tooth is decaying. The decaying process erodes the outer protective coatings of the tooth and bores through to the nerves in the soft centre, causing pain, particularly when anything cold, hot or sweet touches the tooth. Tooth decay (or dental caries) and gum disease are caused by plaque. This is a thin film of saliva and food residue in which bacteria grow. The bacteria thrive in the presence of sugar in the mouth – for example, in the form of refined white sugar, the sugar in dried fruits or even honey – which is one of the reasons why sugar in the diet is so harmful. Teeth can become resistant to the action of bacteria and sugar if they contain fluoride or if they are painted or coated with fluoride as they would be if regularly brushed with a fluoride-containing toothpaste. This is one of the main ways to prevent tooth decay along with good oral hygiene and regular dental check-ups. It is important that children do not lose their first teeth through tooth decay, or through a complication of tooth decay – a **gum boil** (dental abscess) – in which the root of the tooth also decays. The permanent tooth may come through misaligned if a gap is left for too long while the new tooth is developing.

Is it serious?

Toothache is not serious as long as it is treated immediately. If untreated, a gum boil may erupt, causing damage to the underlying permanent tooth, or the loss of a second tooth.

What should I do first?

1 If your child complains of pain in the jaw, **earache** or throbbing, stabbing pains in the mouth, tap her teeth gently with a small metal spoon to see if this identifies the source of the pain.

2 Give your child paracetamol elixir to relieve the pain until you can visit the dentist.

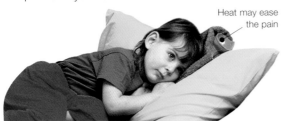

Heat may ease the pain

3 Put a hot-water bottle covered in a cloth or towel against your child's cheek to relieve the pain.

4 Do not apply oil of cloves or anaesthetic jellies as this can cause damage to the gum around the tooth.

Should I consult the doctor?

You don't need to consult a doctor, but you should consult your child's dentist immediately for an emergency appointment.

What might the dentist do?

Your dentist will examine the tooth to determine the extent of the damage. The tooth may only need to be drilled and filled, but if there is a gum boil the dentist will drain the pus from the abscess. If there is no possibility of saving the tooth, it will be extracted, probably under a general anaesthetic, depending on the age of your child.

What can I do to help?

▶ Prevent the development of a sweet tooth by restricting your child's sugar intake. Don't give her sweets, cakes and biscuits, and avoid canned foods and fizzy drinks, which often have a surprisingly high sugar content.

Continued on next page

Continued from previous page

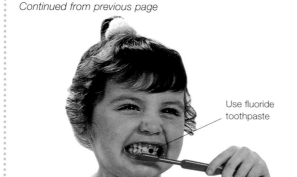

Use fluoride toothpaste

▶ Prevent tooth decay. Use fluoride toothpastes and, depending on the level of fluoride in your local water supply, use fluoride tablets or drops in your child's drinks. Your dentist can provide you with information on this.

▶ Brush your child's teeth yourself once a day or supervise the brushing of her teeth up until the age of six or seven.

▶ Once your child has most of her first teeth (around the age of two), you can start taking her for dental check-ups every six months. Get her used to the dentist from an early age so that the prospect holds no mystery or terror for her.

▶ Encourage your child to drink plenty of water after eating sweet foods. The water will immediately wash much of the sugar off her teeth.

▶ Avoid prolonging the use of a bottle for your baby – get her used to a trainer cup instead.

▶ Ask your dentist about fissure sealing. When your child is about seven or eight, her permanent back teeth can be sealed with a plastic coating to prevent plaque from getting into the biting surfaces.

SEE ALSO:
Earache 122
Gum boil 149

Toxocariasis

TOXOCARIASIS IS A RARE INFECTION caused by the toxocara **worm** that lives in the intestines of some cats and dogs. The eggs of the worm are passed out in the animal's faeces. If a child plays on ground contaminated with faeces, then puts his hands in his mouth, he may ingest the eggs. The eggs hatch and the worms burrow through the intestinal wall into the body and are carried via the bloodstream to the lungs and other parts of the body. They are then coughed up from the lungs; if swallowed, the larvae do not mature in the human intestine, so their eggs are not passed in human faeces. Children show few specific symptoms of the disease.

Is it serious?

Toxocariasis is rarely a serious condition in children, although in rare cases a worm may lodge in the eyes, causing blindness.

Possible symptoms

- **Loss of appetite**.
- **Slight fever**.
- **Bouts of abdominal pain**.
- **Loss of sight**.
- **Coughing and wheezing**.

What should I do first?

If your child has a mild infestation of toxocara worms, you may not even be aware of it. If he suffers from unexplained fever and abdominal pain, it is wise to seek medical advice.

Should I consult the doctor?

Consult your doctor as soon as possible if you think that there is something wrong with your child and you suspect toxocariasis, particularly if you have a pet, or if your child has played on land where animals defecate regularly.

What might the doctor do?

- Your doctor will examine your child and take a sample of his blood for laboratory examination.
- If evidence of worms is found, your doctor may prescribe a special anti-parasite drug, or he may advise you to keep your child away from all animals or possibly contaminated areas for six months while the worms die off.

What can I do to help?

- Encourage your child to wash his hands, especially after playing with animals.
- Worm your dog or cat regularly.
- Train your pet to use its own toilet area well away from places frequented by the family.
- Disinfect any area where your children play if the dog or cat has fouled it. When you go to a public park, if possible keep to the areas where dogs are not permitted.

SEE ALSO:
Worms 263

Travel sickness

TRAVEL SICKNESS OCCURS when the balance organs in the ear are upset by movement. When this sensation of movement doesn't correspond with what the eyes see, it causes confusion in the brain. The problem can result if a child rides a roller coaster or swings at a playground as well as being in a car, boat or plane. Symptoms range from a slight queasiness to **vomiting** and faintness. Children tend to suffer from travel sickness more than adults, though why is not known; most outgrow it by adolescence.

Possible symptoms

▶ **Nausea**.
▶ **Vomiting**.
▶ **Pale, clammy** forehead.
▶ **Weakness or dizziness**.
▶ **Fainting**.

Is it serious?
Travel sickness is not serious, but it is inconvenient. With a young child there is a risk that prolonged vomiting could cause **dehydration**.

What should I do first?

1 If your child complains of feeling sick, looks pale or becomes abnormally quiet while you are travelling, check whether his forehead feels cold and clammy.

2 Tell your child to close his eyes and lay him down if possible. This should minimize the confusing signals being received by the brain.

Should I consult the doctor?
Consult your doctor if your child suffers from travel sickness on even short journeys, or if proprietary brands of travel-sickness medicine do not help.

What might the doctor do?
After questioning you about the symptoms and their frequency of your child's sickness, your doctor may prescribe a drug such as an antihistamine, though some antihistamines can have side effects such as **drowsiness**.

What can I do to help?

▶ Don't make a fuss before you travel. This can make your child more excited and apprehensive.
▶ Prevent travel sickness by giving your child a travel-sickness medicine before you start the journey. There are several good over-the-counter medications available from the chemist.
▶ Give your child a small snack before setting out. Don't let him travel on either an empty or a full stomach.
▶ Take plenty of drinks with you, or check that they will be available en route, to prevent the possibility of dehydration through vomiting. Fresh drinks can also reduce the feeling of nausea.
▶ Carry suitable "sick bags" (strong brown paper bags are best) in case of vomiting.

Tuberculosis

TUBERCULOSIS (TB) IS A DISEASE that causes chronic ill health. It is caused by bacteria, and, if left untreated, can destroy large areas of an affected organ. It most commonly affects the lungs, but can also affect the kidneys and the membranes covering the brain and spine (*meninges*). The disease can take many forms because it is capable of travelling through the bloodstream and affecting any organ in the body. This makes it difficult to diagnose. Tuberculosis has been significantly reduced in Great Britain by means of a pasteurization programme for milk and tuberculin testing of the national dairy herd (cows are the most common carriers of the disease); by a mass X-ray programme to pick up chest tuberculosis in its early stages; by skin testing and vaccination of all adolescents; and by improved drug treatment. However, immigration from areas where TB is still common has recently caused an increase in the number of cases. If a healthy child becomes infected by an adult, this first infection (the primary lesion) hardly ever progresses to anything serious, because the body forms a strong resistance to the tuberculous organism and prohibits its spread by walling it off within a chalky coating. If the child remains healthy and doesn't become reinfected with tuberculosis, there may never be any effects of the disease. If, however, there is a period of malnourishment and illness, the primary lesion may break out of its chalky coating and spread through the blood to affect other organs.

The symptoms of this secondary phase of the disease depend on the organ that is affected. A child may merely be tired and lose his appetite, or, as in the case of TB infection in the lungs, the child will have a dry cough which eventually contains pus and blood.

Is it serious?

Tuberculosis is a serious disease if left untreated. However, there is an efficient public health programme that traces contacts of known carriers of the disease. This means that children who have had contact with someone suffering from tuberculosis are likely to be traced and tested for the disease before serious problems occur.

Possible symptoms

▶ **Tiredness**.

▶ **Weight loss** through loss of appetite.

▶ **Persistent, dry cough** with blood and pus in the sputum if the lungs are affected.

▶ **Headache, fever and coma** if the meninges are affected.

What should I do first?

It is extremely unlikely that you would suspect that your child had tuberculosis from any of the symptoms. However, if you hear of anyone who has tuberculosis and your child has been in contact with them, or if you are advised by the public health authorities that your child may have been in contact with a known TB sufferer, contact your doctor immediately.

Should I consult the doctor?

Consult your doctor immediately if you think your child has been in contact with someone with tuberculosis, or if you are worried about your child's general health or a persistent, dry cough.

Continued on next page

Continued from previous page

What might the doctor do?

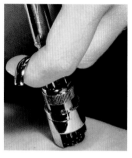

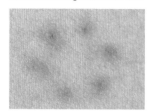

A skin test will be arranged

Marks resulting from skin test

▌ Your doctor will arrange for your child to have a skin test to see if there is an active TB infection or not. If there is, your child will have an X ray and sputum and urine tests to find out which organs the TB is affecting. In the majority of cases, TB can be adequately managed at home. Antibiotics will be prescribed, but rest and a good diet are also essential. Your child will need to be away from school for two weeks after treatment has started. A cure usually takes 6–12 months. There will be periodic check-ups after the treatment is finished to make sure the TB does not flare up again.

▌ Your doctor will ask you for all known contacts of your child so that they can be traced and checked as a possible source of infection.

What can I do to help?

▌ Administer the drugs regularly and keep your child happy and as involved in normal life as is possible.

▌ Make sure your child gets plenty of rest.

▌ Arrange for a friend to come and play with your child regularly. After the drug treatment is started, your child will no longer be contagious and can safely play with friends.

▌ You can get your baby or child immunized against tuberculosis if you wish or if he or she is at risk.

SEE ALSO:
Cough 98
Meningitis 178

Umbilical cord infection

AFTER BIRTH, THE UMBILICAL CORD, which joins the baby to the placenta, is clamped and cut close to the baby's body. It then withers and the remaining stump drops off, usually within 10 days of the birth. You will be advised to clean the navel area and umbilical stump daily since it may become contaminated with urine. The stump will have become infected if it weeps, bleeds, crusts over, discharges pus or appears red or swollen.

Is it serious?

Infection of the umbilical cord is rarely serious and is easily treated.

Possible symptoms

- **Redness and swelling** of the umbilical area.
- **Umbilical stump weeps fluid** which then crusts over.
- **Pussy discharge**.

What should I do first?

Check the stump at every nappy change for signs of infection. If the area seems to be getting red, contact your doctor, midwife or health visitor.

Should I consult the doctor?

Consult your doctor as soon as possible if the stump shows any signs of infection. Consult your doctor or midwife if you are worried about the umbilical cord.

What might the doctor do?

- Your doctor will probably prescribe an antibiotic cream to apply to the cord several times a day. He will also give you advice on daily hygiene.
- If your doctor thinks that infection is spreading along the cord and into your baby's body, your baby will need to be admitted to hospital for treatment with antibiotics.

What can I do to help?

Clean the area thoroughly

- Clean the stump and surrounding area thoroughly at every nappy change. Gently wipe around the stump with a piece of cotton wool soaked in surgical spirit.
- There are anti-infective powders available from the chemist which can be sprinkled on the stump – ask your midwife for advice.
- Place a piece of sterile gauze between the cord and the nappy or fold the nappy below the cord, to prevent urine from contaminating the navel area.
- Put a little salt in your baby's bath water to promote healing. Dry the navel area thoroughly afterwards.
- Allow the stump to fall off naturally. Never pull or twist it in an attempt to remove it.

Urinary tract infection

A URINARY TRACT INFECTION can affect any part of the urinary tract. This includes the kidneys, bladder and urethra (the tube leading from the bladder to the outside). In most cases, the part infected is the lining of the bladder, and the condition is known as cystitis.

Girls suffer from such infections more often than boys because the female urethra is shorter, thus making it easier for infecting microbes to reach the bladder. Young girls sometimes do not clean themselves thoroughly after using the toilet, and if they wipe their bottom from back to front instead of front to back this may bring faecal material near the urethral opening, which could cause infection. Rarely, a minor structural abnormality of the urinary tract is to blame. The most common symptoms of infection are pain on passing urine and the need to pass urine frequently.

Is it serious?
A urinary tract infection is serious.

Possible symptoms

▶ **Pain or burning sensation** on passing urine.
▶ **Frequent urination**, which can lead to bedwetting where previously the child was dry at night.
▶ **Fever**.
▶ **Unpleasant-smelling and/or cloudy urine**.
▶ **Low abdominal pain**.
▶ **Low back pain**.

The urinary system

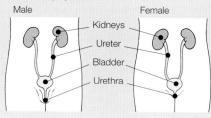

Male   Female

Kidneys
Ureter
Bladder
Urethra

What should I do first?

1 If your child complains of pain when passing urine, check his temperature to see if he has a fever.

2 Check his urine to see if it is cloudy or unpleasant smelling.

3 Give your child plenty of fluids to keep his kidneys flushed out.

4 Place a hot-water bottle against his back if he is suffering from low back pain.

Should I consult the doctor?
Consult your doctor immediately if your child complains of pain on urination.

What might the doctor do?
▶ Your doctor will examine your child and take a sample of his urine for laboratory examination to identify the type of organism causing the infection. Your doctor will then prescribe the appropriate treatment, usually a course of antibiotics.

▶ Your child may be referred for tests (usually kidney scanning) after the first episode of confirmed infection.

▶ If the infection recurs, your doctor may refer your child to a paediatrician for full investigation to see if there is a minor anatomical abnormality.

What can I do to help?
Show your daughter how to wipe herself from the front backwards after using the toilet so that her urethra is not contaminated by her faeces.

SEE ALSO:
Bedwetting 63
Fever 134

Vagina, foreign body in

A LITTLE GIRL IS NATURALLY CURIOUS about her vagina and she will investigate it with her fingers or perhaps something else. Fortunately it is rare for a foreign body to become lodged in a child's vagina, despite such exploration. If, however, there is a foreign body in your child's vagina, there may be symptoms of local soreness and tenderness or, after a day or two, an unpleasant-smelling, blood-stained discharge from the vagina. A discharge with itchiness, especially around the anus, may be an infestation of **worms**.

Is it serious?

Any discharge from the vagina, or soreness of the genital area, should be treated by a doctor, but is rarely serious.

Possible symptoms

▶ **Soreness or tenderness** around the vagina.
▶ **Smelly or blood-stained discharge**.

What should I do first?

1 Ask your child if she or a playmate has tried to push anything into her vagina.

2 Check your child's stools carefully for tiny, thread-like worms.

Should I consult the doctor?

Consult your doctor as soon as possible if you notice any inflammation or discharge.

What might the doctor do?

Your doctor will examine your child to try to determine whether the symptoms are the result of a foreign body being pushed into the vagina. If he thinks there is something there, he may refer you to a paediatric or gynaecological specialist who will perform an internal examination. The specialist will remove the foreign body, treat any infection with antibiotics and prescribe an ointment to relieve soreness or itching.

What can I do to help?

▶ Don't make too much fuss about the incident. It is important that your child doesn't develop an obsession about her genitalia that may affect her in later life.
▶ Discourage your child from using any instruments when playing "doctors and nurses".

SEE ALSO:
Worms 263

Verruca

A VERRUCA IS A WART on the sole of the foot that has been pushed up into the foot by the pressure of walking. It is highly infectious and is spread by direct contact with surfaces where infected feet have been, such as communal swimming pools, showers and gymnasiums. Many verrucae disappear naturally after 6–12 months but, because a verruca can be spread easily and because it can be painful, treatment is advisable.

Is it serious?

A verruca is never serious but it can cause pain and discomfort, depending on where it appears on the sole of the foot.

Possible symptoms

Classic appearance of verruca

▶ **White or brown, flat lump** on the sole of the foot.
▶ **Pain** when walking or standing on the foot.

What should I do first?

1 Wash your child's feet and leave them to soak in warm water to soften the skin.

2 With a clean scalpel (available from the chemist) pare away thin layers of the softened verruca very gently. It is always wiser to take off too little rather than to draw blood.

3 Apply a proprietary brand of wart treatment, obtainable from a chemist. Don't apply the wart treatment to healthy skin. To avoid this, use a corn plaster or a piece of ordinary plaster, with a hole the size of the verruca cut out of it, to protect the surrounding areas. After putting on the lotion, cover the verruca with a sterile dressing and plaster.

4 Repeat the procedure every day until the verruca has disappeared.

Should I consult the doctor?

Consult your doctor as soon as possible if the verruca is painful or if the verrucae are increasing in number, or if self-help treatment fails.

What might the doctor do?

Your doctor may refer you to a special wart clinic under the supervision of a dermatologist. The verruca will be removed either by treatment with a freezing agent such as liquid nitrogen, or by being burned off or scraped out under a local anaesthetic.

What can I do to help?

▶ Cover the verruca with a secure plaster whenever your child goes barefooted; this should prevent the spread of the virus.
▶ Discourage your child from scratching the verruca. He could infect himself elsewhere.

SEE ALSO:
Warts 259

Vision problems

MOST VISION DEFECTS are due to a fault in the eye itself and are not the result of disease or injury. Babies are rarely born totally blind and routine check-ups during a child's pre-school years should detect any defect that could later lead to problems of vision.

Cross-section of eye

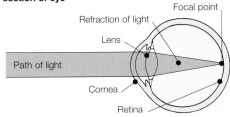

Focal point
Refraction of light
Lens
Path of light
Cornea
Retina

Many defects are caused when the light entering the eye does not focus properly on the retina. If the eyeball is too long from front to back, the images of distant objects will be focused in front of the retina and will appear blurred; near objects will be seen clearly. This is known as short sight. If the eyeball is too short from front to back, the images of both near and far objects will focus behind the retina. All images will be blurred, but near objects will be the worst. This is known as long sight. Short sight usually develops in late childhood and tends to run in families and a child with a parent who is short-sighted should be regularly tested. Long sight is generally present at birth, and can cause eye fatigue as your child strains to focus on objects close to him. Both long- and short-sightedness can be easily corrected with glasses.

Colour blindness is another common condition, especially in boys, and it too tends to run in families. True colour blindness, when everything appears grey, is rare; what most people generally refer to as colour blindness is in fact an inability to distinguish between reds and greens. There is no treatment for this condition but it does not interfere greatly with everyday life.

A **squint** is the other common eye problem. If your baby is under six weeks old and one or both eyes seem to wander slightly, there is no need to worry. However, if the squint persists, you should seek medical advice.

Are they serious?

Vision problems can be serious if they go untreated. Eyes need constant exercise and stimulation to keep them healthy and a disused eye, as occurs in a squint, will deteriorate rapidly. However, early treatment, generally with glasses, occasionally with an operation, should correct most problems.

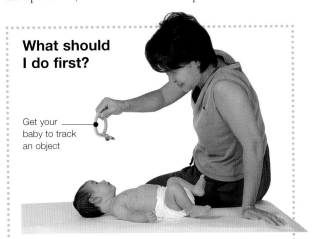

What should I do first?

Get your baby to track an object

1 Although your baby will have regular sight tests, you can check his vision yourself when he's about three months old. Dangle a familiar object about 20cm (8in) from your baby's face and move it slowly to one side. Your baby's eyes should track the object.

2 Be on the alert for any changes in the appearance of your child's eyes, such as the development of a squint, when both eyes do not follow an object together.

Continued on next page

Continued from previous page

3 Be responsive to signs that your child cannot see clearly – if, for example, he is always bumping into furniture or is not able to follow the trajectory of a ball that is thrown to him.

4 Get another eye test done if your child does not co-operate with the health visitor or school nurse at a regular check-up, and the test is not carried out thoroughly for any reason. Often a child who is unable to do the test will cover up the disability with bad behaviour.

Should I consult the doctor?

Consult your doctor as soon as possible if you suspect any defect in your child's vision or notice any change in the appearance of his eyes, if your child complains of sore eyes and rubs his eyes a lot for no apparent reason, or if your child's school performance is poor for no obvious reason. Your child may be having difficulty following his teachers because of some vision problem and may be misbehaving or not concentrating during his lessons because of it.

What might the doctor do?

▌ Your doctor will check your child for sharpness of vision. Your child will be asked to read the letters on a card placed 6m (20ft) away from him. Each eye will be tested separately. A child under three years old will be asked to match figures or pictures placed in front of him with the same object held up for him by the doctor.

▌ Your doctor will check the general condition of your child's eyes with an ophthalmoscope to see if there is any internal eye disorder. If treatment is necessary, your child will be referred to an optician or an ophthalmic surgeon. In most cases, suitable glasses will be prescribed and fitted.

What can I do to help?

▌ Get glasses with plastic lenses – they are lighter to wear and don't break.

▌ Help your child to cope with teasing from his playmates by emphasizing the benefits of being able to see clearly.

▌ Keep a spare pair of glasses as children tend to break frames.

▌ Teach your child how to keep the lenses clean, and encourage him to clean them daily.

▌ Be firm with your child to make sure he wears his glasses as often as instructed by your doctor, particularly in the early weeks when he is still getting used to them.

▌ Tie a piece of elastic around the back of your child's glasses so that they stay on during active play.

SEE ALSO:
Squint 226

Vomiting

CONSULT YOUR DOCTOR IMMEDIATELY if your child continues to vomit over a six-hour period; if vomiting is accompanied by diarrhoea or a fever; or if the vomiting is accompanied by any other symptoms such as **earache**.

Accompanying symptoms	Common causes
Your baby often brings up a little milk during or after a feed, but seems contented, feeds well and is gaining weight.	This regurgitation of a little milk – possetting – is normal and harmless.
Your baby is less than 10 weeks old and has more than once vomited forcibly during, or immediately after, a feed.	He could have **Pyloric stenosis**, *page 205.*
Your baby seems well and hungry but vomits during, or immediately after, his feed.	Solids given before he can chew properly may be the cause. Until your baby is six or seven months old, give puréed foods.
Your baby has a runny or blocked nose, snuffly breathing or a cough.	A **Common cold**, *page 90*, can make your baby vomit if he swallows a lot of the mucus it produces. A **Cough**, *page 98*, may also make him vomit.
Your bottlefed or weaned baby, or child, seems unwell and has passed frequent, watery stools.	**CONSULT YOUR DOCTOR IMMEDIATELY**. Your baby may have **Gastroenteritis**, *page 140*. An older child may have **Food poisoning**, *page 137.*
Your child seems unwell, looks flushed and feels hot.	An infection is the most likely cause. See **Fever**, *page 134.*
When travelling, your child seems pale and quiet and complains of nausea.	**Travel sickness**, *page 248*, is the most likely cause.
Your child complains of a severe headache on one side of his forehead.	He could have **Migraine**, *page 180*.
Your child has abdominal pain around the navel and to the lower right side of his groin.	**CONSULT YOUR DOCTOR IMMEDIATELY**. Your child could have **Appendicitis**, *page 54.*
Your baby is in severe pain and is passing stools that contain blood and mucus resembling redcurrant jelly.	**CONSULT YOUR DOCTOR IMMEDIATELY**. Your baby could have a bowel blockage known as **Intussusception**, *page 169.*
Your child cannot bend his neck forward without pain and turns away from bright light.	**CONSULT YOUR DOCTOR IMMEDIATELY**. Your child may have **Meningitis**, *page 178.*

Vomitting *Continued from previous page*

VOMITING IS THE VIOLENT EXPULSION of the contents of the stomach through the mouth. A baby may posset up small quantities of curdled milk after a feed, but this should not be confused with vomiting. Vomiting has many causes (*see page 257*), but in the majority of cases there is little warning and after a single bout your child should be comfortable and back to normal. Vomiting can be a symptom of a specific disorder of the stomach such as **pyloric stenosis**, or a symptom of an infection, such as an ear infection. It frequently accompanies a fever, and even the **common cold** can cause vomiting if your child swallows enough nasal discharge to irritate his stomach. If your child has a bad cough, this can also cause him to vomit up food that he has recently eaten. Other causes of vomiting include **appendicitis**, **meningitis**, **migraine** headaches, **food poisoning** and **travel sickness**. Some children vomit because of excitement and anticipation but this is usually limited to toddlers.

Is it serious?
Vomiting should always be taken seriously because it can rapidly cause **dehydration**, particularly in a baby or young child.

What should I do first?

1 Put your child to bed and place a bowl for him to vomit into within easy reach.

2 Give your child frequent, small amounts of liquid in the form of a rehydration solution (available in powder form from the chemist).

3 Check your child's temperature to see if he has a fever too.

4 Keep your child cool by wiping his face with a cool, damp cloth.

5 Get him to brush his teeth after vomiting to take away the taste.

Should I consult the doctor?
Consult your doctor immediately if your child continues to vomit over a six-hour period; if vomiting is accompanied by diarrhoea or a fever over 38°C (100.4°F); or if the vomiting is accompanied by any other worrying symptoms such as earache.

What might the doctor do?
❱ Your doctor will diagnose the cause of the vomiting and will then treat your child accordingly.

He will also make sure that there is no danger of dehydration.
❱ Your child may be admitted to hospital to be given fluids intravenously if he is in danger of becoming dehydrated.

What can I do to help?
❱ Give your child plenty of his favourite drinks, but dilute any fruit juices and don't give him milk.
❱ Feed your child bland foods when the nausea and vomiting have passed. Reintroduce solid foods slowly.

Warts

WARTS ARE SMALL BENIGN LUMPS caused by the wart virus. They are made up of an excess of dead cells that protrude above the surface of the skin. They can appear singly or in alarming numbers over all parts of the body, including the face and genitals. If they occur on the soles of the feet, they are known as **verrucae**. Many warts disappear spontaneously in 6–12 months. Warts are spread by direct contact with an infected person.

Are they serious?
Warts are neither serious nor painful.

Possible symptoms

▶ **Hard lumps of dried skin** that appear spontaneously and grow singly or in clusters anywhere on the body.

▶ **Small black dots** within the lumps (these are blood vessels and not dirt).

What should I do first?

1 If your child has a wart, check the rest of his body for others.

2 Try ignoring the warts; they will go away of their own accord.

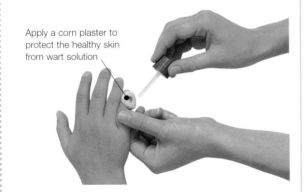

Apply a corn plaster to protect the healthy skin from wart solution

3 If your child wants the warts removed or they appear on a part of the body where they would easily infect other people, try the patent wart cures from your chemist. These work by the application of a weak acid solution to the wart and the daily removal of the resulting burned skin. You should follow the manufacturer's instructions carefully and avoid applying the solution to healthy skin. Don't use patent wart cures on warts that appear on the face or genitals. You may cause scarring.

Should I consult the doctor?
Consult your doctor as soon as possible if you are unsure whether the lumps are really warts. Any growth or lump on your child's skin which you are uncertain about should be checked by a doctor. Consult your doctor as soon as possible if the warts continue to multiply, or appear on the face or genitals and you want them removed.

What might the doctor do?
Your doctor may advise you to ignore the warts, or refer you to a hospital dermatologist. If your child has to attend a special wart clinic, be prepared for frequent visits and some discomfort for your child. Methods of wart removal include cauterization and surgical removal.

SEE ALSO:
Verruca 254

Wax in ears

SOME WAX IN THE EXTERNAL EAR CANAL is quite normal. It is produced by glands in the skin of the canal to protect the ear from dust, foreign bodies and infections, and it appears as golden-brown or rust-coloured waxy crumbs. The wax is usually moved along and out of the canal by chewing movements of the jaw, but in some children an excess of wax is produced as a response to chronic **otitis media** or a dusty environment. Very occasionally wax may collect, dry and block the ear canal, leading to a temporary reduction in hearing.

Is it serious?

An excess of wax is not serious, although it may affect the hearing temporarily until the plug of wax is removed.

Possible symptoms

▶ **Visible build-up of wax** in the ear canal.
▶ **Partial deafness**.
▶ **Feeling of fullness** in the ear or a ringing sound.

What should I do first?

Check your child's ears regularly for wax build-up. Dislodge the wax only if it is at the opening of the ear canal and can be lifted out easily. Never poke anything, even a cotton-wool swab, into the ear canal.

Should I consult the doctor?

Consult your doctor as soon as possible if you cannot remove the wax easily, or if your child seems to be having trouble hearing.

What might the doctor do?

▶ After examining your child's ears with an otoscope, your doctor may syringe his ears with warm water to wash out the wax. This is a painless, though uncomfortable, procedure.
▶ If the wax is hard and compacted, your doctor may prescribe ear drops to soften and dissolve the wax. You may have to return to have your child's ears syringed a few days later if the drops have not dislodged the wax.

What can I do to help?

▶ Insert the ear drops just before your child's bedtime. Lay your child across your lap, or on his side on a bed, and drop the required amount into the ear canal. Ensure he lies still for two minutes so that the drops don't drain out of the ear.
▶ After inserting the ear drops, make an ear plug from cotton wool and leave it in your child's ear overnight. The wax may come out with the ear plug in the morning. If it doesn't, you may have to return to the doctor to have the ear syringed.
▶ Be on the alert for a possible blockage in the future. The tendency to produce an excess of wax is inherited, and blockage may recur after your child has a **common cold** or other respiratory tract infections.

SEE ALSO:
Common cold 90
Deafness 108
Otitis media 198

Whooping cough

WHOOPING COUGH IS ONE OF the most dangerous childhood diseases, especially in babies under 12 months of age. It is caused by the bacterium *Bordetella pertussis*, which causes the airways to become clogged with mucus.

Whooping cough begins as an ordinary cold with a cough. The coughing becomes severe, with spasmodic coughing bouts which make it difficult to breathe. When your child does manage to draw breath during a coughing bout (which can last up to a minute), there is a characteristic "whooping" sound as air is drawn in past the swollen larynx. The breathing difficulties are even greater for babies, who may never develop the technique of whooping to get air into their lungs, an inability which can prove fatal. Sometimes **vomiting** occurs after a coughing bout. The coughing phase of whooping cough can last for up to 10 weeks. The risk of developing a secondary infection, such as **pneumonia** or **bronchitis**, is high after this illness.

Whooping cough has been on the increase because parents have, in the past, chosen not to immunize their children following controversy surrounding the vaccination's possible side effects. However, medical opinion still holds that it is better for your child and for the community if the vaccination programme is continued, though there are some babies who should be placed in a special category and should not be immunized. Ask your doctor's advice.

Is it serious?

Whooping cough is a serious disease, especially in babies, who may become dangerously short of oxygen during a coughing bout. If vomiting is severe, there is also the danger of **dehydration**. A severe attack of whooping cough can damage the lungs and cause recurrent bronchial infections.

Possible symptoms

▶ **Cold symptoms** of a fever, runny nose, aches and pains.
▶ **Excessive coughing**, with a characteristic "whoop" as the child struggles to draw breath.
▶ **Vomiting** after a coughing bout.
▶ **Sleeplessness** because of the coughing.

What should I do first?

1 If your child's cold fails to improve and her cough worsens, put her to bed and seek medical help.

2 If you suspect your baby has whooping cough, consult your doctor immediately.

3 If you suspect your child has whooping cough, do not send her back to school or nursery school until you have seen your doctor.

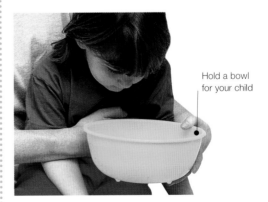

Hold a bowl for your child

4 If your child is having a long coughing bout, sit her up and hold him leaning slightly forward. Hold a bowl so that she can spit up any phlegm.

Continued on next page

Continued from previous page

Should I consult the doctor?

Consult your doctor immediately if you suspect whooping cough.

What might the doctor do?

▶ Your doctor may prescribe antibiotics to reduce the severity of the cough and limit the infectiousness of the child. However, whooping cough is difficult to diagnose during the preliminary stage of the disease, and medication must be taken early to do any good. Your doctor may need to take a throat swab from your baby to diagnose whooping cough because babies rarely whoop.

▶ Your doctor will keep a close check on a baby with whooping cough and if the disease is severe will probably recommend hospital admission to prevent dehydration and to administer oxygen quickly if this should become necessary.

▶ Your doctor will make sure that you know how to hold your child during a coughing attack, and will show you how if you are unsure. He may advise you to raise the foot of your baby's cot and put your baby to sleep on his stomach.

What can I do to help?

▶ During a coughing bout hold your child as you've been shown and keep him calm. Panic will make the breathlessness worse. Hold a bowl under his chin and encourage him to spit up the phlegm into it. This helps to clear the airways.

▶ Put bowls in all the rooms in the house so that he can spit up any phlegm or vomit without worrying about getting to the toilet in time. Clean these bowls in boiling water to prevent the spread of infection.

▶ If your child vomits after a coughing bout, give him small meals and drinks afterwards. This gives him a better chance to keep some food and liquids down and therefore to keep his strength up.

▶ Don't let your child play boisterously while he's recuperating. Exertion will bring on a coughing bout quickly and leave him exhausted.

▶ Keep your child away from cigarette smoke.

▶ Sleep in the room with him so that he is never alone during a coughing bout.

▶ Don't give your child any cough medicines without your doctor's advice.

▶ If, after the whooping cough has cleared up, your child seems unwell and is breathing with difficulty, contact your doctor immediately in case there is a secondary infection, such as pneumonia or bronchitis.

▶ Don't worry if your child "whoops" when he next catches a cold. This is not a return of the disease; your child is simply repeating a habit learned during all those coughing bouts.

SEE ALSO:
Bronchiolitis 72
Dehydration 109
Pneumonia 202
Vomiting 257

Worms

THERE ARE A NUMBER OF WORMS that can live in the human body but the most common in temperate climates is the threadworm. The worm usually enters the body as eggs in contaminated food, which then hatch in the intestine and develop into adults in 15–28 days. The female worms then lay more eggs around the host's anus, which causes itching, especially at night. If your child scratches himself, he can easily pick up the eggs and, by putting them into his mouth, start off the whole cycle again. Threadworms, which are 2–13mm (⅟₁₆–½in) long, are harmless, but they can produce unpleasant symptoms, like the itching around the anus. Threadworms are highly infectious and all the family should be treated simultaneously.

Roundworms are rare but are most likely to infect children in areas where sanitary conditions are poor; they are more common in tropical climates. These parasites are long – 15–35cm (6–14in) – and resemble a white earthworm. The eggs are swallowed with contaminated food or drink and, after hatching in the intestine, the worms lay eggs which are sometimes excreted in the stools. Your child will appear undernourished and he will fail to thrive.

Are they serious?
Worms are not usually serious and are easily treated.

Possible symptoms

Threadworms
▶ **Itching** around the anus, usually at night.
▶ **White thread-like worms** in the stools.
▶ **Sleeplessness** caused by intense itchiness.

Roundworms
▶ **Failure to thrive**.
▶ **White worms** in the stools.

What should I do first?

1 If your child is scratching his bottom, inspect the area about an hour after he has gone to bed. This is when the adult female usually comes out to lay eggs. The worm will look like a tiny piece of white thread.

2 Alternatively, inspect your child's stools for the numerous worms.

3 If you have recently been travelling in areas where infections with roundworm are common, and your child seems unwell and malnourished, inspect his stools for the larger roundworm.

Should I consult the doctor?

Consult your doctor as soon as possible if you find any worms. Consult your doctor as soon as possible if you've been in an area where roundworm is common and your child is not thriving.

What might the doctor do?

▶ Your doctor will prescribe a simple treatment, usually in the form of a pleasant-tasting, soluble powder to be taken by the whole family.
▶ If your child has a roundworm, your doctor will prescribe a drug to be taken by mouth which will paralyse the worm. He may also prescribe a

Continued on next page

Continued from previous page

laxative so that your child can pass the worm easily in his stools.

What can I do to help?

▶ Follow the instructions for the medication carefully. The bowel motions may be loose for 12 hours afterwards, so you may be advised to give the medication early in the morning.

▶ Repeating the dosage may be necessary depending on the type of worm and on the medication taken.

▶ Be meticulous about hygiene. The eggs can be picked up under the fingernails and reingested.

▶ Make sure your child wears pyjamas or pants at night so that, when he scratches, his hands don't come into direct contact with his anus.

SEE ALSO:
Itching 170
Toxocariasis 247

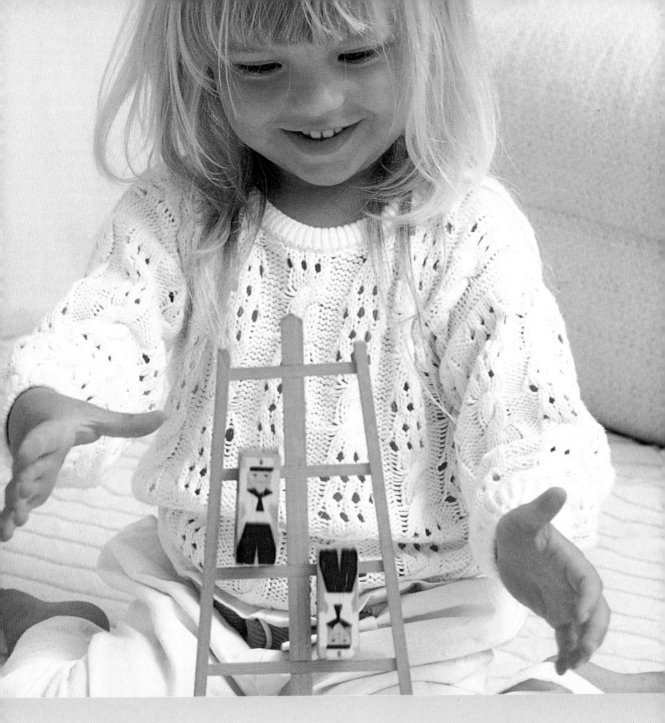

Baby and child safety

Safety around the home

MOST ACCIDENTS OCCUR AT HOME, and more than half of them involve children under the age of five. Many accidents can be avoided if you are aware of the potential dangers. Take time to crawl around your home to gain a child's-eye view of things. Alter the layout and position of items in your home where necessary to make sure that you minimize the chances of an accident occurring. Teach your child self-protection from an early age by making him aware of the dangers. He will not fully understand your instructions at first, and he will probably forget them soon afterwards, but, with persistence, the message will get through. As your child gets older, he will begin to understand the logic of your advice, and will start to do as you say.

However, when your child is young and cannot understand reasoning, there are certain simple, strict rules, such as never touching electric sockets and never playing with sharp objects, that should be observed at all times.

General safety tips

▶ Never leave your child alone for long, no matter how busy you are. Always keep a check on what your child is doing and where he is. Be especially cautious at the end of the day, when you will be tired and possibly preoccupied with the family get-together.

▶ Check all your electrical cords: they are dangerous if frayed or split and should be replaced immediately.

▶ Teach your child that radiators and towel rails are hot to touch. Cover them with towels or seal them off with furniture if necessary.

▶ If you keep a gun in the house, never leave it loaded. Lock it away and lock the cartridges away in a separate container. Television films have made guns more familiar to children and they are now much more likely to use them as part of their play.

▶ Whenever you give your child medicines, read the label carefully to check that you are administering the correct dosage.

▶ Return any out-of-date or left-over medicine to the pharmacy.

▶ Make all upper-storey windows safe by fitting bars or safety catches, depending on the style of window. Don't leave any furniture beneath the window – your child may climb up and attempt to open or lean out of the window.

▶ Fit safety film to large areas of glass that your child could fall against, such as French windows and patio doors.

▶ If you have smooth tiled or wooden floors, use a special polish to make the surface non-slip. Don't let your child run around in stockinged feet.

▶ Put safety covers on all unused electric sockets throughout the house.

▶ Install smoke and carbon monoxide alarms.

▶ Keep emergency numbers by the telephone, especially for your baby-sitter to use.

▶ When visiting grandparents, friends who have no children or on outings, check around the house and garden for possible problems, especially if children don't often visit. Breakable items or sharp objects may have been left in accessible places and cleaning chemicals may not have been put out of reach. Never be complacent; always presume that your child will find trouble if he tries.

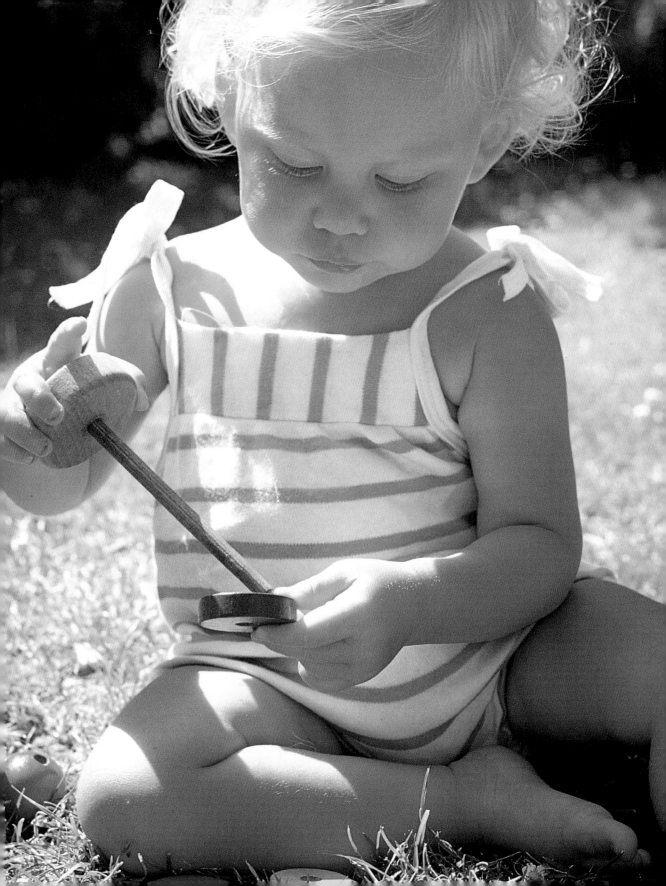

Kitchen

THE KITCHEN IS VERY OFTEN the focal room for the whole household and as such is often full of the bustle of the family. It is potentially dangerous for a number of reasons: from the cooking itself (boiling water and hot fat), from cooking utensils (knives and hot pans) and from the fact that you are preoccupied with food preparation and may not be paying full attention to your child.

▶ Keep all electric flexes out of reach. If they are left dangling over the edge of a work surface your child could pull whatever equipment they are attached to down on himself. Unplug electrical appliances when not in use so that your child cannot start them by accident.

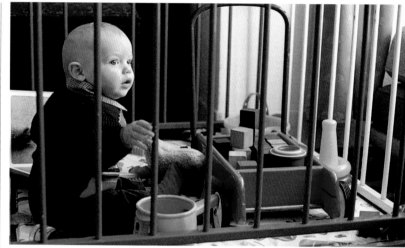

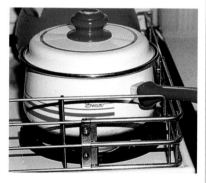

▶ Buy safety guards for your cookers. Point saucepan handles away from the front of the cooker so that your child cannot grab the handle and pull the contents on to himself. When possible, use the back rings.

▶ Keep your iron in a safe place, out of your child's reach; a wall-mounted iron rest is ideal.

▶ Never leave objects near the edges of work surfaces; tuck them well back.

▶ With a young child, arrange a special play area away from your working area so that your child can play near you without becoming a safety hazard.

▶ Clean out your pet's bowls after use, or keep them out of reach.

▶ Keep all sharp knives and forks out of reach.

▶ Use safety film on glass doors and put transfers on clear glass to remind your child that there's an object there.

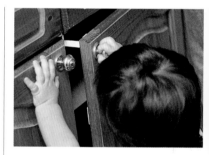

▶ Attach safety catches to all cupboards and drawers that contain dangerous substances. Better still, keep dangerous substances out of your child's reach altogether.

▶ Don't leave hot liquids where your child can reach them – even a cup of coffee can scald badly.

Continued from previous page

Highchairs

Until your child is old enough to sit at the table, a highchair is the most suitable and comfortable way of feeding him. Highchairs are available in a variety of designs, but there are certain safety features that you should look out for, no matter what style you opt for. Choose one that is stable, wlth widely spaced legs. If the tray is removable there should be a strong enough lock or clasp to hold it in position while the chair is being used.

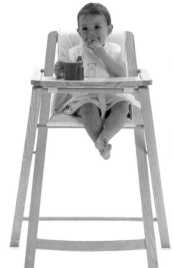

There should be special clips at either side for attaching a safety harness and this should always be used when your child is in the highchair. Never leave your child unattended in the highchair.

**Choose a highchair that
is safe and secure**

▌Make sure your floor is non-slip and free of grease; mop up any spills straight away.

▌Gastroenteritis can be a real risk for a bottlefed baby so sterilize all equipment carefully – milk is a favourite breeding ground for bacteria. Never leave a prepared feed standing at room temperature, or keep the remains of the last feed for the next.

▌Don't store uncooked meat next to cooked meat – one can contaminate the other. Don't store open tins in the fridge; put the remainder into a clean container.

▌Keep a fire extinguisher and fire blanket in case of fire.

▌Secure a swinging or self-closing door when your child is around – he could easily catch his fingers or be knocked over.

▌Don't use tablecloths if you have a toddler. Even a crawling baby can pull a cloth and bring the table's contents on to his head. Keep all items in the centre of the table.

▌Place the highchair out of the way of doors and thoroughfares, and well away from work surfaces.

▌If your child is going through a stage where he rummages through the bin, be very careful with sharp-edged cans. Always put a tin lid back inside the can and squeeze the sides together.

Bedroom

An awareness of safety in the bedroom is especially important in the first year of your baby's life because this is probably the room where your child will spend most of his time – either sleeping, being nursed or being changed.

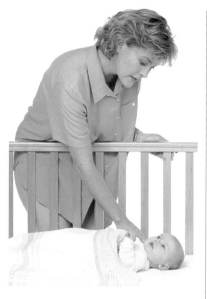

▶ Always put your baby to sleep on his back to lessen the risk of cot death. To raise his head, put a pillow under the mattress to avoid any risk of suffocation. To minimize the risk of choking, use a safety mattress that has air holes through which any vomit can drain away.

▶ Firmly attach mobiles out of your child's reach.

▶ Buy a sturdy cot with rounded edges. If the cot has a movable side rail, make sure it has strong clasps so that your child cannot release it and get his fingers caught. Make sure that the mattress can be positioned low enough so even if your child stands up, he cannot get out of the cot.

▶ Don't leave open electric or gas heaters in your child's room when he is unattended.

▶ Don't overheat the room, as high temperatures increase the risk of cot death.

▶ Use wall-mounted or ceiling lights rather than those with trailing flexes.

▶ Buy non-flammable night-clothes and bedding.

▶ Don't have any lightweight furniture in your child's room – he may topple it over on to himself. Try to buy round-edged furniture.

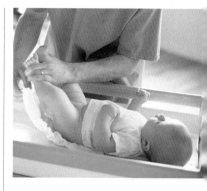

▶ Have all your baby's changing equipment close to the changing mat, but never above it in case something falls on the child. Never leave your child alone on a changing mat that has no sides in case he rolls off.

Bathroom

YOUR CHILD IS MOST AT RISK from falls and poisoning in the bathroom. Electrocution is also a potential danger, but improved building regulations now mean that no power points other than shaver sockets are installed in bathrooms. Only wall-mounted heaters, positioned out of reach, should be used. Portable electric heaters should *never* be taken into the bathroom. Never leave a child under the age of three alone in a bath to answer the 'phone or door: he could go under the water.

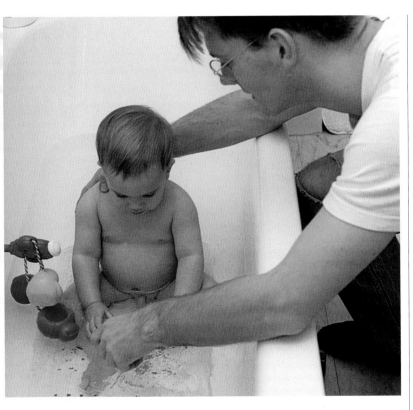

▶ Use a non-slip mat if you have a slippery tiled or polished floor.

▶ Keep the toilet lid closed and never mix cleaners with bleach as this gives off toxic fumes.

▶ Keep all toilet-cleaning chemicals and the toilet brush locked away – don't be tempted to tuck them behind the toilet itself.

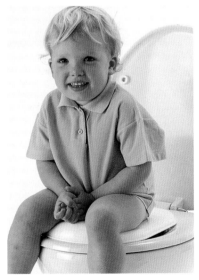

▶ Use a non-slip bath mat.

▶ When running a bath, always put in cold water first and then top up with hot water.

▶ Install a childproof medicine cabinet. Don't put it above the toilet – your child could climb on to the toilet to reach inside the cabinet.

▶ Keep all medicines in childproof containers.

▶ Use safety film on a glass shower door. In case of an accident, the glass will be held in place and will not splinter.

▶ Keep cosmetics out of reach, especially those in aerosol cans.

▶ Use a special toilet seat and step for your toddler so that he does not slip off the seat.

Living room

MUCH OF DAY-TO-DAY LIVING goes on in the living room as well as the kitchen. One of the problems for parents trying to childproof their living room is not only how to make it safe for their child, but how to preserve valuable and much-loved objects from being broken by a child. Initially, it's probably easier to keep breakables well out of reach, but, with time, repeated warnings should work.

▶ If you have an open fire, always use a fireguard when the fire is lit to prevent your child from falling into the flames.

▶ Don't leave anything belonging to your child above the fireplace or resting on a windowsill; he may try to climb up to get at it.

▶ Keep permanent flexes pinned to the skirting board, and position long flexes where they cannot be tripped over or played with by putting them behind furniture or under carpets.

▶ Use safety film on French windows or patio doors.

▶ Keep the television in such a position that the back cannot be touched. It's also advisable to keep any recording, video or stereo equipment out of reach.

▶ Make sure that any carpets and rugs are in good condition, with no holes or turned-up edges which could act as trip wires.

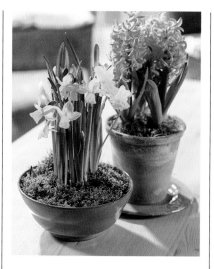

▶ Keep all houseplants high up out of the reach of small children and ensure that none of your houseplants is poisonous.

▶ Don't leave hot drinks, alcohol, cigarettes, matches or lighters where your child can get at them. Don't place heavy objects on low tables.

▶ Keep all breakable items out of your child's reach.

▶ If you have any sharp-edged table tops and there is a risk that your child could run into them, fit plastic safety corners on them.

Hall and stairs

THE TWO MAJOR DANGERS in halls and stairways are the stairs themselves and the possibility that your child could run out of the front door and on to the street. Until your child has the balance to come down a step at a time holding on to the banister, train him to come down the stairs on his bottom. Always stop him from going outside unless he is accompanied by you.

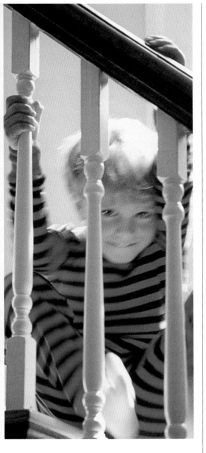

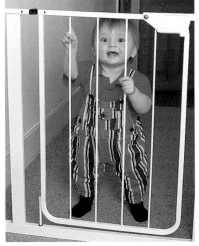

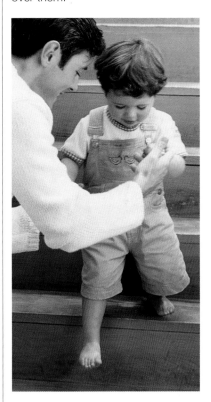

▶ Keep your child's toys as tidy as possible so that no one can trip over them.

▶ Have a stair-gate at the top and/or the bottom of the stairs to prevent your child from climbing up or tumbling down. Stop him if he tries to climb over the gate.

▶ Keep all breakable items, and the 'phone, out of reach.

▶ Make sure that the front door closes properly so that there is no risk of your child being able to pull the door open and escape on to the street.

▶ Keep stairs well lit and keep the stair carpet well maintained to minimize the risk of anyone tripping and falling.

▶ Make sure the banister supports are close enough together to prevent your child sticking his head between them and running the risk of getting it stuck, or of a young child falling through.

▶ If you've got polished floors, don't let your child run around in socks. He could easily fall and hurt himself.

Garden

THE GARDEN CAN BE A dangerous place for a child, not only because it provides the means of escape on to roads, but also because of the machinery that is used to maintain it. There is the added danger, especially for toddlers, that some garden plants are themselves poisonous but nevertheless look like sweets. Although rarely fatal if eaten, they can produce unpleasant effects, ranging from skin to stomach irritation. Never let your child play unattended; keep him away from sharp or prickly plants like roses, and stop him from playing with earth – it may be contaminated with chemicals, or have bits of glass and animal dirt in it. If you have an area in the garden where you keep your car, make sure you know exactly where your child is before your start up the engine and move off.

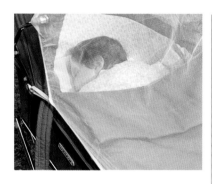

▶ Cover a pram with a safety net to prevent any cat smothering your child.

▶ If you have a pet, clear up excreta before your child has an opportunity to poke, play with or eat them.

▶ Keep all paved areas and steps in good condition and de-moss them regularly to prevent falls.

▶ Pull up mushrooms and fungi as soon as they appear.

▶ Cover drains with wire mesh.

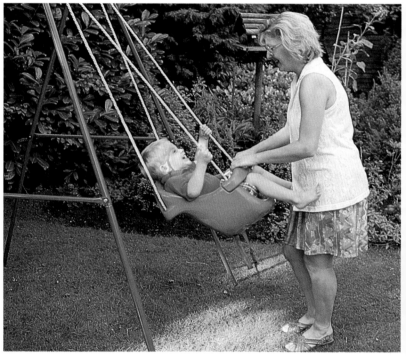

▶ Erect a climbing frame on grass so that any falls are cushioned. Keep all play equipment well maintained – check wood for splinters, ropes for fraying and chain links for good joins.

▶ Empty the paddling pool as soon as your child has finished playing with it. Fit any water-collecting devices with a close-fitting lid so that your child cannot fall inside.

▶ Attach childproof locks to any gates.

Continued from previous page

Poisonous plants

Skin irritation	Mouth and throat irritation	Stomach irritation	General poisoning
Bleeding heart	Daphne	Daphne	Rhododendron
Daphne	Jack-in-the-pulpit	Ivy	Crocus
Poison ivy	Buttercup	Wistaria	Hydrangea
Poison oak	White bryony	Belladonna lily	Larkspur
Christmas rose		Christmas rose	Lily of the valley
Foxglove		Daffodil	Laburnum
		Hyacinth	
		Iris	
		Sweetpea	

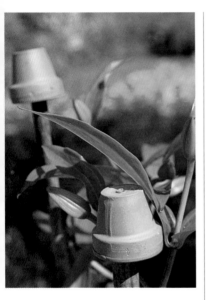

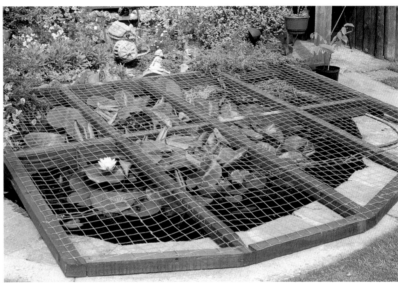

▶ Make sure that staked flowers have sticks that are at least 1.2m (4ft) high. Put a pot over the top of them to make them really obvious and to avoid accidents.

▶ Put deck chairs and garden seats up yourself; don't let your child attempt it – they are notorious for catching fingers.

▶ Erect a barrier or wire mesh around your pool or pond.

▶ Never let your child swim alone and discourage him from running around the pool side – he could slip, bang his head and fall into the water.

▶ Keep all garden chemicals in a locked room or shed and never decant any poisonous substances into old soft-drink bottles.

Road safety

AFTER THE HOME, MOST ACCIDENTS to children occur on the street. It is therefore most important that, from an early age, your child is taught the rules of the road – where it is safe to cross, how to judge distances and where to play safely. The road codes may differ slightly between busy city streets and quiet country lanes but, wherever you are, talk to your child while walking or driving, and explain what you are doing and why.

Never be complacent about your child's road sense: keep reminding him of the rules. Even up to the age of 12 children may have difficulty interpreting road safety; they may always regard a pedestrian crossing as safe, even with fast-approaching traffic; they may be distracted and not think before stepping out on to the road; they will certainly not be able to judge the speed of oncoming traffic, or hear an unseen car.

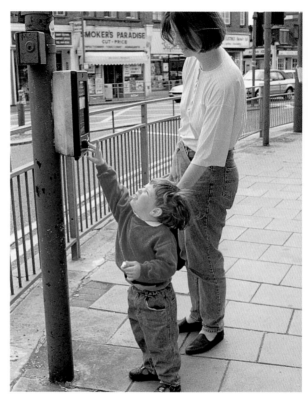

The green cross code

▶ **Find a safe place to cross**, such as a pedestrian crossing, subway or controlled lights.
▶ **Stop at the kerb**, look in both directions and listen for traffic.
▶ **If traffic is coming, let it pass**.
▶ **Look in both directions again** and, when nothing is coming, walk across the road. Keep looking and listening while you cross.

Beware of strangers

At frequent intervals, remind your child of the dangers of talking to strangers. Make up your own code word so that, should you have to send a friend or neighbour to pick up your child, this word can be used. Tell your child never to go with anyone unless they use the code, no matter what the pretext.

▶ Encourage your child to press the button at pedestrian crossings.

▶ Never push a pram out into the road without first checking that there is no traffic coming. Some parents forget that the pram sticks out in front of them by at least 1m (3ft).

▶ Teach your child to wait at pedestrian crossings until the cars stop for him.

▶ When crossing with a pram and an older child, make sure you hold on to the walking child, too. When you know you can trust him not to run away, he can hold on to the side of the pram.

▶ Make the kerb the safety line and make it clear to your child that he's not to cross it without holding your hand.

Points to remember

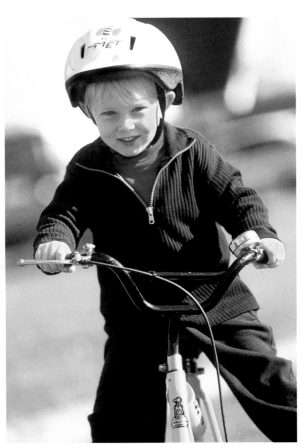

▶ Encourage your child to play or cycle in a garden or park away from pavements and busy roads. Unless you live in a very quiet road with few parked cars, don't let your child play in the road.

▶ Stress that your child must never chase a ball, pet or friend out on to the road without first stopping to look and listen.

▶ Never let your child play near a blind kerb.

▶ Warn your child of the obvious dangers of playing or standing behind parked cars.

Pram safety

When you go out with a pram, never put heavy shopping bags over the handles – they could easily tip it backwards. Instead, buy a pram with a basket underneath. When you park a pram, always put on the brakes, but also point the pram in such a way that, even if the brakes failed, it wouldn't roll into the road. Never leave a child unattended, and never tie a dog to the pram.

What to look for

There should be a safety strap and side buckles for the separate attachment of a safety harness

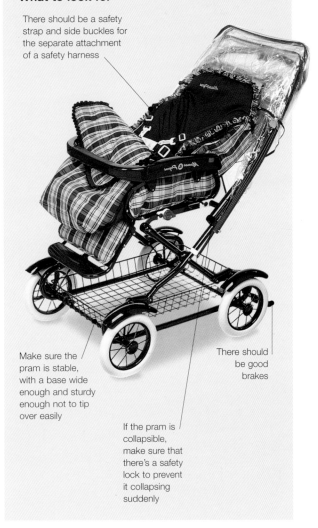

Make sure the pram is stable, with a base wide enough and sturdy enough not to tip over easily

There should be good brakes

If the pram is collapsible, make sure that there's a safety lock to prevent it collapsing suddenly

Car safety

THE SAFETY LAWS FOR CHILDREN travelling in cars differ from country to country but, whatever they are, you should never allow a child under 10 to travel in the front passenger seat. Children are very often more vulnerable than adults in cars because their parents assume that a child travelling in the back is not in danger. This is false. On collision, a child who is not secured in a belt or special seat will be thrown forcefully against the seat or passengers in front or, worse still, through the windscreen. Apart from this basic feature of car safety, there are certain rules that you should observe to make travelling with your child as safe as possible. These are illustrated, below. Even once you have stopped the car, you should still be vigilant: for example, never leave your child unattended, even briefly.

Car-safety guidelines

◗ Be careful when closing car doors. Children invariably leave their fingers in the way and, if you've already put the lock on the door, the effort to release trapped fingers will be even more frantic.

◗ Never be tempted to put a child into the same safety belt as yourself. He will be crushed by the weight of your body in the event of a crash.

◗ A carry cot must lie flat on the seat and its mattress must fit correctly. Make sure that the straps cross the middle of the cot.

◗ Teach your child to get out of the car on the pavement side. Never open the door on the traffic side, even on the quietest street.

◗ Do not put a car seat in the front passenger seat if the car contains an air bag on the passenger side. In the event of an accident, your child could be suffocated.

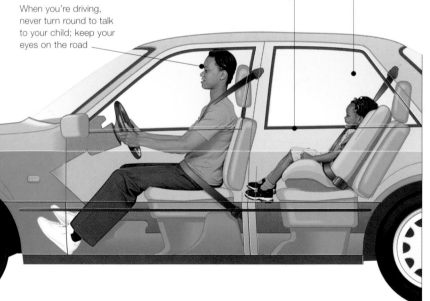

Don't let your child wind the window more than a quarter of the way down, and never let him lean, or put his hand, out of the window

Use the child locks on rear doors until your child is at least six years old

When you're driving, never turn round to talk to your child; keep your eyes on the road

If your child is under the age of 11, or weighs less than 36kg (80lb), a regular seat belt is not the right safety device for him. His pelvic bones are not sufficiently developed to protect the internal organs from the pressure of the belt in the case of a crash. Your child should, instead, be restrained in a special car seat or safety harness. Whatever design you select, make sure that it is approved by the national standards authority, and that you have it properly installed. A baby in a carry cot should be secured to the back seat with restraining straps to prevent the cot from sliding across the back seat, and the straps should be bolted to the car frame. Car seats should also be bolted to the frame. Once your child has grown out of his car seat, he can be strapped in with a safety harness and raised on a booster seat so that he can see out of the window but remain safe.

Safety for babies

Until your baby is old enough to sit up and support his own weight, he will have to travel in either a carry cot, or a special back-facing baby seat. The latter is buckled into an adult safety belt and faces backwards so that, in an accident, any force is exerted against the baby's back and not his pelvis.

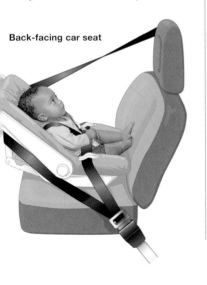

Back-facing car seat

Safety for older babies, toddlers and young children

Once your child can support his head and can sit well on his own, he should go into a car seat. By the time he's about three, or weighs more than 18kg (40lb), he can use a special safety harness, with or without a booster seat. Safety seats come in several styles and sizes – it's important to find the one that best suits your child by shopping around and trying your child out in the ones available.

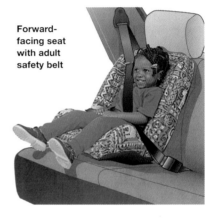

Forward-facing seat with adult safety belt

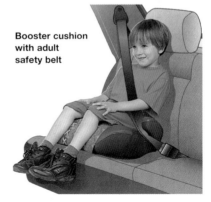

Booster cushion with adult safety belt

Playthings

ALTHOUGH THERE ARE NOW much tougher laws governing the safe production of toys, and the awareness of manufacturers is greatly improving, every year children are hurt and even killed by the toys that they play with. When buying toys or equipment for your child, try to buy those approved by the national safety authority (this will be indicated somewhere on the item by a symbol or number). If in doubt, contact your local consumer association.

Any household is potentially lethal for a child because there is so much that is new to be explored – a couple of minutes away from your child and he could find a shirt button, swallow it and choke. Never give your young child anything to play with that is so small that he might swallow it by accident, or push it up his nose, or into his ear. Make sure there are no sharp edges or projections on any toys, and avoid those made of thin, rigid plastic. On soft toys and animals, check that the eyes and nose, bells and ribbons are well secured and that they cannot be pulled off. Toys are often marked suitable for a certain age – follow these guidelines, and always supervise your child while he's playing if he's under two years old.

Toys and objects

Examine toys carefully before you buy or give them to your child. Smooth-edged, hand-sized, or bigger, toys are safest until your child is old enough to know not to put objects into his mouth. Before giving him household objects to play with, check them over carefully for cracks, sharp bits and splinters. Don't let your child play with pens or other long objects which he could accidentally poke into his eye.

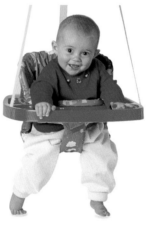

Baby bouncer

Make sure that your child is secured properly into the seat part of the bouncer, and that the clamp at the top is securely fastened to the door frame.

Baby walker

Select a walker with a wide base for stability. Avoid the "X" type of walker – these collapse easily and can trap fingers. Keep an eye on where your child roams, especially if you have any steps or ledges. Babies can build up quite a speed in their walkers, and if they hit a raised threshold, even a carpet ledge, they can tip over, or be catapulted out of the walker.

Paints and pencils

Always give your child non-toxic, edible paints, pencils and crayons to play with. (For your own peace of mind, use non-spill paints, too.)

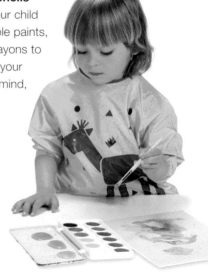

Sports and pastimes

WHATEVER SPORT OR PASTIME your child takes up, you should ensure that he is properly equipped for it and that he is taught the sport's basic rules for safety. For example, if he's skateboarding, bike-riding or roller-blading, make sure he uses the specially set-up areas rather than the road, and that he wears as much protective equipment as necessary. For example, get him to wear the helmet, knee-pads and gloves that are necessary. Almost every child learns to swim and ride a bike, and safety tips for these pastimes are given below.

Bicycle safety

Children under 10 should only ride their bikes in the garden, parks or specially designated areas. They should never ride on the road, not even when crossing it. Nor should they be allowed to ride on the pavement as they are a hazard for pedestrians, especially when going around corners. For your child's first bike, buy one with stabilizers at the back to allow him to gain confidence and general bike sense without having to worry about falling off. If your child has a carrier on the back, tell him it's not for carrying friends as they could easily topple over.

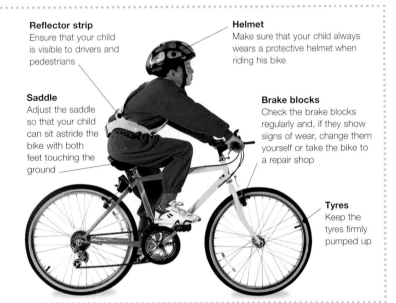

Reflector strip
Ensure that your child is visible to drivers and pedestrians

Helmet
Make sure that your child always wears a protective helmet when riding his bike

Saddle
Adjust the saddle so that your child can sit astride the bike with both feet touching the ground

Brake blocks
Check the brake blocks regularly and, if they show signs of wear, change them yourself or take the bike to a repair shop

Tyres
Keep the tyres firmly pumped up

Water safety

The most important element in water safety is your child's ability to swim. Enquire at your local swimming baths about mother-and-baby groups, and take your child to the nearest pool as often as possible, both to get him accustomed to the water and to encourage him to learn. Never let your child play in or near water without supervision. When you are at the seaside, or swimming in a lake or river, always heed local advice about swimming conditions: never swim when the red flag is flying, no matter how competent your family is at swimming. At the beach, always keep a close eye on your child, no matter how old, and don't let your child play alone with a lilo – it's very easy for either currents or wind to pull your child out from the shore. Because children have less subcutaneous fat than adults, they get cold quickly, so keep swimming times short.

Playground safety

ALL CHILDREN GET BORED PLAYING in their own or a friend's garden and, if there's a playground in your area, they are bound to want to visit it, especially if it's an adventure playground. Part of the adventure of an adventure playground is the sense of danger. However, you must try to help your child to understand his limitations and be cautious. The bravado that comes from being with friends who act like daredevils can easily lead to accidents. Playgrounds usually have special areas for younger children and toddlers. You should keep to these areas if you have young children, as older children play more boisterously.

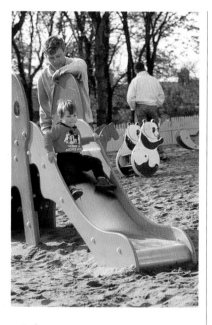

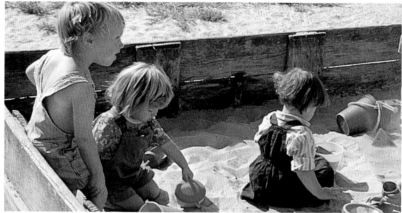

▶ Slides should be no more than 2.5m (8ft) high, preferably constructed on an earth mound so that any fall is broken. The slide should be of one smooth, continuous piece – not jointed panels.

▶ Check that roundabouts have smooth surfaces and that they move round easily. Tell your child never to put his feet underneath the roundabout.

▶ Discourage your child from throwing sand in the sandpit. Sand can scratch the surface of the eye and cause an injury. Make sure that the sandpit is too shallow for your child to bury himself.

▶ Make sure your child has non-slip soles on his shoes and that he is wearing sturdy jeans.

▶ Climbing frames should be built on grass or sand to break falls; they should be completely stable.

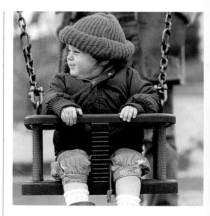

▶ Until your child can hold on properly, always use the box type of swing. Ideally, swings should be surrounded by a fence to prevent children running in front of, or behind, them and being knocked over.

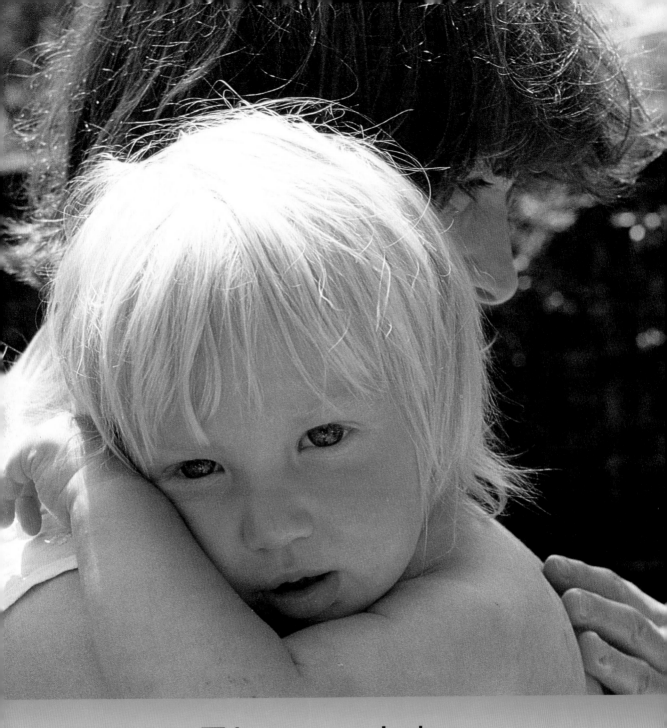

First-aid
techniques

Dealing with an accident

CHILDREN ARE PRONE TO ACCIDENTS because they are naturally inquisitive and often unaware of danger. Although most accidents are relatively minor, it is important that you are familiar with first-aid techniques so that you know what to do in the event of a serious accident. While the information that follows is no substitute for proper first-aid training, it will explain the right way to deal with an accident and enable you to act quickly, efficiently and remain calm. The calmer you are, the more you can comfort and help your child.

On pages 292 to 311 I have described the immediate action and treatment for several emergencies, such as choking, unconsciousness, electric shock, serious bleeding, shock, drowning and burns; other injuries are covered in the A–Z section of the book.

Priorities

Whatever injury your child has sustained, if he is unconscious you must do the following:

1 Make sure that he is breathing (*see page 286*). If he is not, begin mouth-to-mouth ventilation (*see page 288*) before you attend to any other injury.

Note *If a child is breathing, his heart will be beating and there will be signs of circulation (see page 289).*

2 After you have checked his breathing, stop any severe bleeding (*see page 300*).

3 Only when steps one and two have been dealt with should you treat any other injuries.

Examining your child

1 If your child is unconscious but breathing and his injury is not immediately obvious, examine him very carefully from head to foot. Try and keep his head tilted back to keep his airway open (*see opposite*). If possible, get someone else to support his head while you examine him.

2 Always compare one side of his body to the other side, or one limb to the other. Move him as little as possible; slide your hand under his back or his head to make sure there is no sign of bleeding.

Multiple injuries

Your child may have suffered several injuries, and the correct treatment of one may interfere with that of another. If this is the case, treat the injury you consider to be the most serious first, then treat the others as correctly as you can.

Calling for help

Your child will need to be taken to the nearest hospital following any accident resulting in unconsciousness, difficulty in breathing, or injuries such as bleeding, broken bones or burns. You should always call an ambulance if your child needs a stretcher for a broken leg or spinal injury, for example, or if you are on your own and first aid needs to be continued on the way to hospital. However, if speed is very important and there is another adult available who can drive you to hospital, it may be faster if you sit in the back of the car with your child and continue first aid while the other adult drives.

When you ring for an ambulance, give the control officer as much information as possible. He will want to know the extent of your child's injury, the cause of the injury, if it is known, and the age of your child. Also describe any landmarks that will help the ambulance find your house.

Resuscitation

Everyone needs a constant supply of oxygen to survive – permanent brain damage can result after only three to four minutes without oxygen. If your child is unconscious and not breathing, you can carry out various techniques of resuscitation to revive him. These techniques can be remembered as ABC: A for opening the Airway, B for Breathing for your child (*Mouth-to-mouth ventilation, see page 288*), and C for Circulating his blood (*Cardio-pulmonary resuscitation, see page 290*). It is always worth starting resuscitation and continuing until a doctor arrives or your child starts to breathe again on his own.

OPENING THE AIRWAY

The airway consists of the passages between your child's mouth and nose and his lungs. If your child is unconscious, particularly if he is lying face upwards, breathing may be difficult. Air may not be able to get through to his lungs because: the tongue has fallen back and blocked the windpipe; the head has tilted forward narrowing the top of the windpipe; fluid or vomit has collected at the back of the throat and is unable to drain.

IMPORTANT

1 Keep your fingers and hand well away from the soft tissues under a child's chin and along his neck.
2 If you suspect a head or neck injury handle these areas with great care (*see page 309*).
3 Shake the shoulders of a child very gently. *Never shake a baby.*

What should I do?
FOR A CHILD

1 Try and get a response from your child by talking to her or gently shaking her shoulders. An unconscious child will make no response. If there is no response, lay your child on a flat, firm surface.

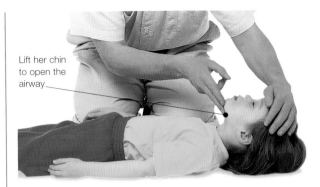

Lift her chin to open the airway

2 Use two fingers to lift her chin and put your other hand on her forehead. Gently tilt her head back. It is in the right position when you can see straight down her nostrils. This action will open the airway. Check her mouth and remove any obvious obstruction (*see page 286*). Check her breathing (*see overleaf*).

FOR A BABY

Babies have short necks and soft windpipes, so do not tilt the head back too far – you could block the airway.

1 Try and get a response by talking to your baby or gently tapping or flicking the sole of his foot. If there is no response, lay him on a firm surface. Check his mouth; use one finger to remove any obvious obstruction (*see page 286*). Do not feel blindly down the throat.

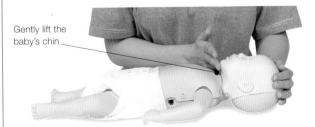

Gently lift the baby's chin

2 Gently lift the chin with one finger. Place your other hand on his forehead and tilt his head back slightly. Check his breathing (*see overleaf*).

Continued on next page

Resuscitation *continued from previous page*

CLEARING THE AIRWAY

If your child is not breathing after you have tilted his head back, take a look inside his mouth to see if there is something blocking the airway.

What should I do?

1 Look into your child's mouth, then quickly but carefully run your finger around the inside of his mouth. If you can see or feel any obvious obstruction, hook out anything you find. Be very careful not to push anything further down his throat.

2 If you cannot see or feel any obstruction, do not use your fingers to probe further down his throat. If you think your child has choked on something, give first aid for choking (*see page 294*).

3 Check your child's breathing again (*see left*).

IMPORTANT

With a baby, do not put your finger in his mouth unless you can see the foreign body clearly and you are sure that there is no risk of pushing it back down his throat and causing a worse obstruction.

What should I do next?

▶ If your child is now breathing, place him in the recovery position (*see opposite*). Remember, if he is breathing, his heart will be beating (*see page 290*).
▶ If your child is still not breathing, begin mouth-to-mouth ventilation immediately (*see page 288*).

CHECKING BREATHING

If your child or baby is unconscious, the first thing you must do before anything else is to make sure he is breathing. Open the airway (*see previous page*) so that his tongue does not fall back and block the air passages, then check his breathing as described below.

What should I do?

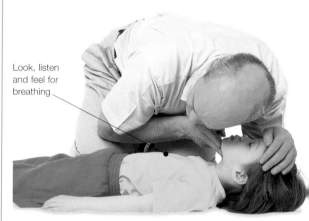

Look, listen and feel for breathing

1 Keeping her head tilted back, place your ear as close to her mouth and nose as possible and look along her chest at the same time.

2 If she is breathing, you will see her chest moving, you will hear her breathing and you will feel her breath on your cheek. Continue to do this for up to 10 seconds to be sure that she is definitely breathing.

3 If she is breathing, even slightly, make no attempt to increase her breathing rate by giving her mouth-to-mouth ventilation. Just turn your child into the recovery position (*see opposite*) while you call for an ambulance. Keep checking her breathing.

THE RECOVERY POSITION

If your child is unconscious but breathing, place him in the recovery position while waiting for medical help. This stops the tongue blocking the throat and allows fluid or vomit to drain from his mouth, preventing choking. Immobilize any broken bones (*see page 70*) and check the airway is open (*see page 285*) before moving your child.

The method below assumes your child is lying on his back. If he is lying on his side or his front you only need to move his head back and bring his uppermost leg and arm up as shown in step 4 to prevent him rolling on to his face.

What should I do?
FOR A CHILD

1 Kneeling beside your child, tilt her head back slightly to open the airway. Straighten her legs. Bend her nearest arm so that it makes a right angle and lay it on the ground, palm facing upwards.

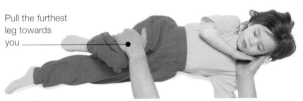

Pull the furthest leg towards you

2 Lay your child's other arm across her chest and hold the back of her hand against her nearer cheek. With your other hand, pull up her far leg just above the knee, keeping the foot flat on the ground.

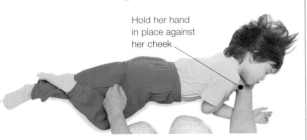

Hold her hand in place against her cheek

3 Keeping her hand pressed against her cheek, pull on the leg to roll your child towards you and on to her side. Use your knees to support her and prevent her from rolling too far forwards.

IMPORTANT

If you suspect back or neck injuries, you must make sure that your child's head and neck are supported at all times (*see page 311*). Place the furthest arm over her chest, not under her cheek (*see step 2*).

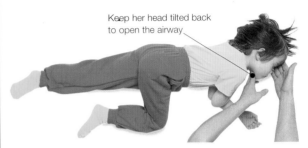

Keep her head tilted back to open the airway

4 Bend her leg at right angles to her body and adjust her arm to prevent her rolling forwards. Tilt her head back to ensure that the airway is still open and that your child can breathe.

FOR A BABY

To place your baby in the recovery position, cradle him in your arms with his head tilted downwards. This prevents him from choking on his tongue or from inhaling vomit.

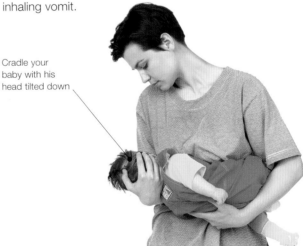

Cradle your baby with his head tilted down

Continued on next page

Resuscitation *continued from page 287*

MOUTH-TO-MOUTH VENTILATION

If your child is unconscious with no signs of breathing (*see pages 285–6*), you must give him artificial ventilation for one minute before calling an ambulance. You should start this wherever the accident occurred, as long as there is no risk of danger. If, for any reason, you cannot put your mouth over your child's mouth, you can close off her mouth and breathe into his nose. For babies, it is easier to place your mouth over the mouth and nose together (*see opposite*).

What should I do?
FOR A CHILD

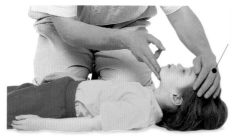

Open the airway by tilting back her head

1 Using two fingers to lift the chin, tilt your child's head back to open the airway and if necessary clear the airway (*see pages 285–6*).

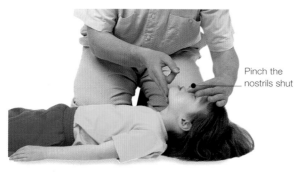

Pinch the nostrils shut

2 Keeping her head tilted back, pinch the nostrils shut with the index finger and thumb of your other hand. Continue to tilt back the jaw with your two fingers so that her airway remains open.

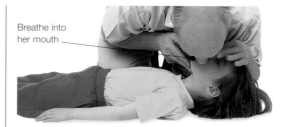

Breathe into her mouth

3 Take a deep breath, open your mouth wide and seal your lips around your child's mouth. Breathe gently but firmly into her mouth until you can see your child's chest rise.

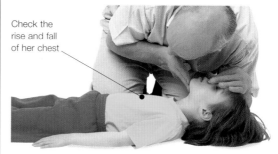

Check the rise and fall of her chest

4 Remove your lips and look along your child's chest to see it fall back. Keep the nostrils pinched. Give a further five artificial breaths, aiming at a complete breath every three seconds.

IMPORTANT

If your child's chest has not risen:

1 Check that the head is in the correct position (*see page 285*); you should be able to see straight down her nostrils.

2 Check that you are pinching the nostrils shut and that your mouth is forming an airtight seal around her mouth.

3 Check the mouth again. Do not put your fingers blindly down the throat unless you can see an obstruction.

Try again; if you are still not successful give back slaps as described for choking (*see page 294*).

---

5 Once you have given your child five artificial breaths, check for signs of circulation and recovery in your child for up to 10 seconds, such as a return of colour to the skin, swallowing, coughing or any other signs of movement.

6 If there are no signs of recovery, give cardio-pulmonary resuscitation (*see page 290*). If there are signs of circulation but no breathing, continue mouth-to-mouth breathing at a rate of one complete breath every three seconds until your child can breathe by herself. As soon as she is breathing on her own, place her in the recovery position (*see page 287*) and stay with her while you wait for an ambulance to arrive.

FOR A BABY

Although the basic breathing techniques for a baby are the same as for an older child, the smaller size of a baby has to be taken into account when giving artificial ventilation. You may find it easier to place your mouth over his mouth and nose together. You will only need to puff a small amount of air into his lungs at a rate of 20 breaths per minute.

Breathe into the mouth and nose together

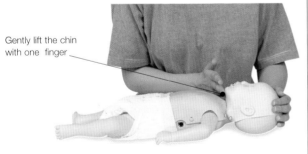

Gently lift the chin with one finger

1 Lay your baby on his back and call his name and tap or flick the sole of his foot to make sure he is unconscious. If there is no reaction, gently lift his chin with one finger and place your other hand on his forehead, tilting his head back slightly (*see page 285*). **DO NOT** tilt his head too far.

2 Seal your lips tightly around your baby's mouth and nose. Breathe into the lungs until the chest rises. Remove your lips and let the chest fall back. Repeat this procedure five times, aiming at one complete breath every three seconds. Look for signs of recovery, such as breathing, swallowing or coughing or a return of colour to the skin.

3 If there are no signs of recovery, begin cardio-pulmonary resuscitation (*see page 290*). If there are signs of recovery but no breathing, continue mouth-to-mouth at a rate of one breath every three seconds. Once your baby can breathe on his own, hold him in the recovery position (*see page 287*) while you wait for an ambulance.

Continued on next page

Resuscitation *continued from previous page*

CPR (CARDIO-PULMONARY RESUSCITATION)

When a child is unconscious and not breathing and his heart is not beating, cardio-pulmonary resuscitation is needed. This technique combines mouth-to-mouth breathing with chest compression, an important device that helps the oxygen you breathe into your child to reach the body tissues and prevent permanent brain damage occurring after only three to four minutes.

What should I do?
FOR A CHILD

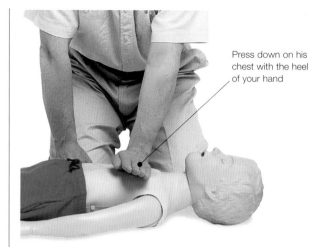

Press down on his chest with the heel of your hand

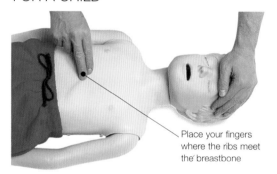

Place your fingers where the ribs meet the breastbone

1 Lay your child down on a flat surface. Kneeling beside him, face his chest. Using your index and middle fingers, find one of his lowest ribs. Slide your fingers up to the point where the rib margins meet at the breastbone. Place your middle finger at this point and your index finger above on the lower breastbone.

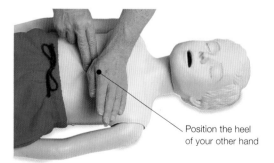

Position the heel of your other hand

2 Place the heel of your other hand on the breastbone, and slide it down until it reaches your index finger.

3 Using the heel of this hand, press down to a third of the depth of the chest. Do this five times quickly in succession at a rate of 100 compressions a minute, counting "one-and-two-and-three-and-four-and-five". Stop and give your child one breath of mouth-to-mouth ventilation by pinching her nose and breathing into his mouth (*see page 288*).

4 Alternate five chest compressions to one breath of artificial ventilation for one minute (approximately 20 times) before calling an ambulance. Continue this while you wait, checking for signs of recovery every three minutes.

5 If there are signs of recovery (*see page 289*), stop pumping the chest. Continue giving your child mouth-to-mouth ventilation until the ambulance arrives or he starts breathing again. Continue to check for signs of recovery and breathing after every 20 breaths. If he starts breathing by himself, stop giving him mouth-to-mouth ventilation and place him in the recovery position (*see page 287*).

FOR A BABY

The sequence for giving CPR for babies is the same as for a child, but the hand position is different and less pressure is required.

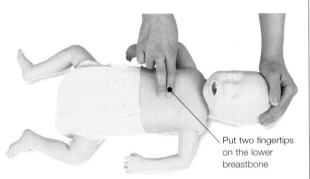

Put two fingertips on the lower breastbone

1 With your baby lying flat on his back on a firm surface, place two fingertips on the lower breastbone, one finger's breadth below the inter-nipple line. Press down at this point to a third of the depth of the chest. Repeat five times in quick succession at a rate of 100 per minute, counting "one-and-two-and-three-and-four-and-five".

2 Give one breath of artificial ventilation by breathing into your baby's mouth and nose (*see page 289*).

3 Alternate five chest compressions with one breath of artificial ventilation for one minute (approximately 20 times) before calling an ambulance. Continue this action while you wait for the ambulance, and check for signs of recovery every three minutes.

4 If there are no signs of recovery, stop pumping. Continue giving breaths until the ambulance arrives, or your baby starts breathing again on his own. Check his circulation and breathing after every 20 breaths. If your baby starts breathing by himself, stop mouth-to-mouth ventilation and hold him in the recovery position (*see page 287*).

Unconsciousness

THE DANGER OF UNCONSCIOUSNESS is that the normal reflexes, such as coughing, that prevent a child from choking while he is asleep do not work properly or do not work at all.

Head injury (*see page 154*), shock (*see page 299*), electric shock (*see page 304*), choking (*see page 294*), convulsion (*see page 94*), diabetes (*see page 111*) and epilepsy (*see page 128*) can all result in a person losing consciousness.

If your child regains consciousness or has been unconscious only for a very short time, he must still be seen by a doctor, even if he appears to be alright. If the unconsciousness was caused by a head injury, your child will need to have a skull x-ray to make sure there is no other injury, such as a fracture.

Levels of unconsciousness

Your child may pass through various levels of unconsciousness, at first appearing very confused, then lapsing into a stupor before becoming completely unconscious. It is essential that you remain with him all the time and, if possible, send another adult to telephone for an ambulance. It is also important to assess the state of your child's awareness and record any changes in his state. This information may help your doctor decide what treatment to give your child later.

IMPORTANT

Any child who has been unconscious or who has a head injury must be seen by a doctor. Do not give him anything to eat or drink beforehand.

What should I do?
FOR A CHILD

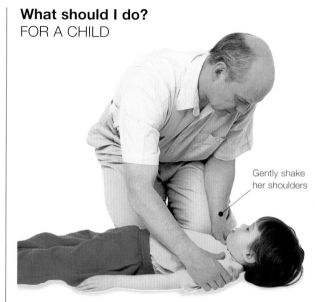

Gently shake her shoulders

1 Establish whether your child is unconscious by gently shaking her by the shoulders. Call her name and ask if she is alright.

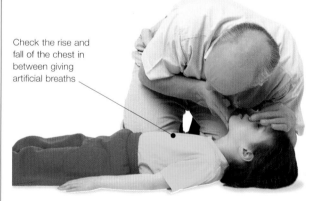

Check the rise and fall of the chest in between giving artificial breaths

2 If there is no response, lift the chin and tilt her head back to ensure that her airway is clear (*see page 285*). Check to see if she is breathing (*see page 286*) and if there are other signs of circulation (*see page 289*). If your child is not breathing, begin mouth-to-mouth ventilation (*see page 288*) and cardio-pulmonary resuscitation if necessary (*see page 290*).

3 If your child is breathing, but making snoring or gurgling sounds, there may be something blocking the airway. Clear the airway (*see page 285*). If she starts to vomit, place her in the recovery position immediately (*see page 287*), but, if you suspect a spinal injury, make sure her head and neck are supported at all times (*see **Important** box, page 287*).

FOR A BABY

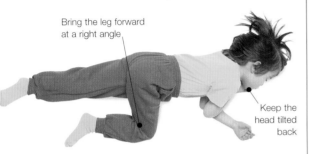

Bring the leg forward at a right angle

Keep the head tilted back

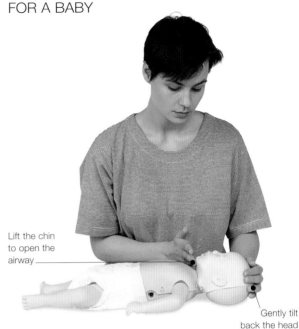

Lift the chin to open the airway

Gently tilt back the head

4 If your child is breathing, keep her head tilted and examine her from head to foot to identify severe external bleeding or major fractures. Treat injuries such as broken bones (*see page 70*), and control bleeding (*see page 300*), then move her into the recovery position (*see page 287*). Again, if you suspect a spinal injury, move her into the modified recovery position (*see page 311*).

Treatment for an unconscious baby is the same as for a child except that you should never shake a baby, and use only one finger to tilt your baby's head back. Puff gently into his mouth and nose when giving mouth-to-mouth ventilation (*see page 289*) and apply only gentle pressure when giving CPR (*see page 290*).

5 If there is fluid coming from your child's ear, position her so that she is lying on the affected ear so that the fluid can drain away.

6 If your child is still not breathing, begin mouth-to-mouth ventilation (*see page 288*) and CPR (*see page 290*) if necessary, then call an ambulance. Check her breathing, circulation and response every 10 minutes.

Choking

Possible symptoms

For a child
- **Coughing**.
- **Grasping the throat**.
- **Redness, followed by blueness in the face** – blood vessels in the neck and face may stand out.

For a baby
- **Obstructed breathing**.
- **Trying to cry, but making strange noises,** or no sound.
- **Blue face**.

SMALL CHILDREN ARE LIABLE TO CHOKE because they may eat something they cannot chew properly, and because they have a habit of putting small objects in their mouths. You must act quickly because, if the object is not removed, your child could stop breathing.

What should I do?
FOR A CHILD

1 Your child may be able to cough up the object on her own. Encourage her to do this, but do not waste time.

2 If this fails, bend her forwards with her head lower than her chest. Give up to five slaps firmly between the shoulders.

3 Check out her mouth and carefully hook out any *obvious* obstructions.

4 If this fails, stand or kneel behind the child. Make a fist against her lower breastbone. Grasp it with your other hand. Press quickly inward up to five times. (This is a chest thrust.) Check the mouth again.

5 If your child is still choking, bend her forwards and give five more back slaps. If this fails, make a fist and place it against her central upper abdomen. Grasp your fist with your other hand, then press into her abdomen in a quick, upward thrusting motion. (This is known as an abdominal thrust.) Do this five times. Check the mouth again.

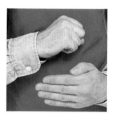
Make a fist against the upper abdomen

6 If the obstruction has still not cleared, call for an ambulance immediately. Repeat steps 2–5 until medical help arrives.

FOR A BABY

1 Lay your baby face down along your forearm, keeping his head low and supporting his chin between your fingers. Give up to five sharp slaps on the middle of his back.

2 If this fails, turn your baby face up on your arm or lap, keeping his head low. Check his mouth and remove any *obvious* obstruction. If the obstruction has not cleared, put two fingers on his lower breastbone, one finger's breadth below the nipple line, and give up to five downward thrusts.
DO NOT use abdominal thrusts.

3 Check your baby's mouth again. If there is no obstruction to remove, repeat the back slaps and chest thrusts three more times. Call for an ambulance immediately. Continue the back slaps and chest thrusts until medical help arrives.

Drowning

BABIES AND CHILDREN can get into difficulty in open water, especially if it is cold or turbulent. Even at home, if a child is left unattended in the bath, there is potential danger. Water does not have to be very deep to endanger a child – a mere 2.5cm (1in) of water is enough to cover a baby's nose and mouth. Although it is essential that you act as quickly as possible, you must make sure you are safe yourself before attempting a rescue. Don't jump into the water unless it is absolutely necessary. Stay on land, if possible, and reach out with your hand, a stick or a branch, or throw a rope or a float.

If your child is unconscious, you or preferably a trained life-saver will have to wade or swim out and tow your child to safety. If he is not breathing, you will have to start mouth-to-mouth ventilation immediately (*see page 288*), even if you are in the water, and as long as you are in no danger yourself. Very young children can hold their breath for a considerable length of time so never dismiss mouth-to-mouth ventilation as too late a resort. Persevere until medical help arrives.

What should I do?

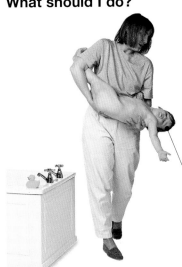

Get your child out of the water as quickly as possible. Carry him with his head low, if possible, in order to reduce the risk of inhaling water or vomit.

Hold him with his head low

If unconscious

1 If he is unconscious lay him down on his back on a coat, blanket or rug. Open the airway (*see page 285*), check his breathing (*see page 286*) and circulation (*see page 289*) and be prepared to give mouth-to-mouth ventilation (*see page 288*) if necessary. You may have to breathe more firmly and slowly than normal in order to get the chest to rise.

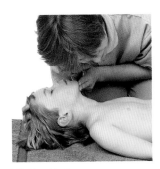

Tilt his chin to open his airway

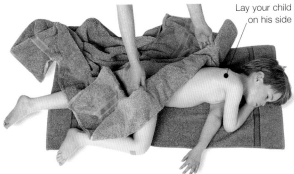

Lay your child on his side

2 As soon as your child is breathing, remove his wet clothes and cover him with a dry towel or blanket to protect him from the cold. Place him in the recovery position (*see page 287*). When he is conscious, give him warm, NOT HOT, sweet drinks.

3 Call an ambulance, even if your child appears to have recovered fully, as any water that has entered the lungs can cause irritation and the air pasages may begin to swell (this is known as secondary drowning) some hours later. Your child may also need to be treated for hypothermia.

Strangulation

STRANGULATION OCCURS WHEN the air passage has been constricted by pressure being applied to the outside of the neck. This could occur accidentally, for example, if a scarf, tie or other item of clothing becomes caught in a piece of machinery. It requires urgent medical attention.

What should I do?

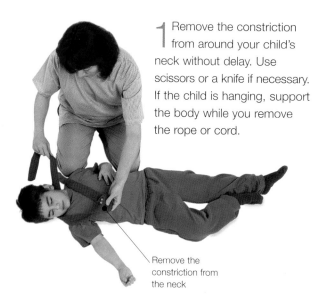

1 Remove the constriction from around your child's neck without delay. Use scissors or a knife if necessary. If the child is hanging, support the body while you remove the rope or cord.

Remove the constriction from the neck

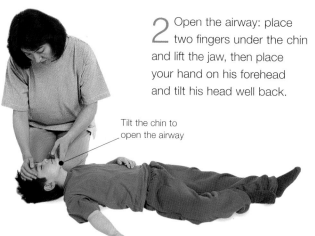

2 Open the airway: place two fingers under the chin and lift the jaw, then place your hand on his forehead and tilt his head well back.

Tilt the chin to open the airway

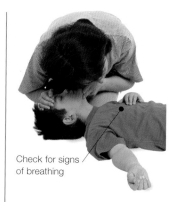

3 Look and listen for breathing for up to 10 seconds.

IF he is not breathing, be ready to give artificial ventilation if necessary (*see page 288*).

Check for signs of breathing

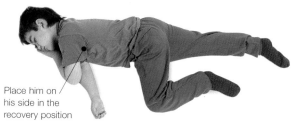

Place him on his side in the recovery position

4 If your child is breathing, place him in the recovery position (*see page 287*). Call an ambulance and keep checking his breathing and pulse while you wait.

Suffocation

THIS OCCURS WHEN there is an obstruction over the child's mouth or nose, a weight on the chest or abdomen preventing normal breathing, or because the child is breathing in smoke- or fume-filled air.

What should I do?

1 Take away the obstruction as quickly as possible. This may restore breathing.

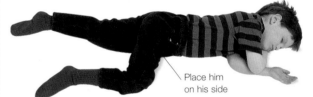

Remove the obstruction from the head

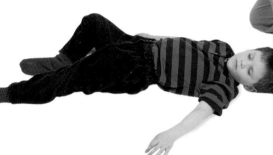

Lift the chin to open the airway

2 Open the airway: place two fingers under the chin and lift the jaw, then place your hand on his forehead and tilt his head back.

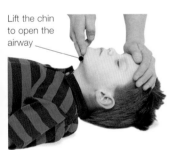

Place him on his side

4 If he is breathing, place him in the recovery position (*see page 287*). Call an ambulance and continue to check his breathing and look for signs of circulation until the ambulance arrives.

3 Look and listen for breathing for up to 10 seconds.

IF he is not breathing, be ready to give artificial ventilation (*see page 288*).

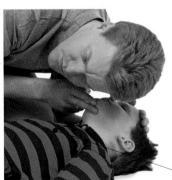

Check for signs of breathing

Diabetes

Possible symptoms
Recognizing low blood sugar

▶ **Weakness or hunger.**
▶ **Confused or aggressive** behaviour.
▶ **Sweating.**
▶ **Very pale face.**
▶ **Strong, bounding pulse.**
▶ **Shallow breathing.**

A CHILD WHO IS DIABETIC can suffer from low blood-sugar levels, a condition known as hypoglycaemia. A diabetic child is likely to be on insulin to control his blood-sugar levels. However, even if he seems recovered after an attack, a doctor should be asked to check the insulin dosage.

What should I do?

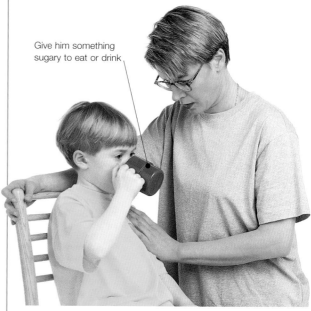

Give him something sugary to eat or drink

1 If your child is conscious, sit him down and give him a sugary drink or sweet food.

2 If he improves rapidly after a sweet drink or food, give him some more and let him rest. If he does not, call an ambulance.

For an unconscious child

If your child loses consciousness, assess his condition (*see page 292*) and be ready to resuscitate. Call an ambulance. If he is breathing place him in the recovery position (*see page 287*). Watch your child's level of consciousness (*see page 292*) and check his breathing rate until medical help arrives.

Shock

Possible symptoms

▶ **Pale, cold, sweaty skin**, tinged with grey.

▶ **Rapid pulse**, becoming weaker.

▶ **Shallow, fast breathing**.

▶ **Restlessness**.

▶ **Yawning and sighing**.

▶ **Thirst**.

▶ **Loss of consciousness**.

MEDICAL SHOCK IS A POTENTIALLY fatal condition that can occur if blood pressure becomes severely lowered after a loss of blood, or if the heart is not working properly. The most likely causes include serious bleeding (*see overleaf*), or a severe burn or scald (*see page 302*). Shock can also be caused by electric shock (*see page 304*), or by dehydration following profuse vomiting or diarrhoea. It can also occur as a severe reaction to an insect bite, such as a bee sting; or to some medicines, a condition known as anaphylactic shock (*see page 306*).

Even if your child is not showing any of the symptoms above, but is bleeding or badly burned, for example, there is a possibility of shock developing. Treat him as described here and get him to a hospital as quickly as possible.

Internal bleeding

When an internal organ is injured in an accident, or a large bone such as the thigh-bone or pelvis is broken, and internal bleeding occurs, shock can result. If your child develops any of the symptoms listed above, even though he shows no obvious signs of injury, if he complains of severe pain in the chest, or is unusually quiet after an accident, treat him as above and get him to a hospital quickly.

What should I do?

1 Lay your child down flat on a blanket, rug or coat, keeping his head low as this improves the blood supply to the brain. Turn his head to one side and reassure him, then treat any injury.

2 Carefully raise his legs on cushions or pillows so that they are higher than his heart. Loosen any tight clothing at his neck, chest or waist.

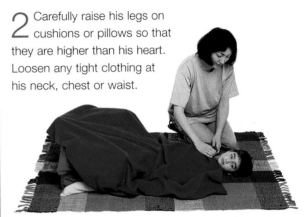

3 Cover him with a blanket or coat, but do not let him get too hot. Never use a hot-water bottle or apply direct heat as this takes blood away from the vital organs. Do not give him anything to eat or drink.

4 Check your child's pulse in the artery in the neck and encourage him to talk. Note any changes in his state and pass this information on to medical personnel.

For an unconscious child

If your child loses consciousness, assess his condition (*see page 292*) and be ready to resuscitate. Call an ambulance. If he is breathing place him in the recovery position (*see page 287*). Watch his level of consciousness (*see page 292*) and check his breathing rate until medical help arrives.

IMPORTANT

Do not leave your child unattended. If possible, send someone else to telephone for an ambulance while you stay with your child.

Bleeding

BLEEDING HAPPENS WHEN ANY of the vessels that carry blood around the body are cut or torn. It can be internal and not visible (*see page 299*). Serious bleeding should be treated as an emergency because, if too much blood is lost from the child's circulatory system, there will not be enough left to supply the body cells with oxygen, and shock can result (*see page 299*). Treat the child as described below and constantly reassure him.

MINOR INJURIES

Most small cuts and grazes can easily be dealt with at home. Sit your child down and gently wash the affected area with soap and water using a gauze pad. Make sure you remove all particles of dirt or gravel then, once the wound is thoroughly clean, protect the cut or graze with a plaster that has a pad large enough to cover the wound. Do not cover cuts with cotton wool or any other fluffy material that may stick to the wound.

SEVERE BLEEDING
What should I do?

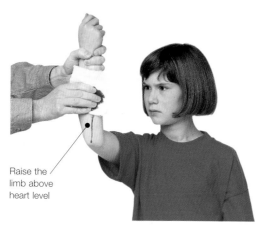

Raise the limb above heart level

1 Use a clean pad or handkerchief, or the palm of your hand, to press firmly on the wound to compress the ends of the damaged blood vessels. Raise your child's limb above the level of her heart.

2 If your child is not already lying down, help her to lie down with her head low. (Put a thin pad under her head for comfort.) Keep the injured area raised and keep pressing on the wound for up to 10 minutes.

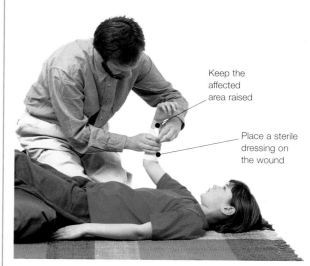

Keep the affected area raised

Place a sterile dressing on the wound

3 Cover the wound with a clean, non-fluffy dressing that is larger than the wound itself, still keeping the injured area raised above the level of the heart. Secure the dressing in place with a bandage, tied firmly, but not so tightly as to cut off the blood supply to the limb (*see page 302*). If any blood comes through the bandage, secure another dressing with a second bandage firmly on top. Where necessary, support the wounded area in a sling (*see page 301*).

4 If the bleeding persists, follow the treatment for shock (*see page 299*). Get your child to a hospital as soon as possible because she may need stitches. Either call an ambulance or get another adult to drive you while you sit with her, continuing first aid if needed.

For dealing with a foreign body embedded in a wound, see opposite.

Embedded object

IF AN OBJECT IS EMBEDDED in a wound, do not try to remove it as this may cause further damage and bleeding. Instead, protect the damaged area from infection with some sterile gauze and rolled-up bandages placed around the embedded object.

What should I do?

1 Help your child to rest. Apply pressure on either side of the object and raise the injured part above the level of your child's heart.

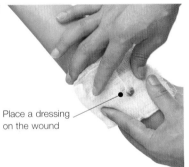

Apply pressure to the affected area

2 Place a piece of gauze over the wound and the object to minimize the risk of infection.

Place a dressing on the wound

3 Use spare bandage rolls to build up padding to the same height as the embedded object.

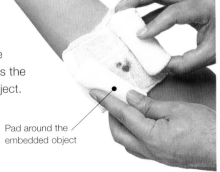

Pad around the embedded object

4 Secure the padding by bandaging over it, being careful not to press on the embedded object. Take your child to hospital.

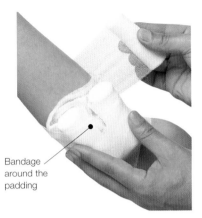

Bandage around the padding

Bandaging around a larger object

If the object is very big, build padding around it and bandage above and below the object.

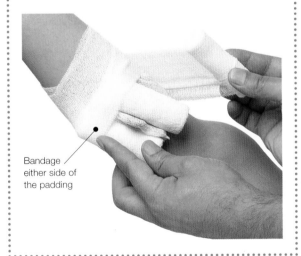

Bandage either side of the padding

Burns

Burns need urgent medical treatment because of the risk of infection and the risk of shock (*see page 299*). There are two main types of burn: superficial and deep. Superficial burns damage the surface of the skin, while deep burns affect the whole thickness of the skin. If fire has caused the burn, you should assume that any accompanying smoke or hot air has affected your child's respiratory system as well.

The most important thing to remember is that only small, superficial burns can be safely treated at home (*see pages 303*). If you are in doubt, consult your doctor. For information on how to deal with electrical burns, see page 304.

IMPORTANT

If one tenth or more of your child's body is injured, call an ambulance immediately. Treat your child as described for shock and lay him on a sheet of non-fluffy material to prevent the burned area from touching the ground.

IF CLOTHING IS ON FIRE

Do not let your child run about in a panic because this movement will fan the flames. Because flames rise, you must get him to lie down on the floor with the burning side uppermost.

What should I do?

1 Lay your child down and douse the flames with water or another non-flammable liquid, such as milk. **DO NOT** do this if his clothes have been set on fire by electricity and he is still near the source – you will electrocute yourself (*see page 304*). Break the contact, if necessary, and follow step 2 instead.

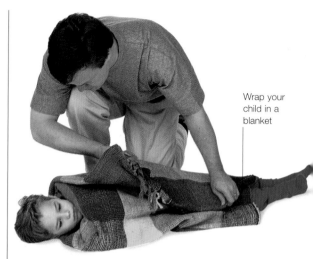

Wrap your child in a blanket

2 If no water or non-flammable liquid is available, lay your child on the ground to stifle the flames and wrap him tightly in a coat or blanket (not nylon or cellular), or other heavy fabric.
DO NOT remove his clothing, or any material that may be sticking to the burned area, as this may cause further damage and introduce the risk of infection. Roll him on the ground to put out the fire.

3 Check your child's airway (*see page 285*), breathing (*see page 286*) and be ready to give mouth-to-mouth ventilation if necessary (*see page 288*). If the burned area is large or deep, call for an ambulance as your child will need to be treated for shock. You can treat him yourself (*see page 299*) while you wait for the ambulance.

DEALING WITH GENERAL BURNS
What should I do?

1 Remove your child from the source of danger, breaking any electrical contact if necessary (*see page 304*).

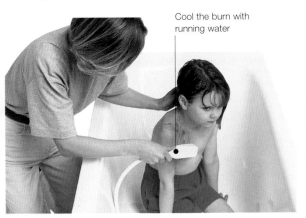

Cool the burn with running water

2 Cool the affected area immediately; hold under cold running water for at least 10 minutes to relieve the pain. If there is no water, use another non-flammable liquid, such as milk.

3 Remove any jewellery, watches, belts or constricting clothing from the injured area before it begins to swell. If the pain persists, cool again. Cut around any material sticking to the skin.

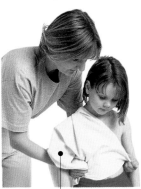

Place a non-fluffy material on the burn

4 Cover the injury with a sterile dressing or clean, non-fluffy material, to protect it from infection, and bandage loosely in place if necessary. To dress a burned hand or foot, use a plastic bag or clean kitchen film. Secure this with a bandage or plaster around the bag, not on the skin.

5 Do not give your child anything to eat or drink and watch for signs of shock (*see page 299*).

CHEMICAL BURNS
What should I do?

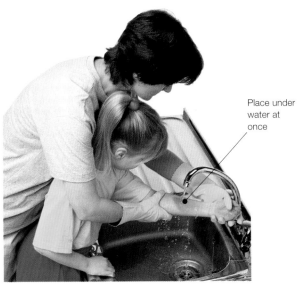

Place under water at once

1 Wearing protective rubber gloves, hold the burned part of the body under cold running water for at least 10 minutes to wash away all traces of the chemical. Beware of fumes.

2 While you are doing this, remove any contaminated clothing very carefully, taking care not to contaminate yourself.

3 Get your child to a hospital, keeping a close eye on her breathing (*see page 286*) and checking that her airway is open (*see page 285*).

4 As soon as possible, seal the chemical container, and ventilate the area where the accident occurred. Be sure to store the container out of your child's reach.

Electric shock

CONTACT WITH HOUSEHOLD ELECTRICITY can cause burns and the shock may cause unconsciousness, or even stop your child's breathing and heartbeat. If your child is still in contact with the electricity, you must switch off the power source or break the electrical contact (*see below*) before touching him, otherwise you will electrocute yourself.

Contact with electricity can also cause burns that may occur not only at the point where the current enters the body, but also at the point where it leaves it. Although these burns look small, they are often deep and carry a serious risk of infection; therefore it is essential that all electrical burns, however small, are seen by a doctor.

BREAKING ELECTRICAL CONTACT

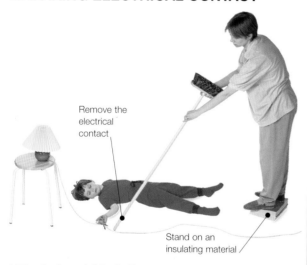

Remove the electrical contact

Stand on an insulating material

What should I do?

If it is not possible to switch off the source of power, you must break the contact immediately. Find something that will not conduct electricity, such as a broom or plastic tube, and push your child's affected area away from the source. Before you do this, make sure your hands and whatever you use are dry and that you are not standing on anything wet or made of metal.

DEALING WITH ELECTRICAL BURNS
What should I do?

1 When the contact is broken, examine your child carefully. If you find a burn, check to see if there is one on the other side of the affected area.

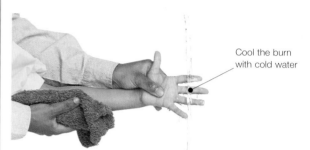

Cool the burn with cold water

2 Cool any burns by placing the affected area under cold running water for at least 10 minutes (*see page 303*). Cover the burns with clean, non-fluffy dressings, then get your child to the nearest hospital.

3 Treat your child for shock (*see page 299*) while you are waiting for the ambulance or during your journey to the hospital.

For an unconscious child

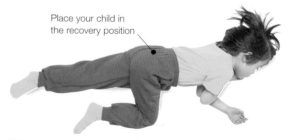

Place your child in the recovery position

When you have broken the electrical contact, if your child loses consciousness assess her condition (*see page 292*) and be ready to resuscitate. Call an ambulance. If she is breathing place her in the recovery position (*see page 287*). Watch her level of consciousness (*see page 292*) and check her breathing rate (*see page 286*) until medical help arrives.

Poisoning

Possible symptoms

▶ **Vomiting and diarrhoea**.

▶ **Burns** around the mouth (if he has taken a corrosive poison).

▶ **Convulsions** for no apparent reason.

▶ **Empty or open container** known to have held a poison or medicine lying near your child.

▶ **Poisonous plant or berries** in his hand or near him if he is unconscious.

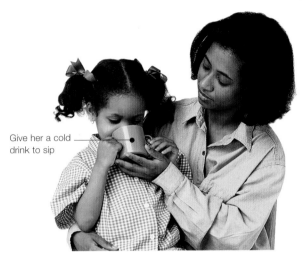

Give her a cold drink to sip

IF YOUR CHILD HAS SWALLOWED something poisonous, or something you think may be poisonous, find the container, if there is one, and read the list of ingredients. Ring your local poison centre, your doctor, or the nearest hospital as soon as you can and tell them what you think your child has swallowed. They will probably be able to tell you whether the substance is poisonous and what you can do while you are waiting for the ambulance or are being driven to the hospital.

What should I do?

1 Ask your child to tell you or point to what she has swallowed. Do this as soon as you realize something is wrong, because she may lose consciousness.

2 Keep a sample of what you think your child has swallowed, for example a few leaves or berries, or keep the bottle, can or container and examine the label. If she has swallowed some pills, count how many are left. Get as much information as possible to help the doctor or hospital staff decide on the most appropriate treatment for your child.

3 If your child has swallowed bleach, weedkiller or some other form of corrosive poison, **DO NOT** try to make her sick. (Anything that burns the gullet going down will burn the gullet again coming up.) Wipe away any residual chemical around her mouth and lips, then get her to sip cold water or milk to cool the burns. Get her to hospital as soon as possible.

If your child is unconscious

Call an ambulance immediately, or get another adult to drive you to the nearest hospital. In the meantime give first aid. Open the mouth and hook out with a finger any drugs or items that you can see. Open the airway, check her breathing (*see page 286*) and be prepared to resuscitate. If it is necessary to give him mouth-to-mouth ventilation (*see page 288*), take care not to get any of the poison on your mouth. If necessary, push your child's lips together and breathe into his nose. Keep checking his breathing and watching for any change in his level of consciousness.

IF he is breathing, place him on his side in the recovery position (*see page 287*) and treat him as described for unconsciousness on page 292.

Anaphylactic shock

Possible symptoms

- **Anxiety**.
- **Red, blotchy skin**.
- **Swelling** of the face and neck.
- **Puffiness** around the eyes.
- **Wheezing**.
- **Difficulty in breathing**.
- **Rapid pulse**.

THIS IS A SEVERE ALLERGIC REACTION that may develop within a few minutes following the injection of a particular drug, the sting of an insect or marine creature or the ingestion of a particular food.

The reaction causes restriction of the air passages. Furthermore, swelling of the child's face and neck increases the risk of suffocation.

What should I do?

1 Call an ambulance. A child with a known allergy may have medication to take in case of an attack. Use this medication as soon as the attack starts. Follow the directions carefully.

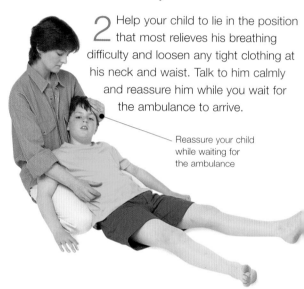

2 Help your child to lie in the position that most relieves his breathing difficulty and loosen any tight clothing at his neck and waist. Talk to him calmly and reassure him while you wait for the ambulance to arrive.

Reassure your child while waiting for the ambulance

For an unconscious child

If your child loses consciousness, assess his condition (*see page 292*) and be ready to resuscitate. Call an ambulance. If he is breathing, place him in the recovery position (*see page 287*). Watch his level of consciousness (*see page 292*) and check his breathing rate (*see page 286*) until medical help arrives.

Hypothermia

HYPOTHERMIA IS A DANGEROUS CONDITION that can develop if the body's temperature drops below 35°C (95°F). It can be fatal, as the functions of vital organs such as the heart and liver can slow down and stop.

The symptoms are not always easy to spot. It is worth keeping a low-reading thermometer so that you can check for low body temperature. A child's body can lose heat just as quickly through wet clothing as through being in water if the temperature is very low.

IMPORTANT

Never use a hot-water bottle or other source of direct heat to treat hypothermia. This loses blood to the body surface, causing heat loss and shock.

FOR A CHILD

Possible symptoms

▶ **Shivering**.
▶ **Cold, pale, dry skin**.
▶ **Listlessness or confusion**.
▶ **Failing consciousness**.
▶ **Slow, shallow breathing**.
▶ **Weakening pulse**.

What should I do?

1 If your child is out of doors, put something dry on top of his wet clothes and carry him to the nearest shelter or into the house.

2 Remove his wet clothing as soon as he is in a warm room and give him dry clothes. Wrap him in a blanket next to someone else. Call the doctor at once.

3 An older child can be put in a bath of warm, NOT HOT, water. When his skin has returned to normal, help him out of the bath and dry him quickly. Wrap him in warm towels or blankets.

4 Dress him in warm clothes and put him to bed, covered with plenty of blankets. Cover his head with a hat and make sure that the room is warm.

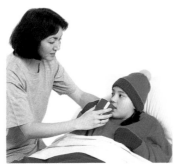

5 If conscious, give him a warm, NOT HOT, sweet drink. Take his temperature or feel the skin every 30 minutes. Stay with him until his colour and temperature return to normal.

6 If your child's temperature does not return to normal, get him to a hospital as soon as you can.

For an unconscious child

If your child loses consciousness, assess his condition (*see page 292*) and be ready to resuscitate. Call an ambulance. If he is breathing place him in the recovery position (*see page 287*). Check his responses and his breathing rate (*see pages 292 and 286*) until help arrives.

FOR A BABY

A baby can develop hypothermia if sleeping in a cold room or if inadequately dressed when it is cold.

Possible symptoms

▶ **Pink and healthy-looking skin** that feels cold.
▶ **Baby is limp** and unusually quiet.
▶ **Refusal to feed**.

What should I do?

Call your doctor immediately. Meanwhile, warm your baby gradually in a warm room. Wrap him in blankets, put a hat on his head and cuddle him so that he is warmed by your body heat.

Heatstroke

Possible symptoms

▶ **Sudden onset of headache**.

▶ **Confusion**.

▶ **Hot, flushed, dry skin**.

▶ **Rapid deterioration in level of response**.

▶ **A full, bounding pulse**.

▶ **Temperature** above 40°C (104°F).

IF THE BODY BECOMES SEVERELY overheated in hot surroundings, heatstroke may occur. Because of prolonged exposure to heat, the body is unable to cool itself through sweating.

What should I do?

1 Lay your child down in a cool place and remove all outer clothing. Put a folded towel or pillow under his head and talk to him calmly.

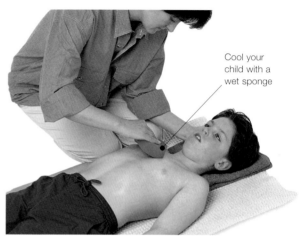

Cool your child with a wet sponge

2 Sponge your child down repeatedly with cold or tepid water to cool him. Leave his skin damp and let it dry in the air.

3 Fan your child by hand or with an electric fan to bring his temperature down.

For an unconscious child

If your child loses consciousness, assess his condition (*see page 292*) and be ready to resuscitate. Call an ambulance. If he is breathing, place him in the recovery position (*see page 287*). Watch his level of consciousness (*see page 292*) and check his breathing rate (*see page 286*) until medical help arrives.

Back and neck injuries

IF YOU SUSPECT THAT A CHILD has a back or neck injury do not move him unless his life is in imminent danger. If you do have to move him, try to do so in "one piece", taking care not to twist or bend the child's neck or spine.

IMPORTANT

Before placing anyone in the recovery position (*see page 287*), always try to assess whether there are back or neck injuries. If you suspect injuries to the spine and neck use the modified recovery position (*see page 311*).

FOR A CONSCIOUS CHILD

What should I do?

1 Call an ambulance. Reassure your child and tell him not to move. Steady and support his head and neck by placing your hands over his ears and keeping his head in line with his spine. Be careful not to pull his neck.

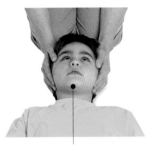

Keep his head and spine aligned

2 Keep his head supported in this position until help arrives. Ask someone to put rolled blankets or towels around his neck and shoulders for extra support.

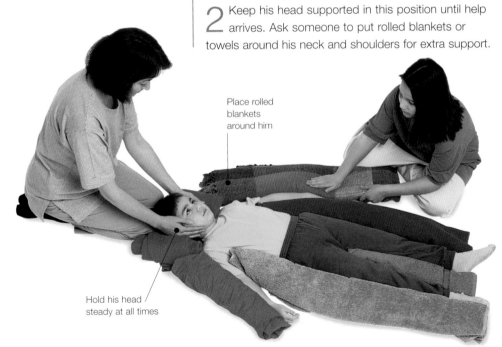

Place rolled blankets around him

Hold his head steady at all times

3 Get a helper to arrange rolled towels or blankets around your child's neck and shoulders and either side of his body while you continue to keep his head steady and aligned with his spine.

Continued on next page

Back and neck injuries *continued from previous page*

FOR AN UNCONSCIOUS CHILD

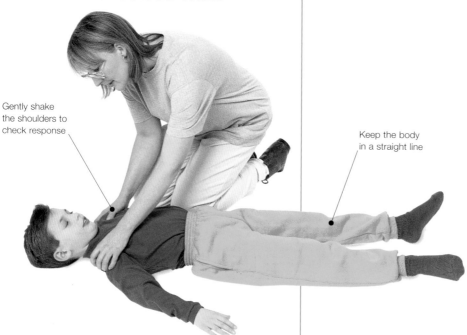

Gently shake the shoulders to check response

Keep the body in a straight line

What should I do?

1 Call an ambulance. Keep your child's head, trunk and toes in a straight line.

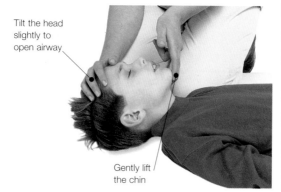

Tilt the head slightly to open airway

Gently lift the chin

2 Place two fingers under his chin and lift the jaw very gently to open the airway. At the same time, gently place your hand on his forehead and tilt the head back slightly to help keep the airway open.

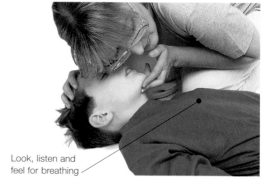

Look, listen and feel for breathing

3 Check for breathing (*see page 286*) and be prepared to resuscitate. If the child is breathing and the ambulance has not yet arrived, gently place him in the modified recovery position (*see opposite*), keeping his head, neck and spine aligned at all times

MODIFIED RECOVERY POSITION
What should I do?

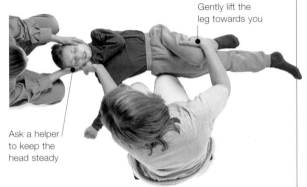

Gently lift the leg towards you

Ask a helper to keep the head steady

1 Ask a helper to support your child's head with her hands. Grasp the thigh of the leg furthest from you. Gently lift and bend the leg. Draw the arm furthest from you across the child's chest.

2 Draw over his knee and ease him round gently. Keep his head and trunk aligned.

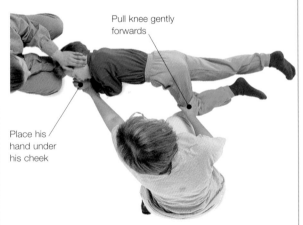

Pull knee gently forwards

Place his hand under his cheek

3 With your child turned on to his side and his head tilted back, support him in this position until help arrives. Monitor his breathing and circulation (*see pages 286 and 290*) and be prepared to resuscitate if necessary.

ROLLING AN UNCONSCIOUS CHILD
What should I do?

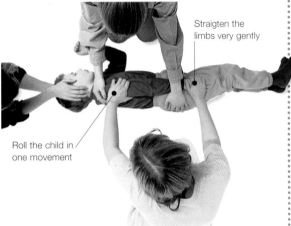

Straigten the limbs very gently

Roll the child in one movement

If the child stops breathing while in the recovery position, use the "log-roll" technique to move him on to his back. It is vital to keep the child's head, trunk and feet in a straight line. You will need helpers to do this safely. While one adult holds the child's head, two others should gently straighten the limbs and roll the child over in one synchronised movement. You can then resuscitate as necessary.

Bandaging techniques

WHEN APPLYING A BANDAGE, try to get your child to help because it will take his mind off his injury. If you are applying a bandage to secure a dressing or support a muscle or joint injury, always start below the injury and work up the limb because the bandage will lie flatter and therefore provide more support. Always leave your child's fingertips or toes exposed so that you can check the circulation in the affected area after applying the bandage.

SLING

These are used to support an injured arm, or the arm on the injured side if your child has a chest injury. Use a triangular bandage as described below. If you do not have one in your first-aid kit, you can improvise using a piece of material or a scarf about 1m (1yd) square, folded in half diagonally.

1 Sit your child down and place his arm across his chest so that his wrist is slightly higher than his elbow.

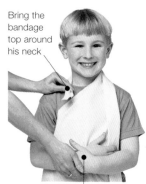

Bring the bandage top around his neck

Get your child to help support his arm

2 Fold up the long edge (base) of a triangular bandage to make a hem and then slide the bandage up through the gap between your child's elbow and his chest. Keep the base parallel to his side and carry the top end over his shoulder and round to the front on the injured side.

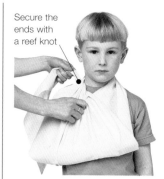

Secure the ends with a reef knot

3 Still supporting your child's arm, carry the lower end of the bandage up and over his arm and tie the ends together in the hollow above his collar bone using a reef knot.

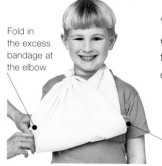

Fold in the excess bandage at the elbow

4 Fold back the corner of the bandage at the elbow and bring the point forward; pin it to the front of the sling.

Keep his fingers free to check circulation

5 Check the circulation (*see below*) in the fingers and, if necessary, adjust or reapply the sling.

Checking circulation

1 Press one of the exposed fingernails until it turns white, then release the pressure. The nail should become pink again immediately.

2 If colour does not return quickly, or the fingers look blue or feel cold, remove the bandage immediately and start again.

LEG/ARM BANDAGE

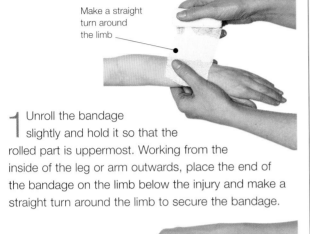

Make a straight
turn around
the limb

1 Unroll the bandage
slightly and hold it so that the
rolled part is uppermost. Working from the
inside of the leg or arm outwards, place the end of
the bandage on the limb below the injury and make a
straight turn around the limb to secure the bandage.

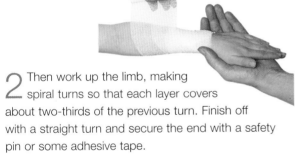

Roll the bandage
up the limb

2 Then work up the limb, making
spiral turns so that each layer covers
about two-thirds of the previous turn. Finish off
with a straight turn and secure the end with a safety
pin or some adhesive tape.

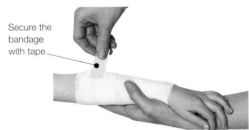

Secure the
bandage
with tape

3 Secure the bandage with hypoallergenic tape. If
you have not got any tape, leave about 15cm (6in)
hanging free – enough to wind once around the limb.
Cut down the centre of the piece of bandage and tie a
knot at the bottom of the split. Wrap the ends around
the limb and tie off on the other side.

ANKLE/HAND BANDAGE

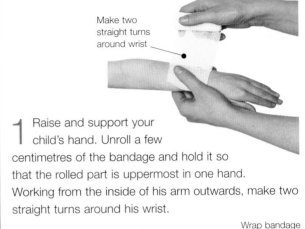

Make two
straight turns
around wrist

1 Raise and support your
child's hand. Unroll a few
centimetres of the bandage and hold it so
that the rolled part is uppermost in one hand.
Working from the inside of his arm outwards, make two
straight turns around his wrist.

Wrap bandage
diagonally

2 Take the bandage
diagonally across the top of your
child's wrist to his little finger, round under
the palm of the hand and up at the base of his
thumb. Make two straight turns around the base
of the injured palm.

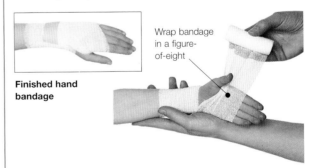

**Finished hand
bandage**

Wrap bandage
in a figure-
of-eight

3 Take the bandage across the back of the hand to
the base of the little finger, then around the palm,
and up between the thumb and forefinger, and across
the back of the hand to the wrist. Repeat the "figure-
of-eight" until the hand is covered.

First-aid kit

KEEP A FIRST-AID KIT in your car and another in an accessible area of your home. You can buy ready-made-up standard kits. You may want to add extra dressings and bandages, and disposable gloves. Make sure your first-aid box is readily accessible and easy to identify, and check the contents regularly. Don't keep medicines in the first-aid box; they should be locked in a medicine cabinet. A well-stocked kit might contain the articles shown below.

Dressings

Plasters (adhesive dressings) are used for minor wounds. Keep several different sizes and shapes. Keep a selection of larger sterile dressings for more serious wounds.

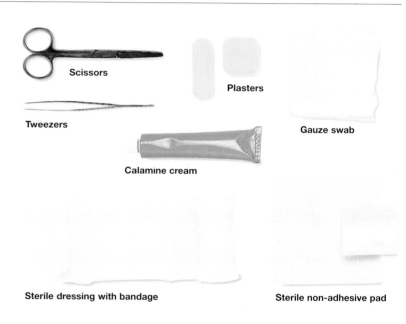

Scissors

Tweezers

Plasters

Gauze swab

Calamine cream

Sterile dressing with bandage

Sterile non-adhesive pad

Bandages

Keep a variety of bandages to secure dressings and support injured joints. Conforming bandages shape themselves to the contours of the body and so are easy to use. Triangular bandages can be used to make slings and for broad- and narrow-fold bandages.

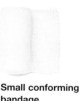

Small conforming bandage

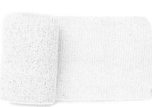

Large roller bandage

Large conforming bandage

Safety pins

Hypoallergenic tape

Crepe roller bandage

Finger bandage

Folded triangular bandage

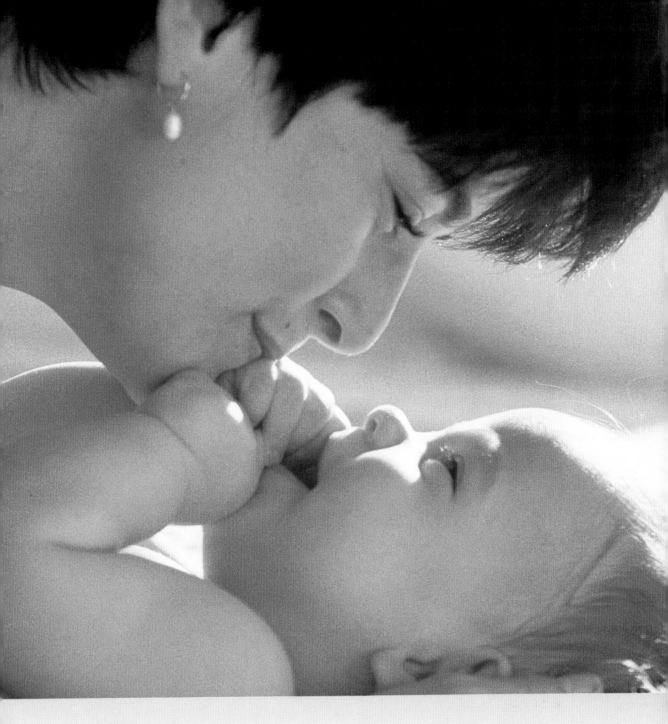

Complementary
therapies

Complementary and alternative medical therapies in childhood

PARENTS ARE KEENLY INTERESTED in using complementary and alternative medicines for their children, particularly parents of children with chronic, recurrent and serious conditions and where a child needs to be nursed in hospital.

If I were the parent of a sick child I, too, would be casting about for ways I could look after my child, outside of orthodox medicine and more under my own control.

The questions I would feel forced to ask myself, however, before I embarked on that route would be:
- do these therapies work; are they likely to be effective for my child?
- do they interact with the mainstay treatments that my child is taking?
- are they safe; could they do my child harm?

No doctor would exempt themselves from taking an holistic approach to treating patients, caring for the whole child – body, mind, emotions and spirit, in the context of the child's and family's values, culture and community. Few would not approve of integrative medicine wherein a broad range of therapies is reviewed, and those with the best evidence of safety and effectiveness are chosen.

It's useful in this context to examine what parents and doctors alike would agree are valuable goals.
1. curing disease
2. relieving symptoms
3. preventing disease
4. promoting wellness
5. reducing stress
6. a happy child
Any treatment can be measured against these goals.

So, for instance, acupuncture may be used in a child suffering from cancer, not to cure the cancer as in goal 1, but to help alleviate pain as in goal 2 or to promote a sense of wellbeing as in goals 4 & 5.

You may like to know that there's quite a wide range of complementary and alternative options which can help your child in different ways.

Metabolic
▶ Infusions, tinctures, creams, lotions
▶ Herbs
▶ Dietary supplements

Lifestyle
▶ Diet
▶ Exercise
▶ Environment – home, school
▶ Mind – body

Physical
▶ Massage
▶ Chiropractic/manipulation
▶ Surgery

Emotional
▶ Acupuncture
▶ Reike, laying on of hands, touch
▶ Prayer and ritual
▶ Homeopathy

Every mother, as well as every paediatrician knows about the consoling nature of home remedies, be they steam inhalations, camomile tea, chicken soup or a few drops of mentholatum on the pillow at night. And we're all happy to use them in mild, self-limiting conditions like coughs and colds. But common sense demands more stringent evidence of safety and efficacy for more serious conditions where, in nearly all cases, safe and effective medicines already exist. So you should bear these points in mind when considering using complementary and alternative medicine for your child.

The safety and effectiveness of complementary therapies is still in question and the list below provides food for thought when considering complementary therapies.

- Yogurt and probiotic healthstore products are often given to children with diarrhoea or as a precaution against it when antibiotics are taken to "support healthy intestinal function" but THE EFFECTIVENESS AND PROPER DOSING FOR CHILDREN REMAINS UNKNOWN.

- For many other dietary supplements such as St. John's Wort and echinacea THERE ARE NO SAFETY OR EFFICACY STUDIES IN CHILDREN.

- Herbs are potent chemicals and there is much evidence that they react dangerously with prescribed medicines and have some serious side effects in adults, let alone children.

- Hypnosis is an effective preventive therapy for migraines, nausea and pain from chemotherapy and some behavioural conditions.

- Massage can be helpful in low birthweight babies, pain, asthma, attention deficit hyperactivity disorder (ADHD) and depression, and it's safe and enjoyable.

- THERE IS NO EVIDENCE AT ALL, on the other hand, that chiropractic is of any significant help for any major childhood disease.

Continued on next page

Continued from previous page

- Some children with nausea and pain are ready to accept acupuncture, some are not, though it's offered in about a third of paediatric pain treatment programmes in the United States – at academic centres. But at the present time THERE IS NO PUBLISHED EVIDENCE THAT ACUPUNCTURE CAN WORK IN CHILDREN AS IT DOES IN ADULTS.

As a doctor, I would always err on the side of safety and caution. No child should be given a supplement of any kind without conferring with a doctor. For a seriously ill child a wise precaution is to seek advice from your pediatrician before using complementary or alternative medicines. Usually you'll get a sympathetic and encouraging response. Your doctor will point you in the direction of remedies they've used themselves along with conventional medicines, and about which they feel comfortable.

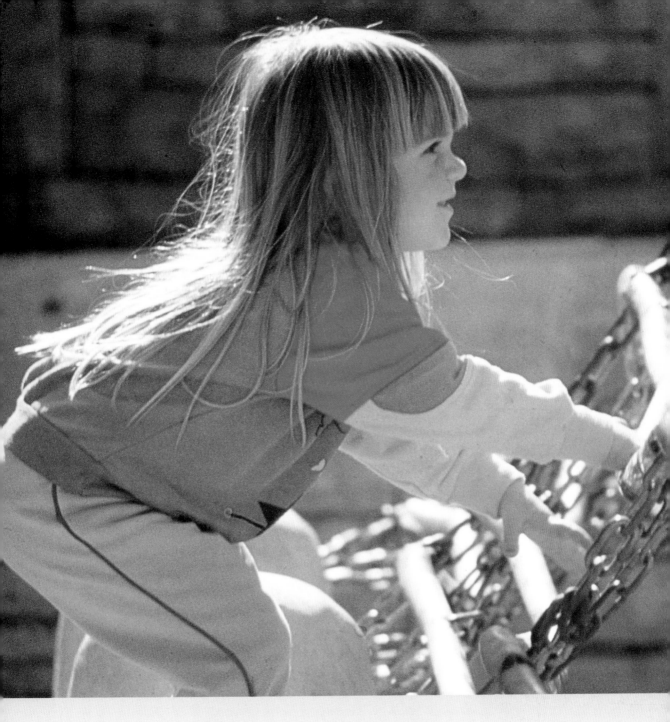

Personal
records

Growth charts

YOUR CHILD WILL GROW and put on weight at his own rate so, while it is interesting to plot his development, do not become obsessive or anxious about it. It is only in the first few months of a baby's life that weight gain should be watched closely, and it will be monitored at your clinic. After this stage, it is regularity of weight gain which is most important.

To use the chart, first weigh your baby. Then go along the bottom axis until you find his age. Look up the vertical axis until you reach your baby's weight. The point where the two axes meet will give you an idea of your baby's progress in comparison to an average figure. You will also find growth charts in your parentheld record book.

Large baby　　Medium baby　Small baby

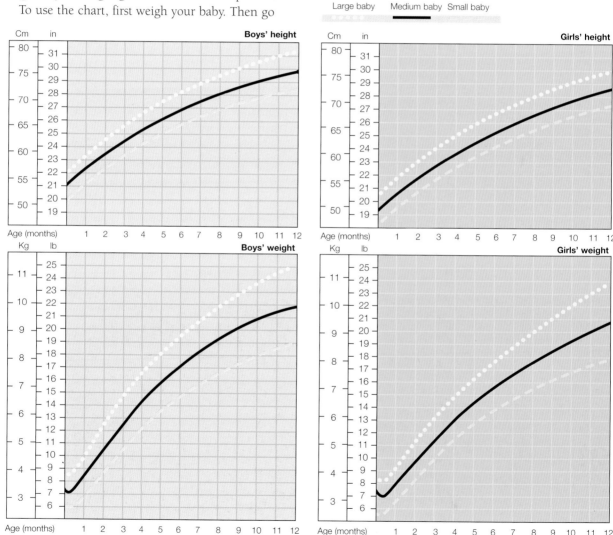

Immunization

THE AIM OF IMMUNIZATION is to protect both individuals and communities from infectious diseases. Every parent should therefore take steps to have their child properly immunized. Even if a disease has been eradicated, it is still necessary to continue immunizing against it to prevent its re-emergence.

Immunization works by preparing the body to repel infection. The body usually has to have an infection once before its defences are capable of responding against it. Immunization does this for us – by means of injection, drops in the mouth or scratching of the skin. The substance introduced into the body is called a vaccine, and the method for doing so is known as vaccination or inoculation.

Most vaccination programmes start at about two months, and you should receive a card asking you to attend your doctor's practice or clinic. Remember to keep a record of dates and type of vaccination, along with a record of your family's medical history. This is necessary to help your doctor determine whether or not your child should have a particular vaccination. With the re-emergence of tuberculosis your doctor may advise BCG immunization for your baby in the first year of life. Similarly, children who suffer from convulsions, who have a family history of epilepsy or who have a long-standing heart or lung disease may be advised to consult a doctor before having a measles or whooping cough vaccination.

It is quite common for a small red bump, the size of a pea, to develop at the site of an inoculation. If, however, your child becomes irritable or develops a fever, or a high-pitched scream, and certainly if your baby has a convulsion, get in touch with your doctor.

The chart (*below*) outlines the commonly recommended immunizations of childhood. The guide to infectious fevers (*see page 322*) lists the symptoms and treatment for some of the most common childhood illnesses; it also lists preventive measures, where applicable. If you think your child has contracted an infectious fever, always contact your doctor to confirm the diagnosis.

Childhood vaccinations

Disease	Time	Reaction	Protection
Hib (Haemophilus influenzae type b), diphtheria, whooping cough (pertussis), tetanus	Injections at 2, 3 and 4 months; repeat at 3–5 years	Child may become feverish; the site of the injection may be sore	Tetanus must be repeated every 10 years to provide continuing protection
Poliomyelitis	Oral vaccine at 2, 3 and 4 months; repeat at 3–5 years	None	Has to be repeated every 10 years to provide continuing protection
MMR: Measles, mumps, German measles (rubella)	Injection at 12–15 months and 3–5 years	Child may become feverish and have a slight rash	Not known how long protection from vaccination lasts
Meningitis C	Injection at 2, 3 and 4 months NB: As this is a recently introduced vaccination, there is a "mop-up" programme to vaccinate older children up to the age of 18	The site of the injection may become red and swollen	Long-lasting protection. As a recently introduced vaccine at the time of publication, it is impossible to be more specific about length of protection

Infectious fevers chart

Disease	Incubation period	Symptoms
Chickenpox (*see page 82*)	7–21 days	Groups of spots that quickly develop into intensely itchy blisters. These appear in crops every three or four days, usually starting on the trunk, then spreading to the face, arms and legs. The spots are usually accompanied by headache and fever.
German measles (*see page 142*)	14–21 days	Slightly raised temperature; a rash of tiny pink or red spots, which starts behind the ears, spreads to the forehead and then to the rest of the body; and enlarged glands at the back of the neck.
Measles (*see page 177*)	8–14 days	The first signs are a runny nose, dry cough, headache, fever with a temperature as high as 40°C (104°F) and white spots inside the mouth and on the linings of the cheeks (Koplik's spots); also, the eyes may be red and sore. These symptoms are then followed by a brownish-red rash, which starts behind the ears and spreads to the face and torso.
Mumps (*see page 184*)	17–28 days	Swelling and soreness of the glands at the sides of the face, just below the ears and beneath the chin; painful swallowing; dry mouth, fever and a headache. In boys, the testes may be swollen and painful; girls may experience lower abdominal pains.
Roseola infantum (*see page 211*)	7–14 days	A fever with a temperature of 39–40°C (102.2–104°F) for three days, with no other symptoms. As the fever subsides, a rash of separate, flat, red or pink spots appears, first on the trunk, then spreading to the limbs and neck.
Scarlet fever (*see page 213*)	1–5 days	Sore throat, inflamed tonsils, fever with a temperature as high as 40°C (104°F), vomiting, abdominal pains, rash of small spots starting on the chest and neck then merging over the body, except the area around the mouth, and strawberry-red patches on a furry tongue.
Whooping cough (*see page 261*)	5–14 days	Slight temperature, runny nose, slight cough, which develops into a compulsive cough accompanied by "whooping" breath.

Treatment	Complications	Immunity	Prevention
Relieve itching with calamine lotion. If your child develops a fever, reduce it by tepid sponging (*see page 31*), then by paracetamol elixir.	In rare cases, chickenpox may cause encephalitis (*see page 126*) or be complicated by Reye's syndrome (*see page 208*).	Lifelong	None
If the child's temperature rises above 38°C (100.4°F), give him paracetamol elixir.	None to your child, but fetal damage could occur in a pregnant woman who comes into contact with your contagious child.	Lifelong	Inoculation at about 13–14 months
Try to reduce your child's temperature with tepid sponging (*see page 31*), then by paracetamol elixir. Prophylactic antibiotics.	In rare cases, otitis media (*see page 198*), pneumonia (*see page 202*) and encephalitis (*see page 126*).	Lifelong	Inoculation at about 13–14 months
Try to reduce your child's temperature with tepid sponging (*see page 31*), then by paracetamol elixir. Liquidize food if eating is painful and give your child plenty to drink.	In rare cases, encephalitis (*see page 126*) and meningitis (*see page 178*).	Usually lifelong	Inoculation at about 13–14 months
Try to reduce your child's temperature with tepid sponging (*see page 31*), then by paracetamol elixir.	Possible febrile convulsions.	Usually lifelong	None
Try to reduce your child's temperature with tepid sponging (*see page 31*), then by paracetamol elixir.	Rare, though scarlet fever can cause inflammation of the kidneys (nephritis, *see page 189*) or of the joints and heart (rheumatic fever, *see page 209*).	Lifelong	None
Antibiotics, which must be given early to be properly effective.	Very rare nowadays, although there's a possibility of bronchitis (*see page 73*) or pneumonia (*see page 202*).	Lifelong	Inoculation at 2, 3 and 4 months

Useful addresses

PARENTS' GROUPS

Bliss (Baby Life Support Systems)
2nd Floor, Camelford House
89 Albert Embankment
London SE1 7TP
Tel: 020 7820 9471
Web: www.bliss.org.uk

CRY-SIS Support Group
BM Cry-Sis
London WC1N 3XX
Tel: 020 7404 5011
*Advice on babies who
cry excessively*

Enuresis Resource and Information Centre
34 Old School House
Britannia Road, Kingswood
Bristol BS15 8DB
Tel: 0117 960 3060
Web: www.eric.org.uk

Foundation for the Study of Infant Death
Artillery House, 11–19 Artillery Row
London SW1P 1RT
Tel: 020 7222 8001
Helpline: 020 7233 2090
Web: www.sids.org.uk/fsid

National Council for One-Parent Families
255 Kentish Town Road
London NW5 2LX
Info line: 0800 018 5026
Web: www.oneparentfamilies.org.uk

Parentline Plus
520 Highgate Studios
53–79 Highgate Road
London NW5 1TL
Tel: 020 7284 5500
Helpline: 0808 800 2222
Web: www.parentlineplus.org.uk

SPECIAL NEEDS ORGANIZATIONS

Association for Spina Bifida and Hydrocephalus (ASBAH)
Asbah House, 42 Park Road
Peterborough PE1 2UQ
Tel: 01733 555988
Web: www.asbah.demon.co.uk

British Dyslexia Association
98 London Road
Reading RG1 5AU
Tel: 0118 966 8271
Web: www.bda-dyslexia.org.uk

British Epilepsy Association (BEACON)
New Anstey House
Gateway Drive
Yeadon
Leeds LS19 7XY
Tel: 0808 800 5050
Web: www.epilepsy.org.uk

British Stammering Association
15 Old Ford Road
Bethnal Green
London E2 9PJ
Tel: 020 8983 1003
Web: www.stammering.org

Coeliac Society of UK
PO Box 220
High Wycombe
Buckinghamshire
HP11 2HY
Tel: 01494 437278
Web: www.coeliac.co.uk

Contact-a-Family
170 Tottenham Court Road
London W1T 7HA
Tel: 020 7383 3555
Web: www.cafamily.org.uk
*Supports parents of children with
special needs*

Cystic Fibrosis Trust
11 London Road
Bromley
Kent BR1 1BY
Tel: 020 8464 7211
Web: www.cftrust.org.uk

Diabetes UK (previously known as British Diabetes Association)
10 Queen Anne Street
London W1G 9LH
Tel: 020 7323 1531
Web: www.diabetes.org.uk

Down's Syndrome Association
155 Mitcham Road
London SW17 9PG
Tel: 020 8682 4001
Web: www.downs-syndrome.org.uk

The Haemophilia Society
3rd floor, Chesterfield House
385 Euston Road
London NW1 3AU
Tel: 020 7380 0600
Web: www.haemophilia.org.uk

Hyperactive Children's Support Group
71 Whyke Lane
Chichester
West Sussex PO19 2LD
Tel: 01903 725182
Web: www.hacsg.org.uk

Kawasaki Syndrome Support Group
13 Norwood Grove
Potters Green
Coventry CV2 2FR
Tel: 02476 612178

Leukaemia Society
PO Box 6831
London N22 3PR
Tel: 020 8374 4821

Meningitis Research Foundation
Midland Way
Thornbury
Bristol BS35 2BS
Tel: 01454 281811
Web: www.meningitis.org

The Muscular Dystrophy Group of Great Britain and Northern Ireland
7–11 Prescott Place
Clapham
London SW4 6BS
Tel: 020 7720 8055
Web: www.muscular-dystrophy.org

The National Asthma Campaign
Providence House
Providence Place
London N1 0NT
Tel: 020 7226 2260
Web: www.asthma.org.uk

National Autistic Society
393 City Road
London EC1V 1NG
Tel: 020 7833 2299
Web: www.oneworld.org/autism_uk

The National Eczema Society
Hill House
Highgate Hill
London N19 5NA
Tel: 020 7388 4097
Helpline: 0870 241 3604
Web: www.eczema.org

Scope (formerly the Spastics Society)
Library and Information Unit
6 Market Road
London N7 9PW
Tel: 020 7619 7100
Helpline: 0808 800 3333
Web: www.scope.org.uk

The Sickle Cell Society
54 Station Road
Harlesden
London NW10 4UA
Tel: 020 8961 7795
Web: www.sicklecellsociety.org

The Terrence Higgins Trust
52–4 Gray's Inn Road
London WC1X 8JU
Tel: 020 7242 1010
Web: www.tht.org.uk

United Kingdom Thalassaemia Society
19 The Broadway
Southgate Circus
London N14 6PH
Tel: 020 8882 0011
Web: www.ukts.org

FIRST AID AND SAFETY

British Red Cross
9 Grosvenor Crescent
London SW1X 7EJ
Tel: 020 7235 5454
Web: www.redcross.org.uk

British Standards Institute
389 Chiswick High Road
London W4 4AL
Tel: 020 8996 9001
Web: www.bsi.org.uk

Child Accident Prevention Trust
4th Floor, 18–20 Farringdon Lane
London EC1R 3HA
Tel: 020 7608 3828

Royal Society for the Prevention of Accidents (RoSPA)
Edgbaston Park
353 Bristol Road, Edgbaston
Birmingham B5 7ST
Tel: 0121 248 2000
Web: www.rospa.co.uk

St Andrew's Ambulance
St Andrew's House
48 Milton Street
Cowcaddens
Glasgow G4 0HR
Tel: 0141 332 4031

St John Ambulance
1 Grosvenor Crescent
London SW1X 7EF
Tel: 020 7235 5231
Web: www.sja.org.uk

COMPLEMENTARY MEDICINE

British Homeopathic Association
15 Clerkenwell Close
London EC1R 0AA
Tel: 020 7566 7800
Web: www.trusthomeopathy.org

Institute for Complementary Medicine
PO Box 194
London SE16 1QZ
Tel: 020 7237 5165
Web: www.icmedicine.co.uk

National Association of Homeopathic Groups
11 Wingle Tye Road
Burgess Hill
West Sussex
RH15 9HR
Tel: 01444 236848

Glossary

Words in **bold italic** denote glossary entries.

Abscess
A localized collection of **pus** that gathers as part of the body's way of fighting an **infection**.

Acute
A term applied to short attacks of a disease or pain.

Allergen
A substance which provokes an allergic reaction in certain individuals.

Allergy
Abnormal reaction of the body to substances called **allergens**.

Amniocentesis
A screening process in which a small sample of amniotic fluid is extracted through a needle from the amniotic sac that surrounds the fetus. The cells and chemicals contained in the fluid can then be examined to detect disorders, such as Down's syndrome or spina bifida. Amniocentesis also determines the sex of the fetus, making it possible to ascertain the risk of some genetic disorders, such as cystic fibrosis. Amniocentesis carries a slight risk of miscarriage and this is lowest at 14–16 weeks when the test usually takes place.

Anaemia
A type of blood disorder in which the oxygen-carrying power, or the number, of mature, healthy cells of the blood is diminished. Lack of **haemoglobin**, the oxygen-carrying agent in the blood, brings about a shortage of oxygen in the body's tissue. Characteristic symptoms of anaemia are pale skin, especially at the tips of the fingers, on the lips and tongue and around the eyes.

Anaesthetic
A drug used to bring about temporary loss of sensation and hence remove pain. General anaesthetics induce unconsciousness and are given in the form of injection or through inhalation. Local anaesthetics are usually given as injections and remove sensation from only a limited area.

Analgesic
A pain-relieving drug. The one most frequently given to children is paracetamol. It is available as a syrup, or elixir, for very young children. Junior aspirin has been withdrawn because of serious side effects, and no form of aspirin should ever be given to a child under 12 except under strict medical supervision.

Anaphylaxis
A very severe, general allergic reaction. Symptoms can range from attacks of asthma and flushing, to collapse and unconsciousness. Where there is severe allergic reaction, caused by a sting for instance, shock may develop.

Antenatal
Literally, before birth; refers to a condition or event during pregnancy.

Antibiotic
A drug used to fight bacterial infection. A prescribed course of antibiotics should always be completed, even if the illness is cured; future treatment with the drug may face greater bacterial resistance if the course is not finished.

Antibodies
Agents of the body's defence system, produced by white blood cells in order to combat an **infection** or an **allergen**.

Anti-coagulant
A drug used to stop the blood clotting.

Anti-convulsant
A drug used to prevent or end convulsions, often in the treatment of epilepsy.

Anti-fungal
A drug used to treat fungal infections.

Antihistamine
A drug used to counter the effect of a **histamine**, a chemical produced by the body as a result of an inflammatory and allergic reaction.

Anti-serum
A **serum** prepared from the blood of a person (or animal) whose defence system has been stimulated to fight an infecting agent or foreign protein, such as snake venom. When given, the antiserum protects against the infecting agent or foreign protein through the **antibodies** contained within it.

Anti-toxin
A substance, produced by the body or injected into it, that nullifies the effects of a **toxin**, a poisonous substance produced by **bacteria** and some plants and animals.

Autoimmunity
A defect in the body's defence system against disease, which causes the body to manufacture **antibodies** that attack and harm the body's own healthy tissue.

Bacteria
A group of organisms, some of

which are harmless and some only harmful when they multiply too quickly.

Benign
The term used to describe unnatural growth that is harmless to surrounding tissue and which will not return once removed.

Biopsy
The process by which a small piece of body tissue is removed for analysis. It is often used to determine if an unnatural growth is *malignant* or *benign*.

Bronchodilator
A drug which widens bronchial passages, and is used in the treatment of asthma. The drug is taken either by nasal inhalation, or orally through a spray.

Carcinogen
A substance that causes or promotes cancer.

Cauterization
The process by which tissue is destroyed, using either a red-hot instrument or a chemical.

Cerebral
Relating to the structure and workings of the brain.

Chorionic villus sampling
A screening process in which a small sample of the developing placenta (chorionic villi) is extracted and analysed for disorders such as Down's syndrome, thalassaemia, cystic fibrosis or muscular dystrophy in the fetus. CVS can be carried out as early as 11 weeks, or at any stage thereafter up to three months, or, in some cases, the middle months of pregnancy. The test is sometimes an alternative to *amniocentesis*,

although it carries a greater risk of miscarriage.

Chromosomes
Microscopic strands which are present within the nucleus of every cell. They carry the genetic information needed to determine the characteristics of an individual. There are normally 46 chromosomes in each cell.

Chronic
A term describing a condition that has lasted, or is expected to last, for some time, while not necessarily being life-threatening.

Cilia
Minute hairs lining the surface of mucous membranes, for example, in the nose. Their waving movement serves a cleaning purpose, clearing dust particles, mucus and *bacteria*.

Congenital
A term applied to a disease or condition present at birth.

Cyanosis
A blueness of the skin, caused by lack of oxygen.

Cyst
An abnormal fluid-filled swelling.

Dermatologist
A doctor who specializes in treating diseases of the skin.

Dialysis
A treatment for kidney failure. Waste products, usually excreted by the kidney, are removed either by cleansing the blood on a dialysis machine (haemodialysis), or by cleaning the peritoneal cavity (peritoneal dialysis) in the abdomen.

Diuretic
A substance that increases water excretion and urine production, thus lowering the body's fluid content.

Drip
The common name for an intravenous infusion (*see* *intravenous*). Liquid, whether blood, saline or *plasma*, is passed from an elevated, sterile container through a vein and into the body. The rate of flow is controlled by the rate of dripping through a transparent container.

Dys-
A prefix meaning difficult, painful and/or abnormal. For example, dyslexia (difficulty in learning to read or spell).

Electroencephalogram (EEG)
A recording of the electrical impulses of the brain, using a painless process called electro encephalography.

Embolism
The sudden blockage of a blood vessel, caused by a blood clot or other foreign solid (known as an embolus).

Endocrinologist
A doctor who specializes in the study of *hormones* and the diseases caused by their disorders.

Endoscope
An instrument enabling a doctor to look into a body cavity, usually the oesophagus, stomach or duodenum. Photographs and tissue samples can also be taken, and some small growths removed, with an endoscope.

Endoscopy
The procedure in which an *endoscope* is used.

Enema
Liquid injected into the rectum, usually to produce a bowel movement or for diagnostic purposes; also the name for this process. The technique is sometimes used to give an **anaesthetic** to a baby or small child, or to give drugs to a child who is vomiting, because the walls of the bowel are so absorbent. An enema should be given only on a doctor's orders.

Excretion
The removal of the body's internal waste matter by natural processes, such as urination, sweating and exhalation.

Febrile
Characterized by fever and a high temperature as in a febrile convulsion.

Follicle
Most commonly, a tiny cavity on the body's surface.

Gammaglobulin
A type of blood protein that includes **antibodies**. Obtained from donated blood, gammaglobulin can be used in the prevention of infections such as hepatitis.

Haematologist
A doctor who specializes in the treatment of diseases of the blood, bone marrow and lymph glands.

Haematoma
A collection of blood under the skin or deep in the tissues.

Haematuria
Blood in the urine, visible either to the naked eye or under a microscope.

Haemoglobin
The oxygen-carrying agent in the blood. It is present only in red blood cells, giving the blood its colour.

Haemorrhage
Bleeding, either externally (from the skin or an orifice) or internally (within a body cavity).

Heaf test
A method of determining tuberculosis **immunity**, using an extract of TB **bacteria**. The extract is applied through a series of light punctures of the skin on the forearm, in the shape of a ring. If the ring becomes a single red patch in about three days, the subject of the test is immune.

Histamine
A chemical released into the body when an allergic or inflammatory reaction takes place (see **allergy**); the most common results are redness, swelling and itching.

Hormone
A chemical released by special (endocrine) glands into the bloodstream. It regulates the activities of certain body organs and tissues.

Hyper-
A prefix meaning "high" or "above" an expected norm. For example, hyperactive (active above the expected norm).

Immune system
The body's own defence system against disease, enabling it to recognize and destroy invading **microbes** (minute **bacteria**, **viruses** or fungi invisible to the naked eye) or foreign tissues, through the white blood cells' production of **antibodies**.

Immunity
Resistance to a disease, developed either by the body's **immune system** when an infection is contracted, or through purposeful intervention, as in vaccination.

Immunization
The process by which the body is prepared, by inoculation, to repel infection

Incubation period
The interval (usually measured in days) between the time a disease is caught – when the germs enter the body – and when symptoms begin to appear.

Infection
A type of illness caused by **microbes** – minute **bacteria**, **viruses** or fungi invisible to the naked eye – invading the body and multiplying within it. The microbes may clog up blood vessels and ducts, and also produce harmful waste products.

Inflammation
A painful, red swelling which is warm to the touch. Inflammation is the body tissue's reaction to a variety of injuries (physical blows, infection, autoimmune disease).

Inoculation
The introduction of a vaccine into the body.

Intravenous
Within, or inserted into, a vein.

Laxative
A type of drug that is used to ease and increase the frequency of bowel movements. Laxatives should be given to a child only on a doctor's orders.

Lumbar puncture
The procedure for taking a sample of fluid from the base of the spine by inserting a needle. This is done under local anaesthetic. The fluid is analysed in order to diagnose certain diseases, particularly those affecting the nervous system, such as meningitis.

Lymph
A colourless liquid which contains white blood cells. Lymph flows in channels, taking nutrients to, and removing waste products from, local cells. The white blood cells in lymph are an important part of the body's defence system against infection.

Malignant
A term applied to a cancerous growth which is likely to spread, and recur, even after removal. A malignant growth is sometimes impossible to eradicate totally.

Membrane
A thin lining or covering tissue of various organs and cavities of the body.

Meninges
The three layers of *membrane* protecting the brain and spinal cord. Meningitis is an inflammation of the meninges.

Metabolism
The body's physical and chemical reactions. Any series of, or single. reactions may be described as metabolic.

Microbes
Minute *bacteria*, *viruses* or fungi invisible to the naked eye.

Mucous membrane
A *membrane* lining a part of the body, such as the mouth or vagina, which secretes a watery or slimy material.

Neuro-
Pertaining to the body's nervous system. For example, a neurosurgeon specializes in surgery of the nervous system.

Neurologist
A doctor who specializes in treating diseases of the brain and those related to the nervous system. Neurologists often work closely with neurosurgeons, who specialize in surgery of the nervous system, principally the brain and spinal cord.

Obstetrician
A doctor who specializes in looking after women during pregnancy and immediately after childbirth.

Oedema
A swelling of the body tissue that is caused by excess fluid content. The condition most commonly affects the ankles.

Ophthalmologist
A doctor who specializes in treating eye injury or disease. An optician, who may or may not be a doctor, detects eye defects and supplies corrective lenses, but does not treat injury or disease.

Ophthalmoscope
An instrument for examining the tissues of the interior of the eye, by shining a light through the pupil.

Orthodontist
A dentist who specializes in treating teeth abnormalities and jaw disorders.

Orthopaedics
The process of curing deformities arising from disease of, or injury to, bones and joints.

Otoscope
An instrument for examining the middle and inner ear, viewed through the semi-transparent eardrum, in order to diagnose disease.

Paediatrician
A doctor who specializes in treating children, usually until the age of puberty.

Paracetamol see *Analgesic*.

Penicillin
The first *antibiotic* to be discovered, used in the treatment of many infections including tonsillitis and otitis media. Penicillin may, however, provoke an allergic reaction (see *allergy*) such as asthma or a rash. If your child is allergic, ensure this is entered on his medical records and that he wears a medic-alert bracelet so that he isn't given the drug.

Physiotherapist
A person trained to give treatment through the use of physical exercise and manipulation. Physiotherapy is often used to help children suffering from arthritis, cerebral palsy, muscular dystrophy, and other neuro-muscular diseases.

Plasma
The liquid (as opposed to cellular) part of the blood, which can be used as replacement fluid in the treatment of shock and burns.

Possetting
In babies, the harmless habit of regurgitating milk soon after, or during, a feed.

Postnatal
A term that literally means after birth, referring to the health of the baby and its mother in the first weeks following birth.

Prophylactic
A substance or procedure that helps to prevent disease (*immunization*, for example).

Psychiatrist
A medically qualified specialist in mental illness.

Psychologist
A non-medically qualified person trained to assess behavioural problems.

Pus
A yellow/greenish semi-liquid substance, made up of decomposed tissue, *bacteria* and dead white blood cells; it is a sign of the body's fight against *infection*.

Sebum
An oily substance that is produced by the sebaceous glands just below the skin's surface. Sebum is the body's own moisturizer, spreading over the skin from the pores. Acne can be caused through a build-up of sebum under the skin's surface.

Secretion
The body's production of substances from special glands or cells. For instance, *sebum*.

Serum
The clear, liquid content of the blood when separated from other blood components, such as clotting substances, which are found in *plasma*. The term is sometimes used loosely as a synonym for *anti-serum*.

Spasm
An involuntary and uncontrollable contraction of one or more muscles.

Stools
The waste matter left over from food, expelled from the rectum.

Tinnitus
An intermittent or continuous ringing, buzzing or roaring sound in the ear, heard only by the sufferer.

Toxin
A poisonous substance produced by *bacteria*, other *microbes*, and some plants and animals.

Tracheotomy
A surgical procedure to restore normal breathing when the throat or larynx is blocked. An incision is made in the neck and a tube inserted below the blockage.

Traction
Means "pulling apart" and is used as a treatment for broken bones, crushed vertebrae, and prolapsed discs. Damaged and compressed parts of the body are held apart and in the correct position until healed.

Tumour
A swelling; usually denotes one caused by abnormal cell-multiplication within the body.

Ulcer
An open sore affecting either an internal or external body surface.

Vaccination
See *immunization*.

Vaccine
A solution made up of an altered, weakened or killed strain of a disease. Usually injected, a vaccine

is designed to stimulate the body's resistance to the disease that has been introduced into it.

Vasoconstrictor
Any substance, whether a chemical produced by the body, or a drug, which causes blood vessels to narrow.

Vasodilator
Any substance, whether a chemical produced by the body, or a drug, which causes blood vessels to widen.

Virus
The smallest type of *microbe*, which invades the body's cells and multiplies inside them, giving rise to contagious viral infections such as influenza.

Index

Acknowledgments

Previous editions

Dorling Kindersley would like to thank: Neville Graham for his skill in bringing both the design and project to a successful conclusion; Rachel Bateson, Jamie MacIntyre Buckingham, Thomas Brown, Isobel Bulat, Sophie Civardi, Aaron and Reuben Fleming, Nellie Frizzell, Nancy and Thomas Graham, Eliza Greig, Josh and Jake Jones, David Louden, JayJay Parkinson, Jack Thomson (and all their parents) for help with referencing; Kathie Gill for proofreading; Richard and Hilary Bird for indexing; Professor Iain MacIntyre and Dr Richard Coombs for medical advice; James Allen, Donald Berwick, Caroline Fraser Ker, Sara Harper and Steve Parker for editorial help; Kelly Flynn, Julia Harris and Brian Swan for design help; Brian Retter and Chris Cope, and, finally, all the staff at Modern Text for their hard work and sense of humour.

Consultant paediatrician

Andrew Whitelaw MD MRCP.

Author's acknowledgment

I am indebted once more to my editor, Charyn Jones, for her tolerance, clearness of vision and the inevitable improvement she makes to my work.

Illustrators

David Ashby, Karen Cochrane, Nicholas Hall, Coral Mula, Andrew Popkiewicz, James Robins, Paul Saunders, Sue Smith.

Revised edition 2001

Dorling Kindersley would like to thank: Bernard Koppmeyer and Simon Roulstone for design assistance; Jane Knott for proofreading.

Photographers

Paul Fletcher 13, 15, 17, 18, 19.
Trish Gant, additional photography.

Picture credits

Jo Hadden.
Marcus Scott.
Melanie Simmonds.
Biophoto Associates: Professor Gordon F Leedale 181cra.
Bubbles: Ian West 274cla; Jim Merrett 268cl.
Corbis: Philip James Corwin 11.
Sally & Richard Greenhill: 268crb, 274c, 282cla, 282crb.
Robert Harding Picture Library: 11, 23, 49, 319; Caroline Wood 315, 322.
Image Bank: 273cl; Tosca Radigonda 270tr.
Meningitis Research Foundation: 178cr; 178cb.
Mother & Baby Picture Library/emap esprit: Emap 1c.
Photos Horticultural: 275c.
Pictor International: title page.
Retna Pictures Ltd: Philip Reeson 277cla.
Science Photo Library: Biphoto Association/SPL 250tl; Dr P Marazzi 163cra.
Harry Smith Collection: 275cl.
The Stock Market: 248–249; 1999 Fuji-Strauss/Curtis 274–275; LWA - Dann Tardif 30–31; Michael Keller 148–149; Norbert Schafer 2–3; Steve Presant 228–229.
Telegraph Colour Library: 273cr; Mel Yates 10-11.
Dr Jean Watkins: 184tr.
The Wellcome Institute Library, London: 196cr, 250tc, 268ca; Anthea Sieveking 265, 273ca, 276tr, 282ca, 283; 271cl.
Elizabeth Whiting & Associates: 272cra.

All other images © Dorling Kindersley.
For further information see: www.dkimages.com